Praise for *The Probiotic Cure*

"Read this book"

"This book is enjoyable to read and easy to understand concerning the power of probiotics. One of the most important things you could do to improve your health is to read this book. The information in it can change your life! I wholeheartedly recommend this book."

–Dr. Richard Snyder, DO
Author of *What You Must Know About Kidney Disease*

⟹◈⟸

"Practical, well-organized"

"*The Probiotic Cure* is a gift to future generations. Martie Whittekin has spent a lifetime studying and utilizing the health benefits of proper dietary regimens and nutritional supplements including probiotics. She brings this firsthand knowledge to an eminently readable book packed with practical, well-organized information that will help readers achieve quantity and quality of life."

–Dr. Robert C. Martin, DC, CCN, DACBN, ABAAHP
Author of *Secret Nerve Cures* and host of *The Dr. Bob Martin Show*

⟹◈⟸

"A must read"

"Martie Whittekin's contributions to human life have proven over time to be truly invaluable. Her insight and knowledge of the microbiome is carefully shared in this articulate offering. This is a must read for anyone living in the 21st century, wishing to be self-responsible for their well-being . . ."

–Danielle Lin, CN
Radio host of *The Danielle Lin Show*

"A much-needed guidebook"

"Almost every radical remission cancer survivor I've studied worked diligently to balance their microbiome, whether by taking probiotic supplements or making their own cultured vegetables. *The Probiotic Cure* is a much-needed guidebook for both understanding the microbiome and taking action steps to balance it."

–Dr. Kelly Turner, PhD
NY Times best-selling author of *Radical Remission*

———◆———

"Life-saving"

"We have more "friendly bacteria" in our bodies than we do our own cells, and it's a good thing! This book explains what these good guys are and how they help run all our systems, starting with digestion, but they live on our skin and everywhere else as well. Modern medicine and agriculture has created a monster by killing these friends off with massive antibiotic use, both directly and indirectly, in our food and water supply. The result is lack of balance and lots more chronic illness. The solution? . . . Check out this book for details which could be life-saving for you and your family."

–Dr. Hyla Cass, MD
Author of *8 Weeks to Vibrant Health*

———◆———

"A game changer"

"The gut microbiome is an endless fascination for me as it is a sort of dynamic 'bodily organ.' It flows, changes, adapts; it is vital to human health yet invisible to the naked eye, and unresectable from a surgical point of view. Promoting a healthy gut microbiome in my patients has been a game-changer in my practice. I am pleased to have Martie Whittekin's excellent reference to help bring it all together."

–Dr. Leslie Mendoza Temple, MD
Clinical Assistant Professor,
Family Medicine University of Chicago Pritzker School of Medicine
Medical Director, Integrative Medicine Program
NorthShore University HealthSystem

THE PROBIOTIC CURE

HARNESSING THE POWER OF
GOOD BACTERIA FOR BETTER HEALTH

Martie Whittekin, CCN

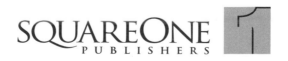

SQUAREONE
PUBLISHERS

The information and advice contained in this book are based upon the research and the personal and professional experiences of the author. They are not intended as a substitute for consulting with a healthcare professional. The publisher and author are not responsible for any adverse effects or consequences resulting from the use of any of the suggestions, preparations, or procedures discussed in this book. All matters pertaining to your physical health should be supervised by a healthcare professional. It is a sign of wisdom, not cowardice, to seek a second or third opinion.

COVER DESIGNER: Jeannie Tudor
EDITOR: Erica Shur
TYPESETTER: Gary A. Rosenberg

Square One Publishers
115 Herricks Road
Garden City Park, NY 11040
(516) 535-2010 ● (877) 900-BOOK
www.squareonepublishers.com

Library of Congress Cataloging-in-Publication Data
Names: Whittekin, Martie, author.
Title: The probiotic cure : how your own bacteria may save you from heart disease, cancer, obesity, and even dementia / Martie Whittekin, CCN.
Description: Garden City Park, NY : Square One Publishers, [2016] | Includes bibliographical references and index.
Identifiers: LCCN 2015045888 | ISBN 9780757004230
Subjects: LCSH: Probiotics—Health aspects.
Classification: LCC RM666.P835 W45 2016 | DDC 615.3/29—dc23
LC record available at http://lccn.loc.gov/2015045888

Printed in the United States of America

10   9   8   7   6   5   4   3   2   1

Contents

PART TWO

Strategies and Tactics for Health Concerns

Acknowledgments

The U.S. ranks very poorly on most measures of wellness compared to other industrialized nations and even compared to some in the third world. And we are losing ground . . . *in spite of spending about twice as much money on medical care as any other nation.* Reversing that trend will require major changes in public policy, medical education, institutional protocols, and in consumers' individual choices. Achieving change requires strong leadership. Thankfully, even one individual can cause a ripple that becomes a wave that eventually helps change the tide. The names below are representative of the many farsighted, brave (change always meets resistance) and diligent (change can be painfully slow) professionals who are guiding us toward smarter, kinder, more effective, and less costly ways to prevent and treat disease.

Everyone knows that MD stands for Medical Doctor. Not as many know that ND stands for Naturopathic Doctor. ND's who attend state-accredited naturopathic medical schools have similarly rigorous academic education as medical doctors and clinic experience, but with a different focus. For example, naturopathic physicians spend less time studying drugs and major surgery and more time learning what keeps the human body well. In addition to the fundamentals of conventional medical treatment, they are also taught how to use natural remedies, such as nutrition, herbs, acupuncture, exercise, psychology, and midwifery. These healers attend one of several great naturopathic schools, such as National College of Natural Medicine in Portland, Oregon. I know the most about Bastyr University in Kenmore, Washington which enjoys similar accreditation as that of the University of Washington. While I was privileged to serve on their Board of Trustees, I came to appreciate the vision, dedication, and sacrifices of Joseph Pizzorno, ND, one of the founders of Bastyr (in 1978). He is also a co-author of important works, such as *The Encyclopedia of Natural Medicine* and *The Textbook of Natural Medicine* (which I believe every MD and DO should be *required* to study).

There is some type of licensing for Naturopathic Physicians in seventeen states, the District of Columbia, and the U.S. territories of Puerto Rico and the U.S. Virgin Islands. The approved "scope of practice" reflects their training and typically allows ND's to prescribe some medications, such as antibiotics, thyroid medication, and other hormones as well as perform minor surgery like suturing wounds. In states like Washington and Oregon where natural medicine has been long-established, naturopaths and mainstream medicine enjoy a productive working relationship. Given the growing shortage of primary care doctors and the increased need for them, I just don't understand why licensing efforts in the other states like mine, Texas, have routinely been squashed. The protectionist instincts of trade associations are likely responsible for the failures, but given the relatively small number of naturopaths, the fear of competition do not seem warranted. *Readers should be aware that the internet is a source of ND certificates that do not require the training discussed above. Certainly some counselors with such short-cut credentials may be skilled, for example, in offering nutrition advice, but much more caution is warranted.*

Of course, not every doctor can go to a school of natural medicine in part because of severe limitations on enrollment. Also, many physicians who already have standard medical degrees and other health professionals are looking for more effective ways to help their patients but cannot take time off to go back to medical school. That brings me to another hero of mine, Jeffrey Bland, PhD. He is a brilliant biochemist, author, researcher, and critical thinker who could surely have relaxed into a cozy tenured spot in any university. Instead he has devoted decades to creating private educational systems that have taught an astounding number of health professionals how to deliver care in a safer, more effective, more practical, and more holistic manner. He launched an international movement and founded the Functional Medicine Institute. A great number of those that he has taught have gone on to teach others

It is hard to know how many tens of thousands of mainstream doctors have quietly complimented their conventional practices with concepts out of the naturopathic or functional playbook. Gastroenterologist Jeffry Fine, MD (who kindly wrote the forward to this book) is an example of a conventionally-trained doctor who was a functional medicine doctor before that discipline had even been given a name. He has added complimentary practices, such as diet and supplements (even probiotics) to his protocols after research and clinical outcomes warranted. Dr. Fine doesn't have a standardized GI treatment because he believes that each patient is unique.

For any system of medicine to be successful, the citizenry must understand and embrace it. That is especially true with natural approaches to health because its success depends on patients taking responsibility and changing behaviors. Therefore, media that educates consumers makes a crucial contribution in this area. For example, two more heroes of mine, Joe and Terry Graedon, are authors of the *People's Pharmacy* books, newspaper columns, and hosts of a long-running syndicated program on National Public Radio. Since long before it became popular, they have helped open the public's minds to natural approaches and home remedies. They calmly acknowledge the important role of drugs, but also ask the tough questions about side effects and alternatives. They call attention to scientific studies and effectively translate them into lay language. (My files are full of clippings from their newspaper columns.) I admire the caliber of scientists and authors that they interview on their radio show and how the duo asks the right questions to illuminate both sides of controversial issues. They have been a major inspiration for my own radio show.

Dr. Mehmet Oz of the popular TV show bearing his name has made it fun to learn about how our bodies work. He has helped his millions of viewers appreciate the importance of nutrition and the role of dietary supplements. Unfortunately, he is a pioneer with arrows in his back. It doesn't matter if a dissident view is correct, those vested in the status quo will circle the wagons and attack. In 2015 a collection of 10 mainstream doctors asked to have him fired from Columbia University where he is a surgeon. One stance that had riled his accusers was that Dr. Oz dared to suggest that Genetically Modified Food (GMOs) should be labeled as such. (In Chapter 6 we'll show why he is right to be concerned.) Dr. Oz exposed his accusers as having financial ties to GMO interests. *USA Today* quoted Dr. Oz as saying "We provide multiple points of view, including mine, which is offered without conflict of interest. That doesn't sit well with certain agendas which distort the facts." Congress called Dr. Oz on the carpet for talking about supplements that they said had not been proven. What the critics fail to mention is that there is no regulatory framework for declaring as "proven" anything except a drug.

Author and television host, Doug Kaufmann, has devoted many years and immense energy to educating his loyal viewers about a common, but often overlooked health threat, yeast. (We discuss yeast in Chapters 3 and 9.) He has collected hundreds of studies proving his point and motivates his audience to make life-changing improvements in their diets. He often shares their impressive testimonies about lives reclaimed.

Former model Carol Alt has made health, nutrition, and alternative medicine concepts sexy on her Fox television show. We need all of these voices plus a lot more at all of these levels if we hope to reverse the discouraging state of health in America.

Any benefit to the effort that may have come from my speaking, writing, and hosting a radio show is thanks to the unwavering support of my husband, Bill. I also depend on my right hand, Darlene Brents and to the loyal radio listeners many of whom have supported me since the show began in 1997.

This book and my prior work, *Natural Alternatives to Nexium, Maalox, Tagamet, Prilosec & Other Acid Blockers,* would not have been possible without the guidance of Rudy Shur, the founder of Square One Publishers (and previously the founder of Avery Publishing). He is a top professional in his field and I'm grateful for his patience in teaching me what constitutes a proper book.

A Word About The Book

This is an exceptionally exhilarating time in the field of health. For most of the relatively short time since the invention of microscopes, scientists believed that bacteria only caused *disease*. We have now begun to appreciate that having a robust, diverse, and well balanced personalized collection of friendly bacteria help us avoid, reverse, or at least improve obesity, depression, heart disease, diabetes, cancer, and many more chronic health concerns of our time. Before we dig in, I'd better define a few terms.

Our body's entire content of living microorganisms, such as bacteria, fungi, and parasites, is variously known as our "microbiome," "microbiota" or "flora." I will use those big picture terms interchangeably.

It is increasingly popular to support the health of our microbiome by ingesting *helpful* bacteria or fungus in the form of "probiotics" or "probiotic supplements." The same species of bacteria that we would normally have had living in us can be isolated for use as supplements. That two-way street leads to a nomenclature gray area. To make this book's important message clearer, at times (as in the title), I may refer to friendly bacteria generically as "probiotics" even if they are beneficial strains already inside us when we are healthy. That is just a less cumbersome way to differentiate them from bacteria that cause disease (the pathogens). Some scientific articles also do that as evidenced by the fact that virtually all of the studies to which I refer appeared in the government database of science in response to the key word "probiotic." The non-harmful bacteria in our systems might be more technically described with terms such as "commensal," "mutualistic," and "symbiotic" bacteria. You needn't worry about fine distinctions among those, but if you are curious, they are defined in the Glossary.

Another source of potential confusion is the word "cure" in the title. Consumers would probably understand the word to mean that a health issue (large or small) is no longer a problem. That is the shorthand sense in which I've used the term. I wanted to quickly attract the consumer's attention to the important news about our microbiome. However, the practice of medicine has a more specific definition and seldom uses the word. Persons who survive pneumonia might be called "cured." However diseases, such as diabetes, arthritis, asthma, heart disease, and cancer, when no longer presenting symptoms are said to be "in remission" rather than "cured." That is because symptoms of those typically chronic conditions can return.

Just to be clear, when I talk about health concerns being improved or reversed I'm saying that *a properly balanced microbiome* is the secret. Science is showing that probiotic supplements often have an important role to play in helping create that balance, but they are usually not solely responsible for the improvement. Furthermore, just as is the case with medicine, if we stop doing what is working, such as diet changes, health problems can return.

Foreword

As a board certified Gastroenterologist with over 23 years experience, I realized the power of probiotics long before it was in vogue to take them. As just one example, I deduced that lactobacillus GG could aid in treatment of lactose intolerance by making the needed enzyme, lactase, within the small bowel. I have used various strains to aid in the treatment of IBS and IBD and a variety of other health issues. I really enjoyed reading this book and I know you will too.

The author, Martie Whittekin, writes from the functional medical point of view, which is refreshing. She has extensively researched the subject matter and all of the information is scientifically based or expert opinion. This book, *The Probiotic Cure*, provides an impressive overview of the important role of probiotics in health and disease in both humans and animals. Various strains of probiotics within fermented foods also have positive effects on one's gut flora and in many cases have been demonstrated to provide a number of positive effects.

Certain bacterial strains discussed within this book have generally encouraging effects, but like anything else, they don't work in every case. The most important factor is maintaining a healthful balance and communication between the human microbiome and human cells because an imbalance in this relationship not only leads to disease but sometimes even to death. As elaborated in this book, each individual's assortment of microorganisms is a unique fingerprint that can be influenced positively or negatively by the food one ingests as well by the probiotics, medicines, and nutritional supplements one consumes.

This book provides a practical guide to navigation of the both the external and internal microbial environment. It also contains a valuable collection of information regarding pathogenic germs, antibiotic, prebiotics, probiotics, and postbiotics in health and specific health complaints.

Every home library should keep this book as a reference. Enjoy the book!

Jeffrey Fine, MD.
Chief of Gastroenterology
for the Medical and Surgical Clinic of Irving
Irving, Texas

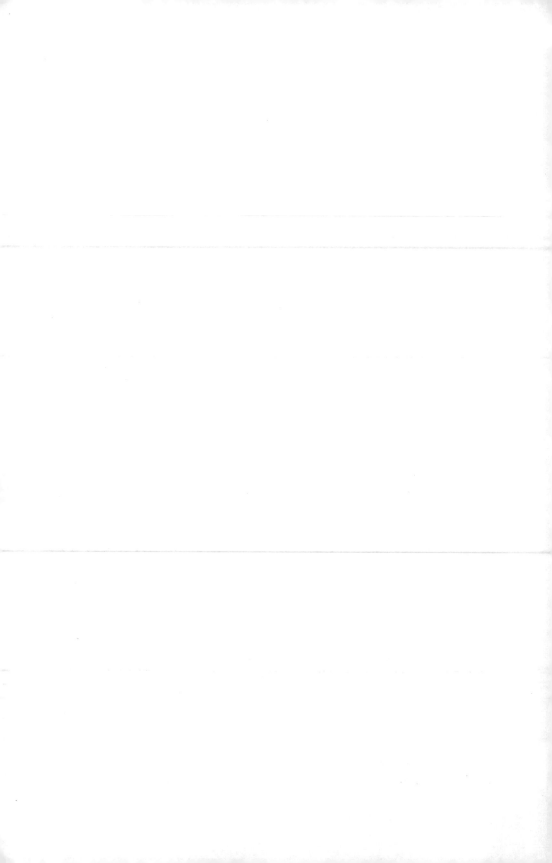

Preface

My interest in probiotic supplements goes back over thirty years, but I now realize that I probably needed their help even as a young child. Certainly I would have benefited when I began suffering with migraine headaches in college. Only someone who has experienced these menaces can relate to the unrelenting pain made all the more insufferable by nausea. During those dark spells I was unreasonably sensitive to well, everything. Every beam of light, faint sound, or smell was another insult and each episode would wipe me out for at least a couple of days.

Each and every doctor that I saw had been trained to simply suggest the latest pain killer. Unfortunately, none of the drugs helped the pain. They did have an effect however—they made my stomach more upset. Because one doc seemed particularly sympathetic, I asked him what he thought might be *causing* the migraines. Looking puzzled, he did his best to respond to my unusual request. He asked: "Have you had your eyes checked?" ("Yes, they are fine.") "Are you under stress?" ("Yes. I am a fulltime student working my way through school, so I'm always under stress, but I don't always have headaches.") The poor guy just sighed and pulled out the prescription pad.

Years later, still suffering with migraines, I happened to stop in a health food store where I spotted a magazine with a cover that mentioned headaches. The article was about migraine triggers like aged cheese and wine. Wait, what? Could there really be something besides a deficiency of pain killers that causes headaches? Avoiding those foods did help a little. One day I was suffering with a particularly awful thumper and in desperation just *stopped eating entirely*. After a day or so of my fasting hissy fit, not only was the headache gone, but also I felt better than I had in a very long time...clearer, more energetic, and even cheerier.

I knew I was onto something, but I needed guidance. Luckily I found Don Mannerberg, MD. He was what we might now call an "integrative" or "functional medicine" practitioner. With his testing and teaching I was on the road to finally getting rid of the migraines. I was also launched on what became a life-long mission to find out if the same kinds of factors that had caused my headaches, might also cause other health issues.

Finding the root cause of a health problem is rather like peeling the layers of an onion. Food sensitivities, mineral deficiencies, low thyroid function, toxins, hormone imbalances, and irregularity had all contributed to my problem . . . but, I had to wonder what had caused those issues? Was my sinus congestion somehow related? I knew nothing of natural medicine back then, but even so it made no sense to me when surgery was suggested to un-stuff my nose. Ultimately, I discovered that behind each of my problems and therefore at the heart of the onion was an imbalance of good and bad microorganisms in my intestinal system. Restoring intestinal balance went a long way toward solving *all* the other issues . . . including that stuffy nose. I was inspired!

Having succeeded with my first client (me), I was encouraged to become a Certified Nutritionist and then a Certified Clinical Nutritionist. The more I learned, the more I was in awe of the tremendous power of friendly bacteria and of probiotic supplements. Humans are actually *super-organisms*, our own flesh and blood cells plus resident communities of trillions of microorganisms.[1] We depend on them for functions so important that they are often collectively described as an "organ" much like our liver or lungs.[2] (Coincidentally, the mass of the microorganisms in just our intestinal tract weighs about as much as a man's liver—3 to 5 pounds.[3]) We are pretty fond of our organs and would never say "Sure go ahead and remove my liver." And yet, folks routinely kill off their microbiome "organ" because they are unaware of the crucial role it plays in their health. My caring doctors were unknowingly in that camp.

Virtually any health problems I had as an adult could be traced back to having been a child during the antibiotic honeymoon. For a time we all believed that the ability of antibiotics to save lives was the whole story. We didn't yet know about the side effects and had not dreamed that they could turn bacteria into antibiotic-resistant superbugs. (There is a hint in the fact that "antibiotic" means *against life*, in clear contrast with "probiotic" which means *for life*.) Blissfully unaware, doctors and parents gave me an antibiotic at the first sign of any upper respiratory something or other and no one noticed that the medicine seemed to start a vicious cycle. For example, I remember having sinusitis, laryngitis, and bronchitis all on top of each other. Later, as a teenager with a few ordinary little pimples, I was prescribed an antibiotic which I took *for a year*. None of us seemed to know that teen skin was likely a sign of a gut imbalance or that the drug surely worsened the problem. Unlikely as it may sound, that drug for my complexion started a chain reaction whose ripple effects lasted for decades.

Many of my clients have had similar histories. I am writing this book in part to help readers avoid the pitfalls that we experienced . . . or if it is too late for that, at least repair the damage. One step is to avoid excess antibiotics. We can do that in part by strengthening our immune systems and an important part of that is paying attention to our flora. There is more good news to share. A healthy microbiota can prevent, cure or at least greatly improve a wide variety of health conditions—even some of the most serious.

Supplemental probiotics help improve bacterial balance and I've been an advocate of them for a very long time. In addition to using them to help myself, my family, and my clients, I wanted to help others spread the good word. As President Elect of the National Nutritional Foods Association (in 1992), I organized a Probiotics Conference in Dallas, Texas so that experts in the probiotics industry could pool the relatively little data known about them at the time.

In my first book, *Natural Alternatives to Nexium, Maalox, Tagamet, Prilosec & Other Acid Blockers,* I provided some basic information about probiotics because acid reflux is one of the many issues I find are helped by them. But today, the scientific information about our microorganisms is simply stunning both in quantity and significance. A search for "probiotics" in PubMed, the government scientific data base, returns tens of thousands of articles. On average, about thirty-five additional submissions appear each week. As you will see in Chapter 2, this cutting edge research is revealing the benefits of our bacteria for an astoundingly wide range of important health concerns.

Recently I attended a Harvard postgraduate symposium on the relationship of diet and the microbiota to health and disease. Presenters were researchers from prestigious universities here and abroad. I was pleased to meet scientists whose work I had studied. It was also simply inspiring to see the scientific cross-pollination among speakers and researchers in the audience. Much of the material presented was so cutting-edge that it was not yet published. I remain in awe of the thoroughness, creativity and diligence these investigators display as they drill down to excruciatingly finer points of how bacteria affect us *and how we affect them.*

Unfortunately, the average consumer does not have access to all this esoteric knowledge. Research has shown that consumers are mainly educated about health factors by product manufacturers. That is a bit of a problem because, clearly, drug companies, supplement makers, and food producers are only interested in providing us with information that will sell their products—whether or not that product is in our highest interest. Consumers can get information on the internet, but as we know, there is a good reason it is sometimes called "the great *mis*information highway"—it is hard to tell a credible breakthrough from a wild tale.

We all know that "pathogenic" bacteria *cause* disease, but there is now simply no question that we need to be just as mindful that beneficial bacteria *protect us* against disease. And we need to develop a sense of urgency about *protecting them* because we are in a race against the clock. Just as medicinal plant species are tragically disappearing from rainforests, the diversity of friendly bacteria that have protected us through the millennia is actually *shrinking*. And we cannot replace them.[4]

We are also at a tipping point between knowing enough to take action and having such a mass of information that it is simply impossible to deal with. Guidance is needed, but most doctors don't quite know what to do with this holistic concept. In fact, a recent study showed that, even among the doctors who believe that functional foods, such as those containing probiotics, are probably good for patients; most admit that they do not know much about them and feel that they should not be involved in counseling patients about them.[5]

We need to find the useful patterns in the jumble of emerging science, translate it into lay language, and condense it into a simple guide to help con-sumers solve problems and optimize their health by optimizing their flora. Because of my personal and professional interest in these astounding bacteria that are essential to our good health (you will soon see why I speak of them so enthusiastically), I aim for this book to be that guide. And I want to do it *now* because I see some disturbing trends emerging. If we are prepared for those developments, then we won't miss opportunities, spend more than is necessary, and potentially hurt ourselves with inappropriate choices.

Just as a note, I have included a number of brand name products through-out this book. I have recommended them on the basis of their effectiveness. It is important to point out that I do not work for any of these companies, nor do I sell any probiotics.

Introduction

The discussion of health-giving bacteria may make more sense if I put it in the context of a much bigger picture. I've listed a number of serious health concerns on the cover and indicated that they might be overcome by helpful bacteria. If that seems a bit bold, it may be in part because we have become accustomed to *managing* diseases and using medicine to *quiet symptoms*. The conventional approach may be common, but that doesn't make it ideal. We can obviously be fooled into complacency by what is around us constantly, but history is replete with examples of times when we did not know until too late that "the parade was out of step."

Fortunately, there may actually be two parades from which to choose. Modern high tech medicine is unequalled in *crisis care*. It excels at putting us back together after an accident and keeping us from falling off the edge with an acute disease. However, when compared to most other developed countries (and even some in the third world) our chronic disease statistics look quite grim. Medications alleviate symptoms, but often at a significant expense and reduced long term wellness. One underlying problem is that conventional medicine is thoroughly trained in those interventions that it may discount the impressive self-healing force of the human body. In fact, we've spent the last several decades trying to defy the laws of nature when it might have been at least as productive to invoke the power of nature. Our microorganisms are an important component of that force.

The approach I will describe in this book is more aligned with healing disciplines that are less mainstream . . . a different parade if you will. According to the Institute for Functional Medicine (functionalmedicine.org), "Functional Medicine *addresses the underlying causes of disease*, using a systems-oriented approach and engaging both patient and practitioner in a therapeutic partnership." I added the emphasis because that is a key point we will come back to frequently. Although functional medicine offers specific training to practitioners, I will use the term "functional medicine" as generic shorthand to cover a broader scope of disciplines that have much in common, such as integrative medicine, complimentary medicine, naturopathic medicine, nutrition-based preventive medicine, and even alternative medicine. These systems have in turn gained valuable insight from ancient gentle arts, such as Traditional Chinese Medicine, Ayurveda from India, and Native American Shaman healing. (Practices that have worked for thousands of years shouldn't be discounted simply because they didn't come out of a white coat Western laboratory.) The functional approach is gaining traction in mainstream medicine as evidenced by the fact that the prestigious Cleveland Clinic has opened a Center for Functional Medicine.

Functional medicine deals successfully with preventing and healing (curing) chronic disease in part because it is personalized. These professionals also tend to view symptoms not as the enemy, but as almost blessings which alert us to an imbalance. Identifying and correcting an imbalance can achieve a sustainable *reversal* or cure of disease. As a bonus, the rebalancing approach can restore health without creating further damage in the process as might often be the case with some mainstream treatments, such as surgery, radiation, and pharmaceutical drugs. An imbalance usually involves an *insufficiency* of one or more factors that the body needs for optimum function and/or *excess* of one or more factors that are interfering with normal function.

A valid treatment yardstick that applies to *any style* of medicine is the "risk versus benefit ratio." Let me use a familiar example of non-steroidal anti-inflammatory drugs (NSAIDS), such as aspirin. The *benefits* include reduction of pain and inflammation. On the other side of the equation, aspirin's *risks* include bleeding disorders, such as ulcers, intestinal bleeding, and hemorrhagic stroke. In fact, Non-steroidal Anti-inflammatory Drugs (NSAID) are blamed for over 16,000 deaths per year. That figure may be higher given that the Food and Drug Administration (FDA) recently required warning labels on non-aspirin NSAID pain killers noting that they increase the risk of heart attack, heart failure, and stroke. (The higher the dose the higher the risk.) Therefore, there is ongoing debate about the risk/benefit regarding these drugs. Tylenol is another example. The drug has been approved to reduce pain, but it is not expected to address the root cause of the pain. Under regulators' view of the risk-to-benefit ratio, Tylenol is *expected* to cause side effects like liver damage (especially when it is combined with alcohol), but that is allowable as long as deaths don't exceed the number that had been predicted.

Probiotics look fabulous when subjected to this same risk-to-benefit test. On the risk side there are really none—probiotics are organisms that are *supposed* to be in our systems—they are a key part of the original plan. Probiotics often help medications work better and reduce their side effects. On the other hand, most pharmaceutical drugs have negative effects on our friendly bacteria. Probiotics are viewed by some scientists as "living drugs."[1] A rapidly developing new field of study is called "Pharmacobiotics." Perhaps that medical sounding term will make probiotics more acceptable to mainstream docs than might be the case with quaint-sounding "fermented foods" and humble "over-the-counter probiotic supplements." Since there is *almost* nothing to say about *risks* associated with probiotics, most of the rest of this book will be about clarifying the *benefit* side of the equation.

The reader may be one of the many who still have no earthly idea what probiotics are. Thanks to massive advertising especially by yogurt companies, the majority of consumers do seem to understand one tiny bit of the story—that probiotics are bacteria which help with constipation. Constipation is indeed a common concern and we will discuss it in the second part of the book. More serious clinically-diagnosed digestive diseases, such as chronic diarrhea, ulcers, and gastrointestinal (GI) cancers, are responsible for over 200,000 deaths annually in the U.S. Probiotics may be an important part of the solution to those as well. But, perhaps even more interesting are "sub-clinical" digestive issues related to an imbalance of microorganisms. (Sub-clinical means they are ones that we don't even know we have.) They are often directly or at least indirectly responsible for many other discomforts, diseases, and deaths that at first seem unrelated to the GI tract.

Readers will learn that the benefits of having a thriving and well-balanced assortment of microbes range from clearer skin and a healthier weight to better control of allergies, asthma, depression, osteoporosis, and potentially deadly diseases, such as cancer, heart disease, and diabetes. For that matter, we should consider supporting the body's team of beneficial microorganisms as a key part of the plan to resolve virtually any type of health complaint.

As I mentioned in the Preface, our collection of probiotic microorganisms is like an organ with functions every bit as health-defining and complex as that of our liver or kidneys. Our team of microorganisms creates hundreds of metabolic substances in our circulation that help direct functions all around the body.[2] Happily, it is not as difficult to create a proper healing community of microorganisms as it would be to say . . . build a kidney from scratch. On the other hand, as we will see, it is also not as simple as buying ones favorite flavor of yogurt with its one or two strains of bacteria. Our systems are home to thousands of species and subspecies of bacteria—*all with different jobs.* And, to make matters even more interesting, each person's assortment is unique to them!

Obviously, no product can possibly contain a bacterial blend that matches a person's highly complex individualized system. That's why this book discusses how simple choices that we make each day support or harm our team of microbes. I also explain some of what is known about the various metabolic jobs that our microorganisms perform. That is not only to heighten the reader's appreciation of their value, but also to make it easier to fathom how they can possibly have such wide-ranging health benefits. As scientists learn more about these mechanisms, they begin to connect the dots to new uses for probiotics. That expanding research will uncover exciting possibilities, but may generate some problems. With a grasp of the big picture fundamentals, the reader will be less likely to be overwhelmed by the massive amount of research data coming down the pipeline. And they may be able to make better choices among a wildly growing list of options.

These are some of the issues:

- It appears that the average consumer ranks probiotic supplements based on how well they relieve constipation. While that is a worthy goal, as you will see, our friendly bacteria can improve so many other aspects of health.

- Some suppliers want us to believe that all probiotic supplements are equally effective and that we should choose based on how many "bugs" you can get for a buck. We are beginning to understand that high bacterial counts are not the same thing as high potency and that there may even be questions about ingesting huge numbers of certain single bacteria.

- Because the field is so new, federal regulators do not control which microorganisms are put in a pill and would only get involved if a pattern of harm emerges. An example of this concern would be a probiotic strain promoted as being "antibiotic resistant." This could lead to trouble since bacteria swap their genetic material and a disease-causing bacterium might acquire this skill.

- Food manufacturers have found that adding "probiotic" to a label is a good marketing tool. Generally speaking, more ways to obtain probiotics is usually better. However, there is a potential concern with this fad of adding probiotics willy-nilly to everything from peanut butter to wine. Probiotic label-decorating may lead to a problem similar to the one that developed when "fat free" was added to labels. The allure of probiotics might distract us from asking if the product is intrinsically healthful.

- It may become increasingly difficult for consumers to become informed about probiotic benefits through the usual channel, which as noted, is the manufacturer. In addition to already strict limits enforced by the FDA on product health claims, in 2014 the Federal Trade Commission and the Department of Justice filed an action against one of Phillips' Colon Health products. Regulators sued to stop the maker from saying that their probiotics defend against occasional constipation, diarrhea, gas, and bloating and insisted that *two randomized, controlled, clinical trials* be required for *every single strain* in a blend. To begin with it doesn't make much sense to prove the strains individually when probiotics work best in diverse teams. Also, such studies are extremely costly. So, if such a ruling prevails, the precedent will have a chilling effect on the creation, marketing, and availability of *all* probiotics. This government overreach exposes its historic bias in favor of drugs. They may not be satisfied until they can classify bacteria as drugs— even though probiotics have been part of our physical makeup for all of human history.

- Pharmaceutical companies see the potential profit to be gained from patenting a particular strain of bacteria for the treatment of a specific diagnosis. They have the vast amount of funding required to do research, achieve drug approval and acquire the right to make claims. Readers of this book may be spared the unnecessary expense of a prescription product because they will have learned that, in most cases, their problem may be solved by building a well-functioning diversity of microorganisms with strains of bacteria that are already available.

- The research focus on single strains may pay dividends. For example, clinical trials are under way on a bacterium that has been genetically modified to have anti-inflammatory benefits for those with Crohn's disease.[3] I will point out later another isolated strain that serves a unique purpose.

My goal in *The Probiotic Cure* is to help the reader harness the extraordinary power of their microbiome and probiotic supplements for the benefit of their short term comfort and vitality as well as their long-term health. There is a lot of ground to cover in Part One before we can get to the how-to's of using probiotics to solve our health concerns and support wellness every day as we will do in Part Two. I first will quickly put our experience with microbes into a historical context in Chapter 1. Then in Chapter 2 I'm hoping to shock readers a bit with a glimpse of the dynamic and breathtaking world of cutting-edge research. Hopefully, an appreciation of the startling power of our microbiota will generate added enthusiasm for the important business of learning the basics of how probiotics work and how to assure that we maintain a wholesome blend of colonies. To understand what we are up against, we take a closer look at the attributes and effects of enemy microorganisms in Chapter 3.

In Chapter 4 we begin to understand the extent of the skills of our ally bacteria. One serious threat to peace in our gut is antibiotics, a double-edged sword. Understanding how to use the drugs in a safer manner is covered in Chapter 5. Chapter 6 reveals other hidden threats to the stability of our microbiome. Then, in Chapter 7, we look at how to recruit additional microbes and feed them well. Chapter 8 explains how to reverse an imbalance of gut microbes and what to look for in selecting a probiotic product as well as how to use them. We can now put these fundamentals to work on basic subclinical digestive issues in Chapter 9. Part Two of the book gives strategies and tips for a variety of common health complaints. The concluding remarks reinforce probiotics' place in the future of medicine.

To provide recommendations that are specific enough to be useful, I will mention brand names occasionally. Please know that I do not work for any of these companies. The products are ones that I know to be of high quality and effectiveness and are often what I use myself and/or give my family members. Unless noted otherwise, they are widely available.

I encourage that the reader not simply jump to the "how to" sections. Understanding more fully how our body functions and how probiotics do their work will prove very useful as the reader's future needs and the landscape change.

PART ONE

Probiotic Basics

1.

The Eternal Internal Battle

I t is a zoo in there! There are teeming forces of friendly microorganisms doing battle with those that would harm us. Although human health and development has depended on microorganisms since we first walked the earth, the whole idea of "farming" our colonies of good bacteria and putting them to work in service to our health is new to almost everyone. So, let's assume nothing and start at the beginning. Bacteria are tiny animal-like organisms (microorganisms) that can be found virtually *everywhere*, from sub-glacial lakes in the Antarctic to the steaming pots of Yellowstone National Park. They are even in the clouds and have an effect on weather. They are versatile and can even make sea animals glow in the dark. Bacteria are so adaptable that they can withstand not only temperature extremes, but also high altitudes, radiation, desert dryness, salty seawater, chemical assaults, and with oxygen or without it. They can be round or rod shaped, smooth or with various types of protrusions. For those of us who are rusty in Latin, one is a bacterium *and two or more are bacteria.*

Today even children know that germs (bacteria) can cause illness and they may have a vague idea that our immune system cells protect us from them. However, even that knowledge is relatively new. Before the age of microscopes, neither bacteria nor immune cells could be seen. Well, that isn't precisely true. Now that we know what we are looking for, we can see a few that are extremely large. Throughout history, because the causes of disease were invisible, humans had to imagine explanations for them, as well as for the forces of healing. From the ancient Romans to our own Native Americans, most of those involved spirits of one sort or another.

A VERY BRIEF HISTORY OF MICROBIAL DISCOVERIES

Having devised a way to greatly increase magnification, an eyeglass maker, Antonie Philips van Leeuwenhoek discovered tiny life in the 1600's that he dubbed "animalcules." Another piece of the puzzle was added by Ignaz Semmelweis, an Austrian physician in the mid-1800's when he noticed that mothers seemed more likely to die while giving birth if their physicians had just performed an autopsy. Although he didn't know exactly what mechanism was responsible, survival statistics improved dramatically when he instituted a strict hand-cleaning regimen in the hospital where he practiced. Unfortunately, that didn't catch on and the battle over hand-washing continues today. In the late 1800's, surgeon Joseph Lister pioneered sterilization of surgical instruments. I'm sure he would be proud to be permanently remembered in the mouthwash name, Listerine. (Sterilization of surgical instruments may be vital, but in Chapter 4 we discuss that getting carried away with sterilizing and sanitizing everything around the home may have a downside.)

About the same time, French chemist Louis Pasteur was trying to figure out why alcohol went bad and discovered that microorganisms were the reason. He is credited with developing pasteurization (obviously named for him) and vaccines to protect against rabies and anthrax. A new era of connecting bacteria *to disease* had begun. As we will cover in Chapter 3, we are now aware of a great many more bacterial illnesses than was imagined in Pasteur's day. Of course, we also know that some bacteria are life-savers and some are merely annoying—for example, they are the reason some people use Odor Eaters in their gym shoes.

Around the same time as Pasteur's discovery, French scientist Claude Bernard declared that there was something quite important about the "terrain" in resisting infectious microorganisms. By terrain he meant something inside our bodies. I've read reports that on his death bed Pasteur declared that "Bernard was right; the pathogen is nothing; the terrain is everything." Whether he said that or not, today we are certainly beginning to appreciate that our condition as host is at least mighty important and that our friendly defenders are a key part of our terrain.

Russian biologist Dr. Ilya Ilyich Metchnikoff earned a Nobel Prize in Medicine in 1908 for progress in this newly discovered microscopic world. He isolated our immune cells called "phagocytes" and determined that they gobble up disease-causing bacteria. He is also considered the father of probiotics, the friendly type of bacteria. He identified the bacterial strains *Lactobacillus bulgaricus* and *Streptococcus thermophilus* and determined that they were protective of our health and presumably increased longevity. The era of connecting bacteria to *health* had begun. Metchnikoff began recommending milk fermented by the bacteria *acidophilus*.

There is typically a forty year lag between a health discovery and its general acceptance. In the case of good bacteria the lag was much longer, perhaps because killing bad bacteria consumed so many resources. Probiotics began to be studied in Europe decades before getting any real attention in the U.S. The late Dr. Kehm Shahani, a professor of food technology at the University of Nebraska, contributed an essay as part of a final report for that Dallas probiotic symposium that I mentioned. He noted that early research on the probiotic *Lactobacillus acidophilus* was done mostly just for the benefit of the dairy industry. The pace of research into probiotics for human use quickened in the 1980's when it was discovered that probiotics could be so valuable for digestive issues. I find it interesting (and a bit discouraging) that as far back as 1992, Dr. Shahani was impressed by past studies showing that probiotics would apparently benefit a wide range of conditions, including cholesterol and cancer. More than two decades later, these topics are being discussed as "new" ideas.

THE SCIENCE OF PROBIOTICS

Dr. Shahani would be amazed and thrilled at the current sophistication and dizzying pace of research on the microbiome. There are articles about beneficial bacteria in journals for virtually every scientific discipline (for example, publications dedicated to heart disease, cancer, diabetes, and psychiatry). Microbes also now have several scientific journals of their own (*Microbes*) and international conferences that attract participants from around the world to discuss the role of microorganisms in health and disease treatment. Perhaps you have heard of the Human Genome Project that mapped the location and function of all the genes in human DNA. While that project has not fulfilled all expectations regarding finding solutions to major diseases, it did stimulate the development of equipment that could analyze DNA quickly and at relatively low cost. That technological advance facilitated The Human Microbiome Project which is a similarly impressive multinational five-year study that has contributed greatly to our knowledge of gut microorganisms by mapping their genes. Previously only about 1 percent of gut bacteria could be identified by culturing them in a lab dish. DNA tells scientists what kind of an environment a specific bacterium needs so they can now culture them and study their behavior. A second phase of the project will focus on our microbiome as it relates to Pregnancy and Preterm Birth, Inflammatory Bowel Diseases, and Prediabetes.

Microbiome and *microbiota* are terms that refer to the totality of microorganisms that are part of us, both good and bad. *Flora* is a more informal way of saying the same thing and as noted earlier I will use those three terms interchangeably. Beneficial microorganisms in the body are sometimes offhandedly called *probiotics*, however the term technically means *ingested bacteria*. It is an easy lapse in precision because bacteria found in healthy people often become available as probiotic supplements and good bacteria can be added to the skin. We are host to trillions of bacterial cells, perhaps 10 times more than our own.[1] It is hard to imagine totals even higher than the government debt—100 trillion in the intestinal tract alone.[2] We walk around in something like a cloud of of our own bacteria and they are all over us inside and out. For example, in a belly button (along with the lint) there is a virtual metropolis teeming with millions of diverse bacteria. Bacteria literally coat our skin.[3] As reported by Associated Press medical writer, Lauran Neergaard, "Scientists decoded the genes of 112,000 bacteria in samples taken from a mere 20 spots on the skin of 10 people."[4] Bacteria also occupy any tissues that are similar to skin, such as those in the sinuses, gastrointestinal tract, vagina, placenta, and even the lungs. A healthily diverse community is comprised of 1,000 species and 5,000 or more sub-species.[5] Some experts say that there are up to 10,000 sub-species. (Imagine the program it would take to help us tell these players apart.)

Each person has a unique assortment of microorganisms and that can explain, for example, why one person metabolizes a drug differently than another. Researchers have decided that the average human hand carries 150 species of bacteria and that only 13 percent of them are common to any two people.[6] That makes them quite literally like a fingerprint. Forensic scientists (criminologists) will be able tell whether it was me or someone else who left a smudge on a glass table. Since the combination of types in each part of the body is somewhat different from that in the other parts, they could tell if it was from my hand or elbow! Even in a person's mouth we won't necessarily find the same bacteria on two different teeth. Scientists discovered, with 70 to 90 percent accuracy, that they could identify the owner of a computer mouse from among 270 people based on the bacteria left behind. And this is kind of scary . . . the mouse had not been used for twelve hours.

There are similarities in bacterial profiles among families and even com-munities.[7] Researchers could tell which persons live in which homes because of the distinctive assortment of bacteria deposited on doorknobs, countertops, and floor—even if they had recently moved into the house.[8] The microbiome of vegetarians differs from those of meat eaters. Interestingly, among human omnivores (those who eat plants and animals), the bacterial assortment is not much different from that of other primates like chimpanzees.[9] While there are differences in the variety and functioning of bacteria between men and women, race doesn't seem to matter much.[10]

Occasionally I will mention individual strain names to show the wide variety that is beneficial or to make a specific point. To name them in all instances would quickly become dizzying and intimidating even to health professionals. Secondly, because it turns out that many strains perform overlapping functions, it might not be particularly useful. And, finally, most often the best results are obtained from a diverse microbiome and from using several probiotic strains together, which we call a "multi-strain" probiotic.

What do all these bacteria do for us that make them so important to life? We've known for a long time that they helped regularity. However, some of the newly discovered functions are quite surprising and exciting. Chapter 4 will delve into more, but just as an enticing preview, probiotics assist with digestion and nutrient absorption, improve immune function, create targeted antibiotics, manufacture vitamins, help detoxification, make powerful substances that protect our cells, reduce inflammation, and provide energy. Even more amazingly, they communicate with our brains to improve our mood and help us decide things like whether or not we are hungry.

As further evidence of their value, if the numbers and diversity of our microscopic partners are deficient, trouble makers can get the upper hand. We call that imbalance *dysbiosis*. The long-term effects are just now being revealed, but here are just a few common short-term symptoms of dysbiosis:

- acne, eczema, skin, and foot problems
- allergies and chronic food sensitivities
- bad breath and gum disease
- constipation or diarrhea
- digestion problems, including acid reflux
- fatigue that is chronic and unexplained
- frequent colds, flu, and infections
- headaches
- joint pain and inflammation
- menstrual or menopausal symptoms
- sleep problems
- ulcers
- weight gain
- yeast overgrowth

There are a *lot* more negative effects. Those conditions obviously generate symptoms that are typically treated with medications and can in fact worsen the underlying dysbiosis and perpetuate a vicious cycle.

CONCLUSION

We obviously depend on our beneficial flora to keep a peaceful balance with disease-causing microorganisms. But, more than that, our microbiome is fundamental to our very nature. The Human Genome Project did not find enough genes to explain everything about us. So, where then do the rest of the instructions come from to make us who we are as unique individuals and to dictate how we will function? Some of that information comes from mitochondria in our cells (tiny energy factories) which are discussed further in the Glossary. But, our friendly bacteria collectively have perhaps 300 to 1000 times the genetic coding that our cells do![11] They preceded humans on earth and wrote the rules we still live by. We are learning that our microbes can help (along with diet and lifestyle) to turn our own good genes ON and our worrisome genes OFF. With all the power that these microorganisms apparently have over our well-being, it is a relief that science is finally taking them so seriously. The next chapter surveys just a few representative areas of that study.

2.

On the Front Lines of Research

I t is not just a happy accident that our microbes support us in so many ways. The beneficial microorganisms that live in and on our bodies profit by helping to keep us healthy. That relationship is a two way street called *synergy* and we learn more about this important relationship every day. The current research is astoundingly sophisticated, but in a way is also showing us that we have a lot to learn. How soon we have all the answers will be controlled in part by limitations of research time and funding. And, of course, a scientist must be inspired to even ask the particular questions we want answered.

SCIENTIFIC INTEREST IN PROBIOTICS FOR AGRICULTURE

Earlier I mentioned that there are thousands of scientific entries into PubMed. Of course, not all of them are investigating the effects of probiotics on human health, at least directly. For example, there is interest in putting bacteria to work producing alternative fuel from plants and wastes. Some studies are basic research into separating cause from effect and into technical aspects of bacterial cell structure, culturing or preserving them. Many relate to agricultural and food production applications. This first list of applications in that category are interesting in their variety and creativity and because they hint at humans uses for probiotics. Beneficial bacteria are used:

- as a preservative for cheese and fresh cut pineapple

- to improve the growth, immune status, antioxidant protection, egg quantity, and meat quality in chickens

- to control fungus in cow feed that is stored in silos

- to provide naturally-produced antibiotics and to reduce the effects of stress on lobsters and sole

- in the place of antibiotics to promote healthy growth in pigs

- for rabbit tummy problems
- for various health benefits for thoroughbred horses, parrots, and pets
- to protect turkeys from aflatoxin (poison) produced by fungus in feed

In the above cases we know for sure the benefits are not just a placebo effect. (As you may know, a placebo effect is where there is no actual benefit from the treatment, but a person still *feels* that they have been helped.) Another indication of measurable benefit is that producers would not spend precious dollars on something that does not work.

RESEARCH INTO MICROBES AND HEALTH

The sheer volume of studies is so vast and dynamic that those I've listed below are just clues to the exotic new world that awaits us. I encourage the reader to at least scan the categories below—even the ones that don't seem to hit close to home because those items contain information about how the body functions and the general ways that our bacteria and probiotics work for us.

Some of the studies below were substantial human clinical trials. Others were quite small or used cellular or animal models of human systems. Procedures differ. Some simply observed the existing microbiome while others intervened with various materials, such as mixed probiotics, fermented dairy, and/or specific strains of bacteria. I don't necessarily differentiate the methodology in each of these areas. The research list is provided mainly to demonstrate that researchers consider probiotics indeed quite powerful and to show which specific issues they currently find promising enough to study.

With this list I don't mean to imply that any single strain or even combination is considered proven to be an ultimate answer for any of these serious health issues—the science is too young. And there is another problem. No matter how many thousands of years a natural remedy has been valued or how many hundreds of studies show benefit, *nothing natural* can legally be called "proven" or marketed as a "cure." That applies even to natural remedies that become commonly used in medical practice. By law, *only drugs* are allowed to *cure* anything. (I'm quite serious.) Also, only drugs are allowed to say that they *prevent* disease. But, never mind because in this book I am not interested in making drug type claims for any single bacterial strain or product, but I instead want to establish the curative nature of a healthy diverse balance of microorganisms in our body. That is the natural plan. That is a simple, effective plan that also doesn't involve memorizing a bunch of Latin names!

Aging

Our calendar age is often not a good indicator of the health age of our cells, tissues, and organs which can be significantly better or worse than what would be expected. Nobel Prize winner Ilya Mechnikov observed that of 36 countries he compared, Bulgarians lived the longest and he connected that longevity with the inhabitants' consumption of yogurt. Studies show clear differences in the microbiome of those living to a ripe old age and animal studies provide important clues to the role that probiotics play in moderating aging influences.[1] For instance, chronic inflammation is high on the list as a major cause of premature aging and probiotics seem to help reduce inflammation.[2] Free radical damage (oxidation) is another major factor in aging. Probiotics in general help create protective antioxidants, and as you will see in Chapter 4, one probiotic strain has been shown to greatly increase a master antioxidant. Even the visible signs of aging, such as sun damage to the skin, seem to be prevented by probiotics.[3] However, many interconnected factors remain to be sorted out. For example, good microbiomes are a byproduct of healthful habits that also extend a lifespan.[4] As we'll see later when we look at feeding probiotics, less healthy food reduces diversity of probiotics and results in elderly that are frailer. Lack of exercise, exposure to chemicals, and many other factors reduce the benefits of gut flora.

Asthma

Even if you don't personally know someone with asthma, you have probably at least heard about the disease in the television commercials for asthma medications. (One always catches my attention when it mentions a particular side effect . . . that it increases the risk of an *asthma-related death*!) Incidence of this potentially life-threatening restriction of airways is rising. There is now scientific speculation that one reason may be an overreaction by immune systems that have not been exposed to the variety of bacteria as was normal in times gone by. For example, children who play outdoors, or are reared on a farm, or who have a dog may encounter more species of microorganisms and therefore have immune systems that are more tolerant of various environmental exposures and less likely to mount an allergic response.[5] Scientists speculate that probiotics at an early age may have similarly protective effects.[6]

Contrary to textbooks which claim that the lungs are sterile, there is a microbiome *in the lungs*. Normally the bacteria seem to be transient and are similar to those that would have come from the mouth or perhaps sinuses. According to Gary B. Huffnagle, PhD of the University of Michigan Medical Center, the gut is important to asthma because it takes a "perfect storm" of antibiotic exposure, yeast bloom, and challenges from the environment to get the allergic reaction that triggers asthma. Antibiotics will be covered in Chapter 5. Yeast bloom and leaky gut and their relationship to probiotics will be found in Chapter 9. Fiber intake seems to help prevent asthma.

Autoimmune Conditions

When the immune system goes beyond attacking pathogens and targets parts of our own body, that unfortunate process is called an *autoimmune* condition. Medical science now believes that one hundred disease syndromes or more are of that type. They are typically referred to as having "no known cause" and "no known cure." Given that our friendly flora are confirmed to support *normal* immune function, it is no wonder that researchers are investigating gut balance and probiotics as an aid for autoimmune issues, such as inflammatory bowel disease, autoimmune thyroid disease, rheumatoid arthritis, type 1 diabetes, and ankylosing spondylitis.[7,8,9,10,11]

Cancer

While cancer is not the number one cause of premature death (heart disease occupies that place), it seems to be the most feared. Unfortunately, progress to find natural solutions to the prevention and treatment of most forms of cancer has been agonizingly slow. We know that hormone imbalances and certain toxins are associated with some cancers and that microbes may be a cause. But, clearly-identified causes of cancer are rare. An exception is that lung cancers are known to be caused by smoking and inhalation of asbestos. Toxins are suspect in many others. I have a copy of a University of Nebraska animal study from 1989 in my files showing that it was already known then that lactic acid bacteria (the most common type of probiotic) detoxified some cancer-causing substances. Progress on the treatment side is also a bit discouraging especially in that standard cancer treatment options obviously carry their own very serious risks. (Surgery can have complications and both chemo and radiation undisputedly can *cause* cancer.) It is refreshing to see advancement in the field of *probiotics for cancer.*

- Colon cancer is the third leading cause of cancer deaths worldwide and there is not sufficient evidence that colonoscopies as currently administered save lives. Science is showing that there is a greater risk of colon cancer when certain strains of bacteria are prevalent. The ideas that gut bacteria can be used as a screening tool and might help prevent or treat colon cancer are promising.[12,13] It is known that our friendly bacteria help suppress pathogenic bacteria that create cancer-causing substances from our digestive bile. Some researchers believe that probiotics help send messages to colon cancer cells to kill themselves (apoptosis).[14] Substances like polyamines, spermine, spermidine, and putrescine that are produced in the colon from the breakdown of waste material are known instigators of cancer. Researchers seem excited that probiotics reduce levels of these substances and therefore protect against colon cancer.[15,16] (Also, consider that those same toxins, if not neutralized, can escape the digestive tract into circulation where they can cause trouble all over the body.) In animal studies probiotics show benefit in reducing colon cancer cell formation and growth.[17] When researchers compared the intestinal microbes of healthy subjects to those diagnosed with colorectal cancer, they found that the cancer patients' microbiomes were less diverse and had smaller populations of the type of bacteria (*Clostridia*) that produce butyrate, a fatty acid that is known to reduce inflammation and colon cancer.[18] When diversity is reduced, usually the strains that make butyrate are the ones that are missing. It is worthy of note that colon cancer patients with above average levels of Vitamin D survive one third longer. Other budding research indicates that probiotics may improve the intestinal tract's sensitivity to vitamin D.

- In a mouse model of breast cancer, fermented milk (a source of probiotics) was sufficient to suppress tumor growth and slow spreading the disease.[19]

- In one interesting study, a number of bacterial strains were found to stop cancer cells from growing and extracts of the cell walls of 3 strains caused cancer cells to kill themselves, but spared healthy cells.[20]

- Our general health and immune function benefits from the many probiotic functions to be detailed in Chapter 4, so it isn't surprising that studies are investigating probiotics for help against other types of cancer. Probiotics and a microbiome-friendly diet are being studied in connection with cancer of the bladder, breast, cervix, kidney, lung, ovaries, prostate, stomach, and uterus.[21,22,23,24,25,26,27]

- The most promising cancer therapies are aimed at stimulating the body's own immune system to go after the malignancy. As we will discuss, that is something that probiotics do.

- Because probiotics seem to help make chemotherapy more effective and reduce its side effects as well as those from radiation, probiotics may soon become a routine partner in treatment of virtually all cancers.[28] Search "cancer" on my website (HBNShow.com) for natural support for cancer treatments as well as useful information about new testing for early detection and fine-tuning treatments.

- As we will discuss in later chapters, a healthful diet is cancer-protective in part because it provides nourishment for a more beneficial class of microorganisms. Nutritionfacts.org is a good source of information showing that plant foods are especially useful. In *Beating Cancer with Nutrition*, Patrick Quillin, PhD explains that sugar acts essentially as fertilizer for cancer; that nutrients in food do not interfere with cancer treatments; and carefully selected nutritional supplements can improve treatment effectiveness and reduce side effects.

Cardiovascular Diseases

Heart disease is the number one disease cause of untimely death in U.S. adults. (Sadly, the number one *non-disease* cause is the total of errors and complications from medical treatment and hospitalization.) Although it doesn't get comparable media attention, cardiovascular disease kills 5 times as many women as breast cancer. Probiotics show benefits for a variety of cardiovascular risk factors, such as the reduction of inflammation and improvement of antioxidant status even among the critically ill.[29] The following are connections between probiotics and specific cardiovascular issues.

Blood pressure

Even modest reductions in blood pressure (BP) can dramatically reduce the risk of stroke. A meta-analysis (that is a study of other studies) blended nine clinical trials that included more than 500 adults. In it researchers found that probiotic consumption improved systolic BP by –3.56 mm Hg and diastolic BP by –2.38 mm Hg compared to control groups. It is important to note, and I will get back to this point many times, a better result was found in studies that used *multiple* probiotic strains compared to those using single strains and when probiotics were used for a longer time period.[30]

Cholesterol

The situation is *far more complex* than this, but in the simplest terms, it is said that high levels of LDL cholesterol are a prime risk factor for hardening of the arteries and heart disease. Statin drugs are prescribed to lower cholesterol, but there are many concerns about their side effects, such as muscle weakness, brain shrinkage, weight gain, liver damage, cataract risk, and an increased risk of diabetes.

Since the research into probiotics as support for healthful cholesterol levels has been going on for such a long time, I find it concerning that we hear next to nothing about that factor. For example, an animal study *sixteen years ago* showed that administration of a lactic acid probiotic reduced total cholesterol by 38 percent and triglycerides (another risk factor) by 40 percent and improved the ratio of LDL cholesterol to the preferred HDL.[31] More recently:

- In 2000, a European human clinical study showed that among overweight participants, milk fermented with various bacterial strains had positive effects on LDL cholesterol and blood pressure.[32]

- A 43 percent reduction in total cholesterol and 12 percent increase in HDL were achieved in rats by use of a probiotic (*Lactobacillus rhamnosus GG*) along with Aloe Vera gel.[33]

- In a human study, supplementation with 2 probiotic strains (*Lactobacillus curvatus HY7601* and *Lactobacillus plantarum KY1032*) for two weeks improved measures of cardiovascular health by reducing triglycerides and increasing the particle size of cholesterol molecules.[34]

- In another human trial, subjects taking capsules containing 2 strains of probiotics (*Lactobacillus acidophilus and Bifidobacterium bifidum*) 3 times a day for six weeks resulted in lower levels of total cholesterol compared to those taking a placebo.[35]

- A recent meta-analysis of 33 clinical studies concluded that probiotics reduced cholesterol among those not on cholesterol medication.[36]

- Probiotics seem to help children that have high cholesterol and post-menopausal women who have metabolic syndrome.[37,38]

Although the focus has been mainly on the *amount* of LDL cholesterol, recent more finely-tuned science shows that the bigger threat is *oxidized* cholesterol. Oxidation is akin to the process that makes iron rusty. (Incidentally, statin drugs also interfere with the body's ability to make a substance, CoQ10, which among other benefits protects cholesterol from that oxidizing process.) One probiotic strain, *Lactobacillus fermentum ME-3*, has been shown to reduce cholesterol oxidation by boosting glutathione. (There is more about glutathione in the inset on page 54.) That strain is sold as a part of a cardiovascular formula that also contains CoQ10.

Many consumers are still worried about cholesterol in food and are apparently not aware that most of the body's cholesterol is made by the liver. One reason that probiotics are good for cholesterol is that probiotics support liver health. Given the drubbing that saturated fat has received for years with implications that it raises cholesterol, it is good to know that even among subjects who already had elevated cholesterol, consumption of full fat (saturated) yogurt or full fat Camembert cheese did not raise cholesterol or blood pressure.[39] Eating full fat yogurt with probiotics also improves the "good" HDL cholesterol.[40]

Some scientists are optimistic that combinations of diet and probiotics will be proven to provide an alternative to cholesterol medication and its side effects.[41] However, so far this research has not changed the practice of medicine. For some time to come it will apparently be up to the consumer to research natural means of achieving healthy cholesterol levels. Balancing gut bacteria seems like a very good place to start.

Heart attack

The reader may not be overly excited to learn that probiotics reduced the severity of heart attack in rats.[42] Likewise, they may not care that probiotics also seem helpful for heart failure in rats.[43] However, heart failure is a very difficult condition to treat in humans and this particular breed is often used in laboratories as models for humans.

Unhealthy gum tissues release into circulation bacterial toxins that have been linked to heart disease. In Part Two we will discuss probiotics for a healthier mouth.

Diabetes

Diabetes is reaching epidemic levels in the U.S. and has become a major problem even among children. Besides Type 2 diabetes' own negative effects, it is a major risk factor for heart disease. It is clearer by the day that we need to move away from eating so many starches, sugars, and soft drinks to help avoid this crisis of blood sugar. But, interestingly, researchers are now connecting diabetes to microorganisms as both potential causes and protectors.

- Scientists discovered that type 2 diabetics had a different assortment of intestinal bacteria than healthy people.[44]

- Insulin is a hormone that the pancreas secretes to lower blood sugar levels. When cells in the body stop responding to it appropriately, the condition is called "insulin insensitivity," a known precursor of diabetes. An animal study showed that not only did a mixture of probiotic strains improve insulin sensitivity but also obesity and fatty liver.[45]

- Transferring bacteria from lean men into those with blood sugar issues resulted in an improvement in insulin sensitivity of roughly 70 percent.[46]

- A review of several studies shows benefit of probiotics for a number of measures of blood sugar control and evidence of benefit for the cardiovascular risk factors that are secondary effects of diabetes.[47]

- At least one line of research is looking into the role of good bacteria in the prevention of *Type 1* diabetes. The theory is that a lack of certain types of fiber plus high fat and high gluten (a protein in wheat, rye, and barley) intake may lead to the growth of the wrong type of intestinal bacteria which in turn generate the diabetes-causing autoimmune effect.[48]

- A review of studies indicates that probiotics help blood sugar issues via various mechanisms, such as reduction of inflammation, reduction of intestinal permeability (also known as "leaky gut" discussed in the Chapter 9), and prevention of oxidation (like that rusty cholesterol).[49] Unfortunately, metformin and other drugs commonly given to diabetics apparently interfere with the microbiota in the intestines.

- Evidence is mounting that implantation of a very large complex of gut bacteria may be a viable treatment for diabetes.[50]

- A clinical trial showed that a combination of probiotics along with their food fiber supply (prebiotic) reduced insulin levels in pregnant women compared to controls.[51]

- Other researchers believe that probiotics will reduce the complications from diabetes.[52]

HIV/AIDS

Acquired immunodeficiency syndrome (AIDS) is caused by the human immunodeficiency virus (HIV) which attacks the victim's immune system. It is spread through sexual contact as well as by the use of shared hypodermic needles. Although transmission rates have recently moderated a bit, AIDS is still a pandemic affecting over thirty million people worldwide. Unfortunately, in the U.S., according to the Centers for Disease Control (CDC), of those infected with HIV, 20 percent do not receive treatment because they do not even know they are carrying the virus. (This is not a case of "no news is good news." Persons who have engaged in risky behavior should get the test.) In the early days after its discovery, the disease was considered to be almost universally fatal. However, with advances in the anti-viral medications, a well-managed patient can now live a relatively normal life.

Over one hundred submissions to PubMed list both "HIV" and "probiotics" as key words. AIDS scientists are showing a lot of interest in probiotics because of their significant positive effect on the immune system.

- Human immunodeficiency viruses attack and destroy a particular immune cell called CD4. Probiotics seem to help maintain healthier levels of these immune disease-fighters.[53]

- Benefit has also been demonstrated to improve HIV patients' inflammation levels, complications, and drug side effects.[54]

- Sadly, children of an infected mother can be born with HIV. A recent study into the use of nutrients and probiotics among children not being treated with medications has shown that they eat better, improve their immune markers, and present milder symptoms.[55]

- It has been demonstrated that intake of probiotic yogurt improves quality of life among AIDS patients in Africa, and probiotic supplements help control the fungal overgrowth that commonly accompanies the disease.[56,57]

The evidence for probiotics helping HIV is certainly encouraging. However, not every study shows benefit.[58] Furthermore, even a friendly microorganism can get out of hand if the immune system is simply not working, and at the same time the bacteria have insufficient competition from other healthy strains. So, for those very ill patients with severely compromised immune systems, it might be best to supplement with blends of *many* bacterial strains or to simply supply foods (prebiotics) that support the whole array of friendly flora.

Infections

Obviously, HIV is only one of a tremendous number of infections, some of them equally life-threatening. Some of the worst are often actually acquired in hospitals, nursing homes, and other healthcare facilities. That includes the three listed in this section. According to the CDC, there were as many as 721,800 *hospital-associated* infections in 2011.[59] The agency reported 98,987 deaths from them in 2002.[60]

Fortunately, our immune cells are quite versatile in that they can fight off both viruses and bacterial invaders. Probiotics support and help instruct our innate immune protection. They also fight those enemies directly by creating selective antibiotic substances called "bacteriocins." Probiotics are even being used in conjunction *with* antibiotics—to increase the drugs' effectiveness and to reduce side effects. Probiotics are being studied for their help with many infections, such as *Clostridium difficile (C-diff)*, *Methicillin-resistant Staphylococcus aureus (MRSA)*, and pneumonia.

Clostridium difficile (C-diff)

The *C-diff* infection causes a type of unrelenting diarrhea that can be lethal because it does not respond to common antibiotics. The nearly half a million annual cases in the U.S. are responsible for 29,000 deaths. Rates are not going down.[61] Antibiotic use is a major cause of *C-diff* and the use of acid-blocking heartburn drugs is also a risk factor. Probiotics have been shown to prevent the disease in animals, especially if a multi-strain is used and when combined with prebiotics.[62] It is thought that among other actions, probiotics may help keep toxins released by the bacteria from binding to the lining of the intestinal tract. Probiotics may also work against these antibiotic-resistant strains by reminding them to pay attention to the antibiotics.[63] Probiotics also seem to reduce the inflammation that is caused by the bug.[64] For ten years a community hospital in Quebec has given every patient who receives an antibiotic a multistrain probiotic. The facility dramatically reduced their incidence of *Clostridium difficile* and continued to have a lower incidence than comparable hospitals in the area.[65] In Chapter 8 we'll talk about the most effective (almost miraculous) medical remedy, FMT (fecal microbiota transplant), which is a way of supplementing thousands of bacterial sub-strains and the protective substances they make.

Methicillin-resistant Staphylococcus aureus (MRSA)

An alarming headline March 2009 in the AARP Bulletin read: "Drug-resistant staph infections kill more people than AIDS." They were referring mainly to *MRSA* which infects 80,000 Americans annually and is responsible for 11,285 deaths. MRSA infections are spread in places where lots of people congregate, such as schools, rest homes, and gyms. Because sports teams have experienced *MRSA* outbreaks, they now disinfect their workout equipment constantly. Sharing cell phones also holds the potential for spreading this germ.

MRSA is known as a "Smart Bug" because it has become immune to our strongest antibiotics. (Perhaps all bacteria are "smart" because they do whatever they need to in order to survive and multiply.) Probiotics show benefits against MRSA in laboratory studies and one strain in particular, *E. faecalis TH10* has been shown to be especially potent. Unfortunately, there are as yet few clinical studies that put probiotics to the test with *MRSA*, but the early ones are promising.[66] Perhaps there is such panic around cases of *MRSA* that all a physician can think of is finding a stronger antibiotic. It seems clear they should consider at least adding probiotics to their *MRSA* protocol because probiotics help offset the damage that antibiotics do to our gut flora.

Pneumonia

This lung disease is most often caused by bacteria or viruses, but can also be caused by inflammation due to medications and autoimmune disease. The Centers for Disease Control reported 157,500 cases of U.S. *hospital-associated* pneumonia in 2011.[67] Unfortunately, the pneumonia viruses and bacteria lurk in hospitals where patients also happen to be in a vulnerable state. Even if a patient is admitted to the hospital with cancer or another disease, pneumonia is often listed as the cause of death simply because it is the *final* insult. A review of studies shows that administration of probiotics reduces the incidence of hospital-acquired pneumonia.[68]

Because stomach acid is a first line defense against invading pathogens, blocking acid production with acid-blocking medications (like heartburn drugs) leads to a documented increase in pneumonia (and *C-diff*). Probiotics are usually part of the solution to acid reflux.

Kidney Diseases

Among many important jobs, kidneys are indispensable for filtering wastes from blood and for maintaining healthy levels of fluids and blood pressure. Probiotics are enjoying some research attention in regard to kidney health.

- Because it is known that probiotics (especially with prebiotics) help detoxify substances that are poisonous to kidney tissue, a double-blind, placebo-controlled, randomized cross-over clinical trial is under way to document the improvement.[69]

- In a previous study, over a one-year period, patients with stable chronic kidney disease experienced a slower decline in kidney function compared to the control group if they were taking supplements of prebiotics and probiotics pills.[70] (Both groups were on a low protein diet.)

- There is preliminary support for the role of prebiotics and probiotics in reducing the cardiovascular risk due to toxins and inflammation associated with chronic kidney disease.[71]

- Most kidney stones are formed mainly of a crystalline substance called *oxalate*. It was found that persons whose digestive tracts contained a certain beneficial bacteria (*Oxalobacter formigenes*) were 70 percent less likely to be recurrent kidney stone formers.[72] Later research implies the reason is that the bacteria help the body handle oxalate in a safer fashion.[73]

Liver Diseases

The human liver is a marvel of engineering that conducts hundreds of vital processes, including, as noted above, making cholesterol. Toxins really gum up the works and when a liver is failing, the only conventional answer is an expensive, scarce, and risky liver transplant. Therefore, it is encouraging to know the various ways that probiotics help the liver function and protect it. The following is a small sample of studies on probiotics for liver issues. In general probiotics reduce toxins.[74] Read more about this in Chapter 4.

Cirrhosis

Cirrhosis is a disease that most often results from chronic alcohol excess. Obviously, avoiding alcohol is crucial in the treatment. An animal study demonstrated the ability of a probiotic to reduce liver damage.[75] One of the condition's most serious effects is "hepatic encephalopathy" which is altered brain function that can include confusion, depression, and eventually a coma. A recent review of six randomized controlled human trials involving almost five hundred patients concluded that "probiotics decrease overt hepatic encephalopathy in patients with liver cirrhosis."[76] Cirrhosis has now been linked to *leaky gut,* indicating a clear connection to probiotic benefits.[77] Alcohol damage to the liver also impairs the immune system, making alcoholics susceptible to infection. It appears that probiotics help with that as well.[78]

Hepatitis

Inflammation of the liver caused by a hepatitis virus can persist without symptoms or it can lead to the familiar yellowing of the skin (jaundice), scarring of liver tissue, and ultimately to cirrhosis. Because of their general immune benefit, it isn't surprising that probiotics are helpful.[79] But here is an interesting twist—probiotics may help the Hepatitis B vaccine work more effectively.[80]

Non-alcoholic fatty liver

For reasons similar to those that lead to diabetes, fat can build up in the liver and hamper its function. Probiotics help with that condition as well, and the hunt is under way to clarify the mechanisms.[81,82]

Mental Health

There is little public discussion about the *prevention* of mental health issues, such as anxiety, depression, schizophrenia, Parkinson's, and Alzheimer's. When they are diagnosed, psychoactive medications are the current go-to treatment. The intestinal tract (where our microorganisms live) is physically pretty far away from the brain and so we would not immediately think about gut health a factor in such conditions. But, many are because in September 2014, the National Institute of Mental Health took action to spur new research on the gut microbiome's role in mental disorders by awarding four grants with a value of up to one million dollars each. There is mounting evidence that schizophrenia, bipolar disorder, and obsessive-compulsive disorder are at least in some cases caused by bacterial infections. Logically, wherever pathogenic (disease-causing) bacteria are a factor, we should consider their protective counterpart, our friendly bacteria.

But, there is more. Inflammation is associated with these mental conditions and our friendly bacteria have been shown to help with that. Bacteria have also been shown to influence the development of emotional behavior, stress and pain modulation systems, and brain signaling systems.[83] Gut bacteria may also generate electrical impulses that communicate with our gray matter. At least in animal studies a blend of probiotics helped slow age-related memory loss.[84] (One day science may connect the dots and show that our friendly microbes make us smarter.)

Studies now seem enthusiastic about the potential for the *therapeutic* use of probiotics with even "major psychiatric disorders."[85] The gut produces so many nerve and brain signaling chemicals that author Michael Gershon titled his book, *The Second Brain*. In *Brain Maker* author David Perlmutter, MD wrote about the connection between our microbiome and some of these issues as well as ADD/ADHD.

An emerging field of science called "psychobiotics" is delving into the intimate relationship between gut and brain and the benefits we can expect to see. The following is a representative sample of research.

Depression

Studies are currently looking into probiotics' effect on a variety of mood disorders, such as depression (as well as on behavior and brain function).[86] Depression is a common side effect of a systemic overgrowth of yeast and as discussed in Chapter 9, probiotics are an important component of a yeast management program.

Autism / Attention Deficit

It has frequently been found that those children with some expression of autism spectrum disorder have differences in their microbiomes. Recent research showed that germ free mice (ones without a gut microbiome and raised in a sterile environment) developed a leaky *blood brain barrier.* When normal beneficial bacteria were implanted, the barrier became less permeable.[87] The blood brain barrier is crucial to protecting the brain from substances circulating in the blood that could damage the delicate neurological tissue. That's why this stunning study opened up a world of questions for me. For example, some parents claim that their child became autistic immediately after they were immunized. They are called foolish because typical studies deny the vaccine/autism connection because the association doesn't show up in the *averages* of the data. However, is it possible that certain children lack the gut microbes that keep the blood brain barrier protective? Their brains might therefore be disproportionately damaged by the mercury and other ingredients in vaccines. Read more about vaccines on page 73.

Study is under way to determine the cause and how probiotics and prebiotics might be used to help prevent and treat this growing concern.[88] I think the results of a recent study are stunning in the possibilities. It showed that giving probiotics to infants reduced the incidence of Attention Deficit Hyperactivity Disorder (ADHD) and Asperger Syndrome by age 13 to zero in the probiotic treated group compared with 17.1 percent of the children in the placebo group.[89] There are anecdotal reports of autism being reversed with the use of fecal microbiota transplantation (FMT), a procedure that will be discussed on page 112. Could autism or even obsessive compulsive disorder be worsened by *Clostridia* or improved with *Bacteroides fragilis* as one study suggested?[90] At least for mice, friendly bacteria can act as anti-anxiety drug. In a more general sense, daily probiotics and prebiotics delivered in yogurt helped *healthy* children to have fewer sick days, but also "improved social and school functioning."[91]

Parkinson's

A recent Swedish animal study is the first to document that the devastating neurological condition Parkinson's disease (PD) may be due to a misfolded protein (α-synuclein) that arises from the intestinal tract and ultimately travels to the brain's movement center.[92] At this point the science hasn't linked probiotics to improving this process, and I could find no studies that have even asked that question. However, because probiotics are involved in protein digestion and protein synthesis, perhaps it is only a matter of time. In other work scientists linked early Parkinson's to leaky gut (increased permeability of the lining of the intestines) which will be covered in a section beginning on page 130.[93]

I did find one study about using probiotics as a remedy for the constipation that typically accompanies Parkinson's disease. The researchers concluded: "This pilot study showed that a regular intake of probiotics can significantly improve stool consistency and bowel habits in Parkinson's disease patients."[94] (Incidentally, a "pilot study" means that more research is expected to follow, but it seems that we are still waiting.)

Schizophrenia

Schizophrenia is a life-altering disease that can be quite hard to manage. Considerable research interest is focused on the link between probiotics, food sensitivities, and this particular mental illness.[95] As a bonus, probiotics may help with GI (gastrointestinal) symptoms associated with schizophrenia.[96]

Psychoactive drugs may cause worrisome side effects, such as the risk of homicidal and suicidal behavior, that can be even more severe when the drugs are first introduced or withdrawn. Therefore, no one should stop taking such medication without professional guidance.

Necrotizing Enterocolitis (NEC)

NEC is the second leading cause of death among premature infants. It is a tragic situation wherein a section of a baby's intestine dies. These tiny babies are not simply smaller versions of full term babies. They require intensive care because many of their systems are not yet fully developed. For instance, their immune and digestive systems are particularly incomplete and vulnerable to damage. Probiotics seem to trigger the formation of blood vessels that are needed to help the newborn's intestines mature, which may be one reason that probiotics help. Infants with NEC have less diversity in their microbiome. A review of several studies confirmed not only the effectiveness of probiotics for the prevention of NEC, but also the safety of probiotics.[97] One study found that probiotics reduced the incidence of infection with drug-resistant bacterial strains in newborns, and another study found them of benefit in preventing all-cause mortality in premature babies.[98,99] Probiotics also seem to help with one common, as yet unexplained, problem, blood loss in their stool.[100]

Pancreatitis

Pancreatitis is a very serious inflammation of the pancreas (a gland that secretes hormones, such as insulin and digestive enzymes). The inflammation is most often caused by alcohol, but it can also be initiated by pathogens, medications, autoimmune disease, and other factors. A study showed that among patients with severe acute pancreatitis, when probiotics were added early in the treatment, inflammation was reduced; gastrointestinal function was restored more quickly; and there were fewer complications and shorter hospital stays.[101] Many functions of probiotics surely help prevent pancreatitis.

CONCLUSION

I don't want to leave the impression that probiotics *always* work. When (and it is rare) a study does not show a benefit from probiotics, typically the term of the study was short (less than eight weeks) and/or it used an *individual* strain rather than a *complex* of strains like those found in a variety of fermented foods.[102] It might be useful to acknowledge what science already seems to be regarded as *well-established*. Large groups of internationally-recognized experts, such as Health Canada, the World Health Organization, and other committees monitor health issues. Many of them have looked at the randomized controlled trials on probiotics, and they have developed guidelines to help medical practitioners recommend them to patients with diseases, as well as to healthy persons. That is important because prevention of disease is always the easiest, most pleasant, and least expensive approach.

According to an article in the journal *Applied Physiology, Nutrition, and Metabolism*, probiotics can be recommended for the "prevention of upper respiratory tract infections and pouchitis" (an infection that can affect patients who have a colectomy). The article goes on to list "bacterial vaginosis [vaginal infections] and antibiotic-associated diarrhea, including *Clostridium difficile* infection, for treatment of atopic eczema in cow's milk allergy, and of infectious diarrhea." The authors suggest that there is also substantiation for probiotic benefits for prevention of high cholesterol, "the management of constipation, reduction of recurrent urinary tract infections, improvement of Irritable Bowel Syndrome symptoms, and reduction of antibiotics side effects in Helicobacter Pylori eradication." The article also commented that probiotics are safe.[103]

The future holds some fascinating uses for bacteria, such as using them to power microscopic nano bio-robots which circulate in a patient's blood to deliver drugs to a certain target. Probiotics are even a consideration for space travel because conditions inside a space ship are not conducive to good bacteria and yet perversely seem to make pathogens more potent. In the near-term just a scan of headings above should give us all sufficient incentive to make sure that our systems always maintain a plentiful and balanced assortment of beneficial microorganisms. There is more motivation on the way in the next chapter as we investigate the many challenges we face from a plethora of pathogens.

3.

The Enemies– Harmful Microorganisms

O ur own human cells and a vast complex of helpful and harmful microorganisms are engaged in a constant tug of war for survival of their own kind. For simplicity, we'll sort microorganisms into the broad categories of "Enemy" in this chapter and "Allies" in the next, but the sections on "Turncoats" and "Double Agents" below shows that it isn't quite that simple. Microorganisms, such as bacteria, viruses, parasites, and fungus, are not intrinsically evil. As mentioned earlier, activities that probiotics do to *help themselves* also happen to *help us*. With pathogens, it is the opposite—what is *good* for their life cycle is *bad* for ours. The more we know about how they operate the better we can protect ourselves and avoid making the serious error of applying antibiotics inappropriately.

BACTERIA

Of all the various types of microorganisms that occupy our bodies, we have had the longest awareness of bacteria. We understandably fear the bacteria that cause disease, and we have been taught to protect ourselves by sanitizing, sterilizing, and pasteurizing the heck out of *everything* to avoid them. If a bacterium gets past those protections and our innate immune defenses, it will most likely to be attacked with powerful antibiotics. However, as we will learn in future chapters, some of these protective efforts carry their own risks.

Classifying Bacteria

We don't even know how many thousands (millions?) of different kinds of bacteria there are, and telling the good guys from the bad guys isn't as easy as we might hope. Sadly, they don't wear tiny white hats or black hats and so we can't always look at the cell's color or shape under a microscope to tell if they will hurt us. Lab technicians may have to analyze their DNA; what factors allow the bacteria to grow; how they behave; what happens when a stain is applied to the culture; and so forth before they can assign a specific name to the bacterium.

When we say "bacteria" we have just begun to describe the organism's pedigree. There is a system for categorizing them (and all creatures) into levels from general to ever more specific detail. The example below of how the system works is the biological classification of a bacterium, *E. coli*, often in news in connection with incidences of food contamination.

Domain: Bacteria

Kingdom: Eubacteria

Phylum: Proteobacteria

Class: Gammaproteobacteria

Order: Enterobacteriales

Family: Enterobacteriaceae

Genus: *Escherichia*

Species: *coli*

Strain: ___?

Sub-strain: ___?

I mentioned that "*E. coli*" is often associated with food contamination scares and the media usually does not go deeper than that level. However, we also need to know what *strain* and perhaps *sub-strain* we are talking about because not all members of the *E. coli* family are pathogenic. The various strains and sub-strains within the genus *E. coli* share only 20 percent of the same genes and kissing cousins may have quite different effects on us.[1] For example, *E. coli Nissle 1917* may be beneficial to us because it scarfs up available iron, and thereby it slows down the growth of a newsworthy pathogen that needs iron, *Salmonella*.[2] (Strain names typically reflect the name of its discoverer, initials and/or numbers.)

One more twist in understanding the names: the letter E. at the beginning of the name may be an abbreviation for "*Escherichia*" as discussed immediately above. But it might also stand for "*Enterococcus*" which is a totally different genus of bacteria. With the explosion of probiotic information, I'll be surprised if even health professionals don't have a difficult time sorting out all the various genera, species, strains, and sub-strains.

Bacterial Disease

Humans have seen the effects of bacterial infections going back at least as far as the discussion of leprosy in the Bible. In the fourteenth century, a pest-carried bacterial disease, bubonic plague or Black Death, killed about *half* of the population of Europe. You have likely heard the names of many modern day pathogenic bacteria, such as Anthrax (a terrorist threat), Botulism, Cholera, Chlamydia, Diphtheria, E. coli, Gangrene, Legionnaires' Disease, Listeria, Lyme Disease, Salmonella, Scarlet Fever, Syphilis, Tetanus, Tuberculosis, Typhoid Fever, and Whooping Cough, plus MRSA, *C-diff,* and many cases of pneumonia discussed previously. We touched on the fact that scientists are also looking at infectious agents, such as bacteria in connection with heart disease, cancer, diabetes, and mental illness.

How Bacteria Cause Harm

The more we know about the effects of these pathogenic bacteria, the better we can understand how probiotics protect us from them.

- They crowd out or otherwise kill our probiotics. (The impact of that will become apparent when we cover all the crucial work that probiotics do on our behalf.)

- Bacteria can simply overwhelm our immune system and do so very quickly. A 2007 Newsweek Magazine article on the human microbiome project declared, " . . . if there were only one salmonella left in the world, doubling every thirty minutes, it would take less than a week to give everyone alive diarrhea."[3] Most will literally "eat our lunch" in that they may consume the same nutrients that our cells and probiotics need.

- They can secrete substances that are poisonous to our cells. The potentially deadly disease botulism is a case in point. *Clostridium botulinum* can be contracted from spoiled food and then secrete a chemical that paralyzes muscles, including those that allow us to breathe. Honey can contain this bacterium. Therefore we are cautioned not to give honey to toddlers because, although adults are able to handle traces of the toxins, the immune systems of children younger than 2 years of age are not sufficiently developed.

Not every reader will have heard of botulism, but it is a good bet they have heard of Botox. It is described as a "cosmetic" because it is used to paralyze the muscles that cause facial wrinkles. I find such a casual use of the botulism toxin a little disconcerting because there are sometimes unfortunate side effects. There are also medical applications for the toxin, such as use with migraines. (I am grateful that I found the natural way to resolve my migraines as discussed in the Preface and didn't have to resort to poisoning my nerves.)

- Some pathogens can eat us—well, not exactly. In the case of the highly pub-licized "flesh-eating bacteria" (necrotizing fasciitis), what actually occurs is that the toxins they release kill tissues.

- Bacteria can cause our defense systems to go into inflammation mode. Inflammation then slows the proper functioning of cells all over the body and causes pain. (Of course, there are other causes of inflammation that we can control, such as smoking and bad dietary habits.)

- Bacteria can cause diarrhea by spurring the body to get rid of the pathogen or its poisonous output. Diarrhea can quickly lead to dangerous dehydra-tion and loss of electrolyte minerals.

- Bacteria may be associated with fever. However, they are not the *direct* cause—fever is one of our body's tools to get rid of the invader. (When medicine is used to reduce fever, it can actually prolong the infection.)

- Pathogenic bacteria hurt *indirectly* if we suffer side effects of medicines used to control the symptoms that they have caused. For example, if a corticos-teroid drug is used to reduce inflammation from a chronic bacterial infec-tion, a person might ultimately suffer bone weakening because that is a common negative effect of the drug. I believe that the functional medicine community more commonly recognizes that anti-inflammatory drugs can actually slow healing.

Fighting Bacteria

Antibiotics are the main weapons used in modern times to tame bacteria. In many cases they can clearly save lives, but these drugs can also have a dev-astating long-term impact on our probiotics and general health. We'll cover that in the next chapter. (In some cases probiotics are becoming recognized as a viable *alternative* to antibiotics.) There are also various ways that we attack bacteria *before* they can get to us. We'll cover avoiding pathogens and sane sanitizing in Chapter 6.

VIRUSES

Most of us have suffered a computer peril called a "virus." That name was adopted because the way it affects the computer's software is so similar to how viruses work in our bodies. We pick up a computer virus by sharing a contaminated flash drive, opening an unknown file, or visiting an unsafe website. The virus (malware code) uses our machine's software to make the computer do things that we don't want it to. The code also duplicates itself and spreads the misery to our friends, family, and business associates. Likewise, disease-causing viruses are pieces of rogue genetic material (like malware code) that insert themselves into our cells and use *our own cellular machinery* to do their dirty work. Our own cells are commandeered to manufacture copies of the virus which can then affect other cells and other people. Viruses seem to be loners, not colony-living entities like bacteria.

Viral Diseases

As we've already established, viruses are responsible for hepatitis and AIDS. Other familiar diseases caused by viruses are Chicken Pox, Ebola, Herpes, Measles, Mono (Mononucleosis), Mumps, Polio, Pneumonia (some), Rabies, Small Pox, and the Norwalk (or Noro) virus that makes the news occasionally as the cause of outbreaks of diarrhea on cruise ships. Cutting-edge research is looking into viruses as causative factors in various cancers, heart disease, and some types of mental illness.

We all know that the seasonal flu is a virus. However, it is less well-known that the common cold and most other upper respiratory infections are also typically viral. It is unfortunate that patients and even practitioners too often assume that those conditions are bacterial. That confusion leads to a great many patients receiving antibiotics for viral illnesses for which they are *useless*. As will be explored in Chapter 5, those drugs (whether necessary or not) usually cause collateral damage.

How Viruses Cause Harm

Viruses are structurally dissimilar from bacteria with different modes of operation and means for causing us trouble.

- If a virus takes over the machinery in one of our cells for its own purposes, then that cell can't do its regular work. What if that cell happens to be, for example, a heart cell? In that case myocarditis can result and lead to heart failure.

- If a virus causes one of our cells to keep reproducing and/or to become immortal, the result could be malignancy. The *papillomavirus* that can lead to uterine cancer is one such example.

- Viruses can cause cells to lyse (explode). Obviously, a trend in that direction would not be good for the function of whatever organ those cells were part of.

- Viruses are known to move genes around among species. For example, a virus could transfer a gene coding for antibiotic-resistance into a bacteria that was previously easy to control.

- A viral infection can simply overwhelm our immune system thereby keeping it from protecting us from other threats and doing its routine maintenance chores. One of those chores is clearing out dead cells and other debris. If the immune system has been sidelined, it may take some time to fully recover from a virus because the immune system must play catch up with cleanup.

- We know that viruses can get into the cells of our beneficial flora. If they damage them, we would lose all the fantastic benefits they would ordinarily provide.

- Just as noted above with bacteria, if a virus causes symptoms, we can fall prey to overtreatment and any side effects of the medications.

Fighting Viruses

Preventing a viral illness is obviously better than fighting one and we cover strategies for doing that in Chapter 6. Failing prevention, antiviral medications are the conventional treatment. The drugs can be specific for a particular type of virus—for example, the medicine used for Hepatitis is different than the one for HIV. Tamiflu (oseltamivir) is a more general anti-viral that makes the news whenever a flu epidemic threatens. Its potential side effects include incontinence and seizures. We are always advised to take anti-viral medications (even natural ones, such as herbs and homeopathics) at the first sign of the illness or at least within the first two days. The immune system can more readily eradicate them at that stage and not just because there are fewer of them.

When a virus first arrives, it wears just a coating of protein or fat around its genetic material and is therefore easier for the immune system to identify and engulf. Once viruses become hidden inside one of our own cells, it understandably slows the immune system response. Fortunately, many beneficial bacteria, including some probiotics, can often see through the virus's disguise. They basically say to our immune soldier cells, "Hey, look, that's a bad guy. Destroy!" Kimchi, a Korean dish of fermented cabbage, cruciferous vegetables, and healthful spices, contains a probiotic strain (*Lactobacillus plantarum*) that has been shown to have substantial anti-viral activity against a flu virus.[4] Probiotics are even being researched as a way of preventing viral contamination of foods.[5]

Beneficial Viruses

Surprisingly, there are some viruses that *help* us. It is now known that viruses can infect and make pathogenic bacteria sick in the same way that they make us sick. These viruses, called "bacteriophages," become volunteer aides to our immune armies.[6] They reside, for example, in the mucous layer that coats tissues, such as the lining of the mouth, nose, lungs, eyelids, urinary tract, and digestive tract. I don't believe that we yet know any practical way to harness this resource, but the hunt is on.[7] In an unusual twist, a trial is being conducted to determine if a modified form of *herpes simplex* virus (the one that causes cold sores) might stimulate the immune system and be more effective than the standard treatment for melanoma (the deadly variety of skin cancer).

FUNGUS/YEAST

Fungus is a giant category, at the same high level of the hierarchy as bacteria, plants, and animals. Molds, yeasts, and even mushrooms are in this kingdom. (For convenience, I'm going to use "fungus" and "yeast" interchangeably throughout this book. Again, back to Latin, "fungi" is the plural.) They are sort of like plants, but perhaps even more similar to animals. For one thing, their cell walls contain a substance (chitin) that is also the main component of the shells of insects and crustaceans like the lobster. Fungi can be microscopic or form underground networks involving acres of soil. Like the categories we've discussed before, some fungi cause disease and some are helpful.

Fungus-Related Diseases

Mildew in the shower grout lines is just a pest, but black mold (*Stachybotrys*) that can grow in walls after a leak or flooding can actually make people so sick that they have to remodel or *move*. Many familiar health annoyances are due to members of the fungus family: athlete's foot, cradle cap, diaper rash, dandruff, jock itch, ringworm, and thrush for starters. Women are often annoyed by the very uncomfortable effects of a vaginal yeast infection that is common after a round of antibiotics. Those infections are often not taken too seriously, but they might be signs of something much more insidious.

Too often mainstream medicine doesn't pay serious attention to yeasts until they can actually see them, such as when a critically ill person begins to have a thrush coating in their mouth and throat. However, a *covert* (subclinical) overgrowth of yeast can occur almost anywhere in the body, including the sinuses, lungs, and gut. From those locations they can be responsible for causing or at least worsening a myriad of health problems which the average doctor seldom associates with yeast.

A chronic yeast infection may be behind the following issues:

- asthma
- carb cravings
- chronic sinus congestion
- depression
- digestive problems of various kinds (including bloating, constipation, gas, heartburn and rectal itching)
- fatigue
- feeling spacey
- food sensitivity
- headaches
- inflammation (generalized)
- insomnia
- loss of voice
- memory problems
- mood swings
- numbness
- obesity
- PMS
- prostate infection
- rashes of all sorts
- sinus congestion
- sore muscles or joints
- vaginal itching/burning/ discharge

The full list is much too long to include here and there is probably much we still do not know. Yeasts may well contribute to serious trouble, such as auto-immune diseases, cancer, diabetes, and heart disease. Hopefully I've conveyed the general idea of their potential negative impact. We'll get back to yeast in Chapter 9.

How Yeast Cause Harm

Yeasts are structurally and functionally quite different from bacteria or viruses. They also cause trouble in different ways.

- Yeasts generate poisons called "mycotoxins." An extreme example is *aflatoxin;* a mycotoxin produced by a type of mold, Aspergillus, that proliferates on grains. If ingested, aflatoxin burdens the liver, suppresses immune function, and is a powerful carcinogen. Fungus expert, Doug Kaufmann, co-authored a shocking journal article that included compelling evidence that mycotoxins' contamination of the food supply has a much bigger role in causing cancer than was previously thought.[8] He advised that peanuts and grains (especially corn) stored in silos show higher levels of mycotoxins. Aflatoxin has been found in the milk of cows fed grain that was contaminated with it. Yeasts in the human gut put mycotoxins into circulation, potentially affecting every cell in the body. Unfortunately, like with bacterial toxins, cooking does not destroy mycotoxins.

- Yeasts do what is good for their survival and that may include making the host person crave foods that the fungi prefer. Those foods, such as refined carbohydrates, may increase the host's risk of obesity, diabetes, heart disease, cancer, and Alzheimer's disease.

- When yeast numbers reach a critical mass, they can change, grow something on the order of roots (hyphae), and become aggressive parasites. They are a prime suspect as the cause of leaky gut which is an increased permeability of the membrane lining the intestinal tract. This is a big deal because the intestinal membrane is supposed to *assist* nutrient absorption and *prevent* the absorption of pathogens, toxins, and incompletely digested foods. Therefore, when that membrane is compromised, all manner of things can go wrong. (Leaky gut and remedies are discussed in Chapter 9.)

- Initially, yeasts can keep our immune system occupied and distract it from other protective jobs. However, when yeasts become a *chronic* infection, it seems that the immune system may assume that they belong there and give up fighting.

- When yeasts begin to get the upper hand, they can crowd out our beneficial bacteria and deprive us of their functions that we will discuss in the next chapter.

- As is the case with disease caused by bacteria and viruses, if a fungus causes symptoms, medication used to treat those can bring on unwanted side effects.

We'll cover what to do about yeasts more thoroughly later, but of course, probiotics are a significant part of the answer to controlling them. Even extracts of probiotics can slow down yeasts.[9] In wine production and a number of animal studies, probiotics help detoxify the potent mycotoxin poisons and limit the damage they do.[10,11]

Friendly Fungus

Baker's yeast, shitake mushrooms, and truffles come to mind on the helpful side. Yeasts are also used to create antibiotics. One variety of yeast, *Saccharomyces boulardii*, is even considered a probiotic. Because yeasts are not damaged by antibiotics, this yeast helps keep pathogenic yeasts from taking over the digestive tract when an antibiotic kills off too many of a person's protective probiotic bacteria. It is kind of a placeholder in that regard and seems helpful for Irritable Bowel Syndrome.[12]

TURNCOATS

We've seen that we can't classify all bacteria, yeasts, fungi, and viruses as "enemies" because a specific member of that class might be our friend. Beyond that, a *formerly* "neutral" party or even a "friend" can become an enemy if it appears at the wrong location, the wrong time, or in the wrong quantity. Not surprisingly, we call those "opportunists."

An example of such an opportunity might be when immune-suppressing drugs are given to an organ transplant recipient. The immune cells are then off duty, leaving the microorganisms to do as they like. (Think in terms of what can happen in a junior high school class if the teacher is away for very long.) The cases of usually helpful probiotics becoming an opportunistic problem are such rare exceptions that a single one can inspire a journal article.[13] Thankfully, cases of opportunistic infections also seem to be relatively easy to treat. It is also quite reassuring that studies report not only the excellent safety record of probiotics for the vast majority of people but even safety in populations that were theoretically at high risk of such opportunistic complications.[14]

Location in/on the body is a factor. Approximately 25 percent of the bacteria in the adult gut are members of the genus *Bacteroides*.[15] The predominant species in that genus goes by this name: *Bacteroides thetaiotaomicron (BT)*. This type of microorganism serves us well by digesting components of carbohydrates and making other nutrients available. In doing so, it seems to be sort of predigesting food not only for humans, but also for other probiotics to consume. *BT* assists in maintaining the adult intestine's important mucous barrier. It also seems quite important for infants during the transition between breast milk and solid foods. It is even believed to signal the infant's gut to develop the blood vessels it needs, but that were not yet present at birth.[16] However, I've *not* seen this bacterium listed as a component of a probiotic product blend. That may be because, if it gets out of the gut, it can become *an opportunist* and cause infections, such as on the skin.[17]

Even geography seems to be a factor in bacterial behavior. *Treponema*, a genus of bacteria seems to provide a real service to some tribal groups, such as hunter/gatherers. Those populations benefit from this strain's ability to extract food energy from extremely fibrous foods. That is a survival factor in times of lean hunting and shortage of higher calorie foraged foods. However, some varieties of *Treponema* are regarded as pathogenic in industrialized cultures.

DOUBLE AGENT

The strain of bacteria *Helicobacter pylori (H. Pylori)* is quite a puzzle. This microorganism inhabits stomachs worldwide—without incident. In fact, it has been suggested that *H. Pylori* may even offer some sort of protection. For instance, people *without H. Pylori* have higher rates of esophagus cancer. (The esophagus is the tube that connects the mouth and stomach). *Lack* of *H. Pylori* is also associated with an increased risk of asthma and similarly, children without it seem more prone to acid reflux and allergies.[18] Then there is the interesting fact that eradicating *H. Pylori* may lead to weight gain.[19]

We needn't Google "*H. Pylori* supplements" because there are none. This bug is also considered a major cause of stomach cancer and stomach ulcers. It also is blamed for gastritis (inflammation of the stomach) and is associated with other complaints, such as rosacea and morning sickness.

How can a bacterium be a good guy and a bad guy at the same time? I suspect that the difference is in the people and their behaviors. Before I propose reasons for these seeming contradictions, I should point out that the term "associated with" in studies just means that two factors often show up together. It doesn't mean that one necessarily *causes* the other. It is quite possible that the secret to *H. Pylori's* apparent double life is that both positive and negative effects were caused by something else.

- **Cancer of the stomach.** The *H. Pylori* strain does not cause stomach trouble in most people worldwide. Perhaps it seizes an opportunity in persons who do not have sufficient stomach acid to defend against *H. Pylori* organisms multiplying out of control. (Low acid can be due to advanced age or use of heartburn drugs.) Lack of stomach acid also destabilizes the pH of the intestinal tract which in turn is not good for helpful microbes that might otherwise help protect against malignancy. *H. Pylori* might also create more damage when the person is undernourished and lacks nutrients that the body needs to keep the lining of the esophagus in good repair.

- **Asthma and allergies.** Lack of probiotic diversity has been shown to increase asthma and allergies in children. So, perhaps asthmatic/allergic youngsters never acquired a normal protective flora which might ordinarily have happened to include *H. Pylori*. (More in Chapter 7 about how that can happen.) I'm suggesting that the real culprit is not the absence of *H. Pylori*, but the coincidental lack of microbiome diversity.

- **Weight gain.** Was the weight gain really caused by the eradication of *H. Pylori* per se or more likely because the antibiotics used to wipe it out also wiped out various beneficial strains that had been providing a slimming effect? (See Part Two for more on weight loss and probiotics.)

To summarize, *H. Pylori* seems to live peaceably in well-nourished people who have normal stomach acid and a robust diversity of beneficial bacteria. That would explain why in ethnic populations around the world, *H. Pylori* is rarely a threat. Those folks are not as sanitized and medicated as we are, and they are also more likely to eat fermented foods which contain probiotics. *H. Pylori* may not be a double agent after all but just another opportunist. Given that probiotics and even foods like broccoli sprouts seem to control *H. Pylori*, it seems we might want to think twice about using strong antibiotics to eradicate it.[20]

CONCLUSION

Before we get to the good news of probiotics, I should mention that the pathogenic bacteria, fungi, and viruses covered above are not the only microorganisms that threaten our health and well-being. We didn't discuss protein blobs called "prions" probably best known as the cause of mad cow disease. Then there are parasites, such as tape worms and protozoa like *Giardia lamblia*. (Incidentally, lactic acid bacteria make selective antimicrobials (bacteriocins) that among other functions seem to help against *Giardia*.[21] Animal studies indicate that the spices ginger and cinnamon are helpful against this parasite.) Probiotics have been shown to be useful against other pathogenic parasites.[22] It is interesting to note that scientists now believe that even some parasites may have beneficial effects. For example, as strange as it sounds, it has been suggested that a reduction in risk to Alzheimer's disease may be related to having increased numbers of certain intestinal parasites. Parasites are a little outside the scope of this book, so I provided a good reference in the Resource section.

All of these enemies and potential enemies have found ingenious ways to use our systems to support themselves. But, we cannot be cavalier in our efforts to destroy them because we might inadvertently do our health more harm than good if in the process we also destroy our allies. In the next chapter, it will become more obvious what a loss that would be.

4.

Our Allies–
Helpful Microorganisms

Until I had to describe them for this book, I never really considered that pathogens are not *intrinsically evil*. After accepting that concept, I was forced to also accept that conversely, our probiotic bacteria are not *intrinsically good*. We just happen to benefit greatly from the behaviors that probiotics use to survive and reproduce. (For a fascinating and inspiring example of bacteria cooperating with a sea animal, search the web for a TED talk by Princeton Professor Bonnie Bassler.) As we co-evolved with them over the millennia, we became dependent on their genetics and didn't develop certain abilities that they were already handling for us. It is estimated that our microbes perform over 20,000 functions for us. While each of our cells contains 6 feet of coiled genetic material, our microbiome contains 300 to 1,000 times more genetic information. That means that without them we are actually missing substantial chapters of the body's instruction manual.

As I mentioned in the Introduction, probiotics perform complex, sophisticated functions for us similar to those accomplished by any one of our organs. They support us throughout our lives—even from *before* birth. For me, the most exciting part of this chapter is the impressive list of all the specific jobs the helpful microorganisms in our systems perform for us. But, we really should first cover a few big picture basics.

PROBIOTIC BASICS

It has only been in the last few decades that we could go to a natural food store and buy a bottle labeled "Probiotics." Where did we get them before that? Where do they live in us? Who are they exactly? How do they come back after a disease or drug wipes them out? We'll cover those questions in this section to create a context.

Acquiring Our Microbiome

In Chapter 7 we will discuss current issues involved in our acquiring bacteria from our mother in the womb, from traditional childbirth, and breast feeding.

But, at this point I just want to make the point that the mother has been exposed to a shrinking diversity of useful microbes and has fewer types to donate to the infant than was the case in the past. (Interestingly, the father's seminal fluid also normally contains a number of beneficial bacteria. Imbalances may be a factor in fertility.) After we are born, we come in contact with probiotic strains from contact with animals and foods in our environment and of course other persons. For example, a kiss lasting just ten seconds can transfer eighty million bacteria from one person to another.

Concentrations of Microbes

Although there are bacteria all over us, something like 80 percent of them live in our intestinal tract. Of those, roughly speaking, 83 percent reside in the large intestine (colon) where the diversity of bacterial species is the greatest. (Many thought that the colon mainly just absorbed water, but it turns out that a lot more is going on there.) Because the small intestine is harder to access, there has been less exploration of the species, functions, and output of its microbiome, but apparently the small intestine is home to about 9 percent of our total. In spite of stomach acid, 8 percent live in the stomach. As you can imagine, it is tricky business discovering which strains are where and in what quantities because they are not visible even with a colonoscopy camera. Our bacteria are very specialized for function. It has been shown that the microorganisms in any part of our body are more similar to that body part in another person than they are similar to the strains on a different part of our body. Some strains are long term residents while others are like tourists that improve the economy and then move on. Cataloging is made even more complex because many of our probiotics cannot be cultured in a laboratory petri dish.

The Starter Kit

We are so dependent on our bacterial teammates that nature even provided us with a starter kit of probiotics for re-inoculation just in case a disaster (like dysentery) flushes them away.[1] Surprisingly, the location of that starter kit is our appendix. That little pouch at the junction of the small and large intestine was previously thought to be at best useless—probably just an oversight of nature. At worst it was viewed as an unnecessary risk for *appendicitis,* a potentially fatal infection of the appendix. Today we know that the appendix contains a treasure—a sampling of the different types of our probiotics. Proving the point, it has been observed that removing the appendix increases the risk for an inflammatory bowel disease (such as Crohn's disease). We can only wonder what it means that a healthy appendix contains a greater variety of bacteria than does the colon.[2]

Understanding Our Probiotics

Of the probiotics that can be cultured in the laboratory, we know that 99.9 percent are of a type (anaerobes) that do not require oxygen or might even be harmed by it.[3] According to the impressive *Human Microbiome Project*, "More than 90 percent of all bacterial phylogenetic types (phylotypes) belong to just two of the 70 known divisions (phyla) in the domain *Bacteria:* the *Bacteroidetes* and the *Firmicutes*."[4] You won't find either of those names on the label of your favorite yogurt or even a probiotic supplement that boasts over 20 probiotic strains. That is because "phyla" are general categories at a high level in the biological classification structure that we reviewed in the previous chapter. Most probiotics are in groups known as *lactic acid bacteria* which fall within the phylum *Firmicutes* or are *bifidobacteria* in another phylum *Actinobacteria.*

The phylum *Bacteroidetes* is present in the gut in substantial numbers and as we will see under weight loss in Part Two, they are more numerous in thin people. I don't want readers to think that they need to learn the following strain names or should use them as a shopping list. But, just for the record, these are a few genus names that turn up fairly frequently in studies of probiotics: *Bacillus, Bacteroides, Bifidobacterium, Enterococcus, Escherichia, Lactobacillus, Leuconostoc, Pediococcus, Prevotella, Ruminococcus, Saccharomyces, and Streptococcus.*[5,6] We might do a double take when reading "*Streptococcus*" because we thought that was what causes strep throat. However, just as was the case regarding *E. coli* in the previous chapter, each of these genus names represents a *very* big grouping of individual strains and sub-strains. In those details is where the rubber meets the road of determining friend from foe.

Which names appear in studies may seems less relevant when we remember that there are perhaps 5 to 10 thousand subspecies, and that each person has a different blend and even that varies with diet changes. As we will see in following chapters, we can grow the kind of probiotic colonies that we need right in our own gut by feeding them properly and by not killing them off. Probiotics have also become the stuff of commerce, and some subspecies are "owned" by whatever scientist or company isolated them.[7] Sometimes that strain is important, but in most cases there are other strains that perform the same job.

PROBIOTIC BENEFITS

There will be more health benefits discussed throughout the remainder of this book, but we've *already* covered a great many. We've talked about research indicating that our beneficial bacteria may in one way or another help the following conditions:

- allergies
- antibiotic resistant bacteria
- asthma
- autoimmune conditions
- bacterial diseases
- blood pressure
- cancer
- cellular energy
- cholesterol
- cirrhosis of the liver
- constipation
- diarrhea
- eczema
- fatty liver
- fungal infections
- heart health
- hepatitis
- irritable bowel
- kidney disease
- mental health
- pancreatitis
- parasites
- pneumonia
- premature aging
- pre-term infant distress
- ulcers
- viral infections
- weight loss

We are just beginning to understand that the mechanisms used by our allied bacterial armies to create all these health benefits are quite numerous and widely varied. I've grouped them into broad categories hoping to make them easier to follow.

Immune Related

We know that our immune system is vital to keeping us alive and well. However, it is not widely appreciated that the bulk of our immune system (70 percent or more) resides *in the gut!* Not surprisingly, there is a very close relationship between the beneficial microbes that live there and the immune system.

- It is in the best interest of our friendly bacteria to get rid of bad bacteria and yeasts that compete with them for space and resources. To that end probiotic strains create sophisticated, highly selective antimicrobials called "bacteriocins" which target *only their enemies (which are often ours)*, not their friends. There are a great variety of these substances, sometimes named for the type of bacteria that produces them. For example, Salivaricins are produced by *Streptococcus salivarius*, a strain of bacteria isolated from Malaysian subjects who, perhaps not coincidentally, eat a lot of fermented foods.[8]

- Probiotics apparently help our inborn immune system identify trouble and signal immune cells to go after pathogens. This function is called "cross talk," and the effect is increasingly being shown even in human trials.[9]

- Probiotics may also signal immune cells to calm down. That would reduce autoimmune and allergic reactions.

- Probiotics seem to teach antibiotic-resistant bad guy bugs to pay attention to the drugs and obediently die.[10]

- As discussed in Chapter 2, probiotics can signal cancer cells to stop functioning. They also can slow the proliferation of, for example, colon cancer cells.[11]

- Native bacteria can send a message to intestinal cells, telling them to produce an antibacterial protein, Ang4.[12]

- You may have heard of "stem cells." Those are our own generic, *nonspecific* cells that can become whatever type of cell the body needs. Our friendly bacteria are thought to signal immune type stem cells to tell them what particular variety of cells is required at the moment.[13]

- Pathogens can cause more trouble if they escape the intestines into blood circulation. Probiotics seem to keep them from crossing the mucous membrane barrier.[14]

- Probiotics can bind up pathogenic microorganisms, keep them from spreading and speed their removal from the body in feces. As an example, in a mouse study, the friendly yeast, (*S. boulardii*) was shown to facilitate the expulsion of the disease-causing bacteria, *Salmonella*, and reduce its infiltration into the liver and spleen.[15]

- This same probiotic yeast was shown in an animal study to slow tumor's ability to grow new blood vessels (angiogenesis), thereby slowing the spread.[16] A similar effect has been seen with lactic acid bacteria.[17]

- Pathogenic bacteria can band together and hide from both immune cells and antibiotics in a protective coating called a "biofilm." The plaque formed on teeth is an example. Lactic acid probiotic bacteria can help prevent those biofilms.[18]

- Good bacteria deprive bad microorganisms of a place to set up shop simply by taking up space and competing for nourishment.

- Probiotics can encourage vaccines to work better.

- Even friendly bacteria that typically live on our skin help protect us from nasty topical infections.

Detoxification Related

Toxins are substances that interfere with functions in the body. They can be from external sources, such as environmental pollution, smoking or chemicals in foods, and body care products. Or they can originate from sources inside

our bodies, such as mycotoxins produced by yeast overgrowth; the breakdown of foods that have stayed too long in the intestinal tract; or from perfectly normal metabolic reactions that were not completed properly. Whatever
the source, if they gum up the workings of a cell, that cell cannot fulfill its
mission to the organ and the system of which the organ is a part. Probiotics
play an important role in detoxification.

- Probiotics help detoxify chemicals that can cause cancer. For example, compounds (processed meats are one source) can cause cancers of the stomach,
  kidney, and colon. Lactic acid bacteria can decrease their concentrations by
  up to 50 percent.[19]

- A probiotic given to goats bound up and reduced circulation of mutagenic
  chemicals that can cause DNA damage and cancer.[20]

- Glutathione is considered a master detoxifying agent. We discussed it in
  regard to cholesterol in Chapter 2, and it will reappear later under antioxidants. Gluthione helps reduce mercury levels in the body. Added amounts
  of it can be made by at least one probiotic strain. See the inset on page 54
  for more details.

- Preliminary tests show that probiotics may limit the absorption of pesticides and toxic metals.[21]

- The circulation of toxins can cause trouble for any cell in the body. One animal study on a lactobacillus strain showed reduced circulating toxins.[22]

- Kidney researchers are especially interested in the prospect of probiotics
  reducing the toxins that burden kidney function.[23]

- As noted in regard to organisms in the fermented food kimchi, they have
  even been shown to help detoxify the hormone-disrupting plasticizer
  bisphenol A (BPA).

- As mentioned in Chapter 2, probiotics help prevent kidney stones. One
  way they do that is by degrading the offending oxalates from the diet.[24]

- Waste materials, such as dead cells, can become toxic by clogging body
  processes. Probiotics appear to help clean house by clearing up cellular
  debris.[25]

- Constipation allows toxic substances to linger in the system and become
  absorbed into circulation. As we will cover in the second part of the book,
  probiotics help avoid constipation in several ways, including contributing
  to the bulk of stool.

- By digesting fiber, probiotics create fuel for the cells that line the digestive tract. An energized intestinal wall is better capable of moving the digestive process along. The vitality of that gut lining is also very important to blocking the absorption of substances that can harm us if they get into circulation. That will become clearer when we discuss leaky gut in Chapter 9.

Nutrition Related

The saying goes, "You are what you eat." But, that is not quite the whole story. We are what we *eat, digest, absorb,* and *don't eliminate.* We need the help of probiotics for all these steps. Whether or not a dietary supplement, such as glucosamine for example, will have the desired effect may well depend on whether or not the person has the right microbiome to process it. We might be more accurate to say that "We are what our bacteria eat."

- The digestive tracts of newborns are quite immature, not just in size, but also in function. A sufficient microbiota signals the intestines to create the more complex circulatory system that is required to absorb nutrients especially from sources other than breast milk.

- It is agreed among scientists, but little known and appreciated by consumers that probiotic strains manufacture vitamins, such as K_2, Biotin, Folic Acid (including the active methylated form 5-methylenetetrahydrofolate), and other B Vitamins.[26] (Vitamin K_2 helps make sure that calcium goes into bone rather than into plaque in our arteries. We definitely want hard bones and soft arteries.)

- There have been research hints that our bacteria might make small but potentially life-saving amounts of vitamin C. It also seems likely that they help convert various vitamins into their more active forms.

- Since virtually every cell in the body has receptors for vitamin D, it isn't surprising that the vitamin is now enjoying a great deal of attention for helping many health issues. The cells in our bodies must have receptors ready to accept nutrients. Probiotic strains can increase the receptor sensitivity at least in the case of vitamin D.[27] Among persons with low cholesterol, a probiotic supplement seemed to increase blood levels of vitamin D.[28]

- Polysaccharides are chains of sugar molecules hundreds or even thousands of atoms long that are part of carbohydrate foods, such as fruits, vegetables, and grains. The human digestive tract can make fewer than one hundred enzymes for breaking down polysaccharides compared to bacteria that can make many hundreds.

- Flavones are important health-protective substances in fruits and vegetables. The absorption of these from orange juice was shown to be improved by supplementation with *Bifidobacteria longum R0175* for four weeks (but not short term).[29]

- Fiber is especially challenging for humans to digest, but it is easy work for certain bacteria. As noted under detoxification (*see* page 49), they digest fiber into substances that keep the lining of the gut healthy, and that in turn is critical to the absorption of nutrients.

- While processing our sources of fiber, such as grains, they also reduce anti-nutrients, such as phytates, which make minerals less available.[30] Probiotics have also been shown to improve the absorption of minerals, such as iron.[31]

- By digesting lactose (a sugar in milk), probiotics help individuals who are lactose intolerant avoid discomfort and gain the food value from dairy products.

- By digesting proteins into their component amino acids, probiotics not only help utilize protein, but by doing so can also protect against food sensitivities that can be triggered if fragments of undigested protein are absorbed.

- It is a very common misconception that carrots contain vitamin A when, in fact, colorful vegetables contain certain carotenoids that must be *converted* into vitamin A in the body. We know that most vitamin A comes from the small intestine, but even today there seems to be a good bit of confusion about *exactly how* that happens and the source of the enzymes involved. It has been rumored that probiotics make vitamin A, but I have not yet found documentation for that. However, it is known that our gut bacteria help *extract* carotenes from the plant materials. I suspect that in the future we will see that they also assist at least indirectly with the conversion of those into vitamin A.

Antioxidant Related

Oxidants (or free radicals) are unstable molecules (like electron hot potatoes) that can wreak havoc on all parts of our cells and even our DNA which can in turn lead to cancer. They can start a damaging chain reaction which we might visualize as a room full of mouse traps with a ping pong ball sitting on each one. If one is tripped, pretty soon the balls fly in every direction tripping other traps. Free radicals can be generated by toxins, radiation, and even the body's normal use of oxygen. Antioxidants protect us against oxidants.

- Probiotics have long been assumed to have antioxidant capacity which one lab study was able to measure.[32]

- In an animal study, the combination of probiotics and their food supply (prebiotics) was found most effective in preventing oxidant-caused pre-cancerous changes in cells.[33]

- Glutathione (GSH) is considered to be the master antioxidant. See inset on page 54.

Inflammation Related

Inflammation is a normal protective function of the body that kicks in to repair injury or disease. However, it is supposed to do its job and then subside. When inflammation becomes *chronic*, it is no longer helpful, and in fact it is considered to be a major contributor to virtually every degenerative disease visited upon modern man. Probiotics help normalize inflammation in several ways.

- Hundreds of studies credit probiotics with reducing inflammation in the digestive tract. One way that happens is that they reduce harmful microorganisms that create inflammation.[35]

- By helping to detoxify chemical substances that cause inflammation, gut flora seems to be a factor in protecting against metabolic syndrome, a cardiovascular risk factor.[36]

- Food sensitivities create inflammation and probiotics help by digesting foods to the point that they are no longer able to cause those reactions.

- The absorption of anti-inflammatory nutrients, such as magnesium and flavones, is improved by probiotics.

- Since free radicals worsen inflammation, probiotics help by providing antioxidant protection as noted on page 52.

- Probiotics help prevent the excessive permeability of the gut lining (leaky gut) which in turn keeps inflammatory molecules from getting into circulation.

Neurotransmitter Related

Neurotransmitters are chemical messengers in the brain. Most mental health issues are blamed on insufficiencies or excesses of these signaling molecules. Typically, psychoactive medications are used to change balances of neurotransmitters. For example, a class of depression drugs called "serotonin reuptake inhibitors" keeps levels of one such neurotransmitter, serotonin (the so-called happy hormone), artificially high in the brain by blocking its

Glutathione

Glutathione (GSH) is a substance made in the body, but not always in suffi-cient quantities for the challenges that we face—especially as we age and/or are exposed to toxins. These are among its known benefits: increases energy; activates lymphocytes (a type of immune cell); improves athletic performance and recovery; slows the effects of aging; reduces muscle and joint discom-fort; improves skin, mental focus, and sleep quality while reducing the effects of stress. Low levels of glutathione are linked to serious health issues, such as heart disease, cancer, and diseases of the nervous system, such as Alzheimer's and Parkinson's.

Glutathione can have all of those downstream benefits because of its upstream actions. It is considered the emperor among antioxidants. For one thing, it recycles or regenerates other antioxidants, such as vitamins C and E and coenzyme Q10. As the master antioxidant, it is also a component of or generator of dozens of detox enzymes, such as one that you may have heard of, SOD (superoxide dismutase). As noted earlier, glutathione prevents oxi-dization (like rusting) of LDL cholesterol. GSH regulates and enhances immune function, lowers inflammation, and is required to make and repair our DNA, a critical function. GSH also detoxifies pesticides, insecticides, fungicides, and heavy metals (such as mercury, lead, arsenic, and cadmium).

GSH is depleted by alcohol and other toxins, stress, and age. By age 80, glutathione levels have typically declined by about 60 percent. That is doubly

breakdown. We know that probiotics help restore neurotransmitter balance naturally and that they send messages to the brain affecting hunger, satiety, pain, nausea, discomfort, and perhaps even joy and sadness. In addition to the studies cited in Chapter 2, there are other areas of research referring to these chemical messengers in the brain.

- Melatonin is a brain chemical that helps with sleep cycles and jet lag, and it is being studied for major benefits with cancer, including breast cancer.[37] Melatonin is generally said to come from the pineal gland in the brain, but interestingly, 400 times more of it is created in the intestinal tract from the amino acid l-tryptophan.[38] It has been found that when probiotics are given, melatonin levels increase and irritable bowel symptoms are reduced.[39] It is not clear yet exactly what role probiotics play in making or protecting cells that make melatonin, but it certainly can't hurt to maintain a healthy gut environment.

unfortunate because during that time oxidation challenges have gone up dramatically. Glutathione levels are difficult to boost in the body because it is relatively rare in food and it is not easily absorbed from ordinary supplement pills. Levels can be improved somewhat by consuming more of what it takes for the body to make it. The amino acid (part of a protein) that is usually limiting its production is cysteine. Cysteine is found mainly in animal products but also to some extent in broccoli, garlic, lentils, oats, onions, red peppers, and wheat germ.

As noted earlier, one strain of bacteria, *Lactobacillus fermentum ME-3*, has been shown to increase glutathione levels dramatically by promoting its synthesis and reducing its loss.[34] It also improves the ratio of *active* GSH to *inactivated* GSH by 49 percent and recorded a 26 percent increase in total antioxidant activity. Most probiotic bacteria display multiple activities and *ME-3* is no exception. It was also shown to: have anti-microbial activity; increase levels of the enzyme that detoxifies organophosphate agricultural insecticides; reduce gut membrane permeability; and to withstand exposure to stomach and bile acids. The only time that supplemental glutathione might theoretically be discouraged is with certain types of cancer treatment.

Lactobacillus fermentum ME-3 has been marketed in Europe for some time and recently became available in the U.S. in three combinations, that include nutrients for detoxification, cardiovascular support, and immune support. See Resources, page 207, for details.

- There really is a "gut feeling" or "gut reaction." Several other brain-active substances (such as gamma-aminobutyric acid or GABA, serotonin, catecholamine, and acetylcholine) are produced in the gut with the help of bacteria.[40] These substances are known to have positive effects at least in the gut which contains more nerve cells than the spinal cord.

Oxygen and Energy

We all know the importance of oxygen to our survival—our brains can suffer damage after only a few minutes of oxygen deprivation. Beyond that, the ability to absorb oxygen into the blood not only helps performance and endurance, but also our immune function because immune cells use oxygen as a weapon. Probiotic strains assist with this key factor.

- Four weeks of supplementation with a multi-strain probiotic increased the distance athletes could run in the heat.[41]

- A Japanese study of long distance runners found that their blood oxygen levels (VO_2Max) improved by over 29 percent when they were supplemented with probiotics. It was also noted that muscles worked better because there was less lactic acid build-up.[42] As interesting as these results were I was surprised I could not find follow up studies. (I wonder if some sports teams are using probiotics, but they are keeping it a trade secret.)

- In a study of race horses, it was found that probiotic supplementation improved oxygen uptake.[43]

- Fatigue is the most common complaint at the doctor's office. It is believed that our friendly bacteria may create up to 10 percent of our total energy. So, not surprisingly, people often say that their energy improves when they take probiotic supplements. Many indirect pathways listed above might help explain that phenomenon, but probiotics also seem to also have a direct role in energy metabolism. For one thing, probiotics may help maintain the health of the mitochondria, the little energy factories inside our cells.[44]

- Our bacteria can digest fiber into a particular short chain fatty acid (propionate) that when transported to the liver, helps release a steady supply of glucose. That helps keep our blood sugar from falling too low. (Low blood sugar causes fatigue, along with fuzzy thinking, headaches, dizziness, and shakiness.)

Cholesterol Related

The more that the positive effects of probiotics on cholesterol levels are noticed, the more interest is generated in learning the specific ways they deliver the benefit. Scientists speculate that probiotics may lower cholesterol by several mechanisms, such as binding up cholesterol, incorporating it into the bacteria's cell membranes, and converting cholesterol into other substances.[45] Probiotics seem to speed the processing (hydrolyzing) of bile salts providing another means of reducing cholesterol levels.[46] And, this factor is so important that I must stress it—the oxidation of cholesterol is perhaps the biggest concern with cholesterol and probiotics help protect against that as previously discussed under Antioxidants.

CONCLUSION

It isn't hard to imagine how various combinations of the above mechanisms could boost the health of *any* of the body's system. Take cardiovascular health as a handy example. Not only do probiotics reduce cholesterol and produce antioxidants to protect it from oxidizing; they also reduce inflammation which is another risk factor; improve immune function to fight infections that damage the circulatory system; and help the absorption of heart protective nutrients like magnesium. The puzzle pieces come together to form a beautiful and healthy picture.

Bacterial species tend to specialize. However, just because a study demonstrates that a particular strain carries out a certain function, that doesn't mean there aren't others that will also do that same job.[47] There is some redundancy among strains and much of their work for us is done by *teams* with each strain contributing a part. That's why we need to maintain a broad diversity of bacterial strains as a base even if we also want to use a particular strain like ME-3 for a special purpose. The gut microbiome is rather like a symphony orchestra and an orchestra wouldn't sound good with only oboe players. Maintaining stability of our microbiome involves not only building cultures but also protecting them from damage. Antibiotics are a potent destabilizer of gut harmony. The next chapter digs into that thorny issue.

5.

The Heavy Artillery–
Antibiotics

A s we saw in Chapter 3, pathogenic bacteria can cause many life-threatening illnesses, a fact that has made humanity understandably very grateful for the availability of antibiotics. Antibiotics can also be a life-saving necessity when a patient's immune system has been suppressed as would be the case with an organ transplant. And antibiotics allow doctors to perform high tech procedures, such as hip replacement and other invasive surgeries, including mastectomies. There is even a growing trend to use antibiotics as an alternative to the standard surgical treatment for appendicitis.

But, we've come to know that these weapons have limitations and a dark side. In order to use them effectively we must understand the potential risks and how they work. Otherwise, we might not only create short and long-term health problems for ourselves individually, we may actually cause all humanity to lose the life-saving benefits of antibiotics. Let's start at the beginning and end with questions about taking probiotics with antibiotics.

THE DAWN OF THE ANTIBIOTIC ERA

In 1928, Sir Alexander Fleming, a Scottish biology, pharmacology, and botany expert, accidentally discovered penicillin as a byproduct of a mold. Great excitement ensued and surely scientists envisioned a world without disease. Indeed, antibiotics have saved untold millions of lives and we are comforted that we can reach for them in the critical cases I just mentioned. It is likely that in the excitement of the discovery of antibiotics, no one realized that antibiotics had side effects or could they have imagined the serious problem that we have today. Many bacteria have grown resistant to antibiotics' control.

ANTIBIOTIC SIDE EFFECTS

Antibiotics are *mycotoxins*, which as noted in regard to aflatoxin, are by definition, *poisons.* That may account for some of the immediate antibiotic side effects, but there are also longer range problems most of which may be due to the fact that they *kill our protective bacteria.* "Broad-spectrum" type antibiotics kill the broadest range of pathogens, but also the greatest variety of those with probiotic benefits. It just stands to reason that by damaging good guys, antibiotics might well produce the *reverse* of any of the probiotic benefits that are discussed in this book. Indeed, some of the antibiotic side effects listed below do look suspiciously similar to what happens when the diversity and balance of beneficial bacteria in our microbiome are depleted.

Scientists just recently determined how antibiotics actually work—they create chain reactions that fatally damage the DNA of the pathogenic bacteria.[1] Unfortunately, they apparently also damage the DNA of the internal probiotics and the mitochondria, those little powerhouses in our cells. With a typical course of antibiotics, after two to three days the *volume* of microbes refills, but not necessarily the same *diversity.* Yeasts often take advantage of the vacancy and can become durable residents for months or even years causing chronic health problems that we will discuss in Chapter 9. Even more alarming, sometimes a life-threatening pathogen gets the upper hand. (It may be something like a garden. If you mowed it all down the weeds seem more likely to return than the vegetables.) I attended a lecture given by Gary B. Huffnagle, PhD where he noted that when antibiotics are given, not only do yeasts increase, so do some bacterial strains (for example, *bacteroidetes* and *enterococcus*) and at the same time lactic acid bacteria (which seem protective against allergic disease) decrease.

There are many different kinds of antibiotics, each with its own specific intended therapeutic effect. But, all also have unintended consequences—some more numerous and/or serious than others. It is beyond the scope of this book to look at the side effects of the individual brands or even the many categories of these drugs, but I'll give a few examples to make the point. Some of these undesirable effects are common, while others are fairly rare. (Of course, if one of these happens to you, "rare" is no longer a meaningful term.)

- Antibiotic use is associated with breast cancer and prostate cancer in a dose-dependent manner. The fact that the association is "dose dependent" is incriminating, but it would take a different type of study to *prove* that they are a cause.[2] Other work shows that frequent antibiotic use is associated not just with higher breast cancer risk but also with reoccurrence and mortality from the disease.[3]

- A large study showed that antibiotics increase the risk of diabetes. A single course of the drugs did not affect risk, but the risk of diabetes increased up to 37 per cent for those having had more than five courses.[4]

- Amoxicillin is the most prescribed antibiotic. These are some of the immediate side effects commonly reported:

  - agitation
  - anxiety
  - back pain
  - behavioral changes
  - bleeding gums
  - chest pain
  - confusion
  - convulsions
  - cough
  - dizziness
  - drowsiness

  - GI symptoms (including nausea, vomiting, diarrhea, constipation, pain bloating, and something disgusting-sounding called "black hairy tongue")
  - headache
  - insomnia
  - joint inflammation
  - kidney and liver problems
  - meningitis (aseptic)
  - muscle aches

- Antibiotics of the Fluoroquinolone class (Cipro, Avelox, and LEvaquin are examples) are linked to severe long-term side effects which now include aortic aneurysm and hallucinations. A 2001 article in the Annals of Pharmacotherapy, by Jay Cohen, MD described 45 cases of severe neurological symptoms. Of the subjects, 93 percent sustained injuries, such as agitation, impaired cognitive function, intractable insomnia, hallucinations, psychosis, acute manic episode, joint or muscle pain, or tendon rupture.[5] In 2008, the FDA (Food and Drug Administration) began requiring "black box warnings" on that class of antibiotics because of the risk of tendon ruptures.

- More than one study shows that Z-Pack (Azithromycin) increases the risk of fatal heart attack among those already at risk. This is an example of a tough risk/benefit call because the drug does reduce deaths from pneumonia in the elderly.[6]

- An article in *Sports Health* stated: "Routinely used antibiotics have been linked to tendon injuries, cardiac arrhythmias, diarrhea, photosensitivity, cartilage issues, and decreased performance."[7]

- *C. Difficile*, as discussed in Chapter 2, is a potentially lethal diarrhea. It typically occurs immediately after a course of antibiotics. Therefore, the antibiotics and their disruption of microbiome balance are assumed to be the cause. Some strains of this disease are now unresponsive to control by even very strong antibiotics.

- Combining some antibiotics with some cholesterol lowering drugs increases risks of muscle and kidney damage, especially in older persons.

- Increased deficiency of vitamin K1 (which affects clotting) is frequently noted along with concerns about bleeding connected to antibiotic use.[8]

- Antibiotics reduce vitamin K2.[9] As mentioned in Chapter 4, this form of the vitamin is crucial for helping calcium get into bone rather than lining the arteries. Since it is made by probiotic type strains, this is a good example of how antibiotics create trouble indirectly.

- The risk of skin allergy in children is increased when infants are given antibiotics.[10]

- Children repeatedly given broad spectrum antibiotics in the first two years of life have a higher risk of becoming obese in childhood.[11]

- When the antibiotic tetracycline is used in young children or pregnant women, it can result in permanent tooth discoloration in the children. *Tetracycline that is beyond its expiration date becomes toxic and can cause kidney problems.*

- Speaking of pregnancy, birth control medications can *fail* when used along with antibiotics.

THE ANTIBIOTIC RESISTANCE PROBLEM

As noted earlier, bacteria long ago evolved to survive environmental hazards like extremes of temperature and pH. It has become a modern survival factor for bacteria to mutate into varieties that are not stopped by antibiotics. You could say that antibiotics have become a victim of their own success because of overuse. Drug-resistant infections, such as antibiotic-resistant tuberculosis, are now a global crisis. An antibiotic-resistant infection can turn a minor operation into a major medical problem. In addition to the *C-diff* and MRSA mentioned in Chapter 2, a relatively new serious concern is infection with *Carbapenem-resistant Enterobacteriaceae* (CRE) which can be lethal for up to half of those infected. *Klebsiella* and *E. coli* are other examples of bacterial species that can develop resistance to the carbapenem class of antibiotics. Foreign travelers returning infected with drug-resistant *shigella* is a growing issue.

Even scarier, it is possible for *any* pathogenic bacteria to acquire genes for antibiotic-resistance. As more strains develop resistance, we stand to basically lose the protection of our arsenal of antibiotics needed for life-threatening conditions.

According to studies reviewed by the Pew Charitable Trusts, "Drug-resistant infections cost the U.S. health care system up to $26 billion annually and prolong hospital stays by more than eight million days."[12] Worse yet, each year, of the two and a quarter million sickened by antibiotic-resistant infections in the U.S., 37,000 people die as a direct result. When basic antibiotics fail, stronger and riskier drugs are used. For example, doctors sometimes resort to Colistin, an antibiotic that was previously abandoned because it was so toxic to the liver.

Pharmaceutical companies are responsible to make profits for the benefit of their shareholders. The problem of antibiotic resistance has been made worse because drug companies aggressively market broad-spectrum antibiotics and promote uses for them that are not approved by the FDA. It also seems that developing *new* antibiotics is not a financially attractive investment. The FDA often has created fast track rules for approval of drugs, such as new antibiotics. The drugs will now be subject to less safety and efficacy data. In 2013, the U.S. government agreed to give GlaxoSmithKline (GSK) $200 million to research stronger antibiotics.[13] That plan still seems to me to be a short term strategy. Without some fundamental changes in the way we deal with disease, the bugs will just become immune to the new drug and we will be back to square one. Incidentally, GSK said they would be careful to not allow overuse of their new super-antibiotic. But, based on history, isn't that expecting the fox to guard the hen house? Stock holders don't usually like their businesses to work at *reducing* income.

SOURCES OF ANTIBIOTIC RESISTANCE

We have seen the growth of antibiotic resistance since at least the 1960's, but the authorities have been agonizingly slow to take definitive action. Antibiotic resistance is clearly the result of the *misuse* of the drugs. As will become obvious, controlling the problem will require help from a variety of sectors, including doctors, hospitals, farmers, government regulators, the public, and those foxes guarding the hen houses.

Doctors' Offices

Colds, influenza, and most other common upper respiratory infections are caused by *viruses*. Antibiotics do *not* kill viruses and there is no evidence that taking an antibiotic for a cold will help anything.[14] Sinus infections are also typically caused by fungus or viruses, neither of which responds to antibiotics. And yet, Amoxicillin is the antibiotic most often prescribed for sinus infections. A study showed it had not relieved symptoms in three days.[15] Even when sinusitis is caused by bacteria, the newer recommendations are for "watchful waiting" for three days, not the use of antibiotics.[16]

A 2010 article in the journal *American Family Physician* stated, "Although 90 percent of bronchitis infections are caused by viruses, approximately two-thirds of patients in the United States diagnosed with the disease are treated with antibiotics."[17] Several issues seemed linked together. For example, it was observed that children given antibiotics for upper respiratory problems have more subsequent visits to the doctor.[18] That apparently results in even more antibiotics.

The trend seems hard to reverse. It had been determined that the use of broad-spectrum antibiotics for children's inner ear infections had grown alarmingly to a rate of 45 percent of visits in 2004.[19] Official practice guidelines in 2004 recommended a significant reduction. Unfortunately, as late as 2010 the use of antibiotics had not declined.[20] According to a study in the *Journal of the American Medical Association*, an hour of education for practitioners combined with a year of personalized audits and follow up greatly improved adherence to antibiotic guidelines for their intended purposes. Even so, antibiotics continued to be prescribed for viral conditions.

Patients and parents can help doctors by not requesting antibiotics, asking for the most narrowly targeted drug and the shortest course possible. They should also be aware of a factor called "decision fatigue," whereby at the end of the day a doctor is 26 percent more likely to prescribe an antibiotic whether it is needed or not.[21]

Hospitals

According to the Centers for Disease Control (CDC), "Studies indicate that 30 to 50 percent of antibiotics prescribed in hospitals are unnecessary or inappropriate."[22] We might expect hospitals to be more careful than the average doctor, but hospitals are businesses and they make money when they dispense drugs. In 2014, Medicare began assessing financial penalties for hospitals with a record of failing to prevent infections (for example, at IV or catheter sites). I worry that hospitals might give out even more antibiotics in the name of preventing infections. Given that antibiotic-resistant infections cost 3 times as much to treat, that gives hospitals a third subtle disincentive to slow the overuse of antibiotics. I'm not sure how Medicare could determine a hospital's contribution to antibiotic resistance so that they could penalize that, but we can hope they find a way.

Agriculture

Most consumers are unaware that antibiotics play such a huge role in food production. There are some alarming facts that illustrate the situation.

- Antibiotics, such as Streptomycin and Oxytetracycline, may be sprayed on fruits like blueberries, apples, and pears to act as pesticides. Also, if an antibiotic-treated animal's manure is used as fertilizer on vegetable crops, the antibiotics can then contaminate the produce.

- According to the FDA, "In 2011, drug makers sold 29.9 million pounds of antibiotics for use on industrial farms."[23] That is the most ever reported.

- In 2009, the agency reported that about 90 percent of the farm antibiotics were sold for use in food animals' feed and water.[24] That means that the drugs were not used to treat existing diseases, but used to cause animals to put on weight faster and to *anticipate* diseases that might possibly develop as a result of crowded unnatural conditions. Roughly 4 times more antibiotics are sold to feed *healthy animals* than are used to treat *sick humans*.

- Industrial farms in the United States use about 6 times more antibiotics per pound of meat produced than is used in Denmark which is the world's leading pork exporter.[25]

- This unnecessary farm use increases the odds that antibiotic-resistant strains will form and be passed on to us. For example, scientists monitoring poultry in grocery stores found some of it to be contaminated with antibiotic-resistant bacteria that make it hard to treat human urinary tract infections.[26]

- We might not think of shrimp as being farmed, but these days most are. Foreign producers use antibiotics to control shrimp diseases and although antibiotics are theoretically not allowed by FDA in imported shrimp, Consumer Reports found residues in many samples. They also detected that antibiotic-resistant bacterium *MRSA* in some samples.

- Functional medicine practitioners and nutritionists are concerned about our exposure to *secondhand* antibiotics in our food—not only for the direct harm to us, but also because they harm our microbiome.

This antibiotic overuse debate has raged for over three decades—health experts on one side and industries on the other. In the 1970's, when the threat from drug resistant germs first became apparent, the FDA tried in vain to ban frivolous uses of antibiotics. Unfortunately, big money lobbying efforts foiled their plan. (We would think the U.S. Food and Drug Administration would have more power than trade groups, but for the most part we would be wrong. The FDA gets their marching orders and budget from Congress and industry money gains access to tell legislators their side of the story. It seems that folks like you and I must get really riled up and join together into large groups to get anything that vaguely resembles the hearing big industries can arrange.)

In 2012 the FDA stated its intent to phase out the use of antibiotics for *nonmedical* purposes over a three-year period.[27] In 2013 to further their goal, FDA asked the drug makers to voluntarily remove from labels any suggestion that the antibiotics work to promote growth. We can only hope their efforts are more successful this time. It is possible to eliminate antibiotics as growth promoters for livestock. The European Union has already done so. It might help that a number of studies now show that *probiotics* may be even more effective than antibiotics for agricultural purposes and are certainly safer.

Maybe antibiotic overuse will be reduced due to an executive order issued by President Obama in the fall of 2014. The resulting task force developed a strategy that set ambitious goals to be achieved by 2020. I hate to be skeptical, but the war on cancer launched in 1971 comes to mind—we are still waging that somewhat unsuccessfully. In the case of antibiotic overuse, the required steps are at least a lot less elusive. The problem is mainly finding the political will to go against the big money interests.

WHAT CONSUMERS CAN DO TO HELP

Although I described the challenge we have making Congress pay attention to our concerns, we have more power than we usually give ourselves credit for. These are some actions the average person can take that will add up to a big difference.

Vote with Dollars

When consumers put pressure on sellers, such as grocery stores and restaurants, the suppliers are compelled to listen. Chipotle is an example of a restaurant chain that has already made the switch to antibiotic-free chicken, and Chick-Fil-A and McDonalds are on a multi-year plan to do the same. Apparently, that involves some work with the producers to insure a sufficient supply of these undrugged birds. The ripple effects of consumer pressure have caused Perdue, a giant producer of chicken, to institute stringent cleanliness procedures that start with the fertile eggs that are grown for their use. The company has pledged to use only antibiotics that are not also used for humans. That is an important start.

Avoid Antibiotics When Possible

In the next chapter we talk a bit about avoiding infection which is an important preliminary step. Also, just being aware that antibiotics don't treat conditions caused by viruses and yeasts may help patients resist the temptation to request an antibiotic and to question if a prescription offered is really necessary. Furthermore, it is useful to know that totally wiping out pathogens

Balancing Probiotics and Antibiotics

It is obvious that we must thoughtfully reduce our use of antibiotics, but sometimes they are necessary. So then the question becomes how to use probiotics to lessen the impact of the drug. These are the questions I'm most often asked on the subject.

Q. Can probiotics be taken with antibiotics?

A. People always seem a little worried that probiotics might somehow cancel the needed action of antibiotics. A study on the treatment of *H. Pylori* is a case in point. Researchers found that when compared to placebo taking probiotics two weeks prior to taking antibiotics made the treatment more effective and greatly reduced side effects. Patients were instructed to take the probiotics two hours earlier or later than the antibiotics because antibiotics can kill probiotics.

Q. Do I finish the antibiotic before starting the probiotic?

A. In this case folks worry about *wasting* the probiotics. No. Don't wait. We want to try to stay even—that is avoid being depleted of good bacteria and having bad species gain ground.

Q. How long do probiotics need to be taken after finishing a course of antibiotics?

A. Because people and antibiotics differ so greatly, there is no one answer for this. It often takes many months to reestablish a full rich complement of gut bacteria, especially after taking a broad-spectrum antibiotic. But, ideally, probiotics should be supplemented every day all the time anyway.

Q. What kind of probiotic to take along with an antibiotic?

A. In addition to whatever probiotic a person might usually take, I recommend taking an additional supplement of the friendly yeast, *S. Boulardii*. Since this one is not a bacterium that the antibiotic can kill, it makes a good place-holder. Prebiotics and Postbiotics are good to take with an antibiotic because the drug does not kill them either. As we will see in Chapter 8, they provide almost as much benefit as probiotics themselves.

may not even be a good goal. Our health thrives when we have about five good guys for each one pathogenic or opportunistic microorganism. Why not *zero* bad guys? It seems that a small population of them may keep our immune capacity sharp and keep any other strains from growing out of control. In some cases you may not be able to avoid an antibiotic. When this occurs there are a number of things that can be done. *See* inset on page 67.

Follow Prescription Directions

Failing to complete the recommended length of an antibiotic prescription can cause harm. That is because not taking all doses increases the chances of developing antibiotic-resistant germs and increases the risk that the infection might return, requiring yet another round of drugs.

Dispose of Unused Medications Properly

Hospitals, clinics, pharmacies, and consumers are encouraged to never flush drugs down the drain or the toilet. Some folks say to mix waste medications into used litter from the cat's box. That might discourage drug abusers from digging them out, but by going into the trash in any form they will eventually end up in a land fill. From landfills the medications leach into the ground water which is then used in agriculture and for drinking water.[28] Unfortunately, municipal processing of tap water is not set up to remove medications. Visit FDA.gov and search for "drug disposal" for advice.

Be Careful of Antibacterials in the Home

The Consumer Reports on Health periodical (4/14) pointed out that home cleaning products like antibacterial cleansers promote antibiotic resistance. Washing with plain soap and water or using alcohol gels does not have that effect.

Be Informed and Speak Out

The Pew Charitable Trusts have done some great work on the issue of antibiotic misuse. Visit their website for resources and current news, SaveAntibiotics.org. (That website is truly a public service, but it is easy to be fooled. A website that looks like it is for protection of wetlands could well be a front for the gas and oil lobby. Many disease websites are established to sell medications or legal services. Of course, profit-driven sites can offer good information, but it pays to be cautious. In this book I aim to direct you to responsible sites.)

It wouldn't hurt to add this issue to a list of concerns that you discuss with your Congressperson and Senators. What they want most is to be re-elected and they *should* welcome your input.

CONCLUSION

We really must save the heavy artillery, antibiotics, for serious emergencies and not wear them out on minor illnesses and ones for which they don't offer benefit. Even more importantly, we have to stop the spread of antibiotic resistant germs with wanton agricultural use. When we must use antibiotics ourselves, supplementing probiotics can minimize their side effects.

Scientists are working to find antibiotics that rather than attempting to kill bacteria instead interfere with their ability to communicate the signal to attack. Meanwhile, wouldn't it be great if there were antibiotics that offered fringe benefits and not side effects? And ideally they would target *only* the harmful bacteria, not our good guys. And what if this miracle "drug" could adapt so that the disease-causing bacteria would not become immune to them? Even better, what if this fancy antibiotic could also get rid of viruses and unhealthful yeasts? You may have guessed that I've just described *probiotics*. Watch for "pharmabiotics" a new name some scientists use to describe the use of probiotics *in place of antibiotics*. New reviews of studies show that probiotics reduce the number and duration of upper respiratory infections. A French study following up on those showed that the general use of probiotics would eliminate millions of sick days, dramatically reduce antibiotic use, and save untold millions of dollars just in France alone.[29]

6.

Lesser-Known Threats to Probiotics

U nfortunately, antibiotics are far from the only threat our beneficial bacteria face. We can unwittingly kill them off doing what seems perfectly normal. And we get no warning (on labels or otherwise) of threats to our essential microbes that lurk in medicines, foods, lifestyle choices, and everyday products that we use around the home. It seems that virtually everything we do can affect our probiotic colonies for good or ill.

THREATS FROM CONDITIONS AND TREATMENTS

Significant threats to the well-being of our probiotic team lurk even in actions that we are encouraged to take by our guides in the health care arena. There are many more examples of *unintended consequences* whereby we desire one of the benefits of a recommendation, but are unaware of potential collateral damage.

Other Drugs

Antibiotics are the poster child of medications that are hard on friendly bacteria, but they aren't alone. This is an example of why I've applied Audi's current tagline, "Challenge all Givens" in this book. We are expected to fill prescriptions without question, but noted pharmacist/author, Suzy Cohen, says that virtually *all* medications have the potential for harming our friendly flora and even some of the pills' so-called "inactive' ingredients do harm.

- Treating chronic pain with non-steroidal anti-inflammatory drugs (NSAIDs), such as aspirin and ibuprofen) is a known risk for death from intestinal bleeding. It appears that the risks may go well beyond that since these drugs act as *antibiotics* and would suppress the normal healthy flora.[1]

- Often, as we saw with antibiotics, medications can poison probiotics directly. With others the damage is indirect. For example, acid-blocking heartburn drugs allow pathogens to get past the stomach to compete with them. Also, the drugs alter the normal pH of the gut environment, and therefore define the assortment of microorganisms that feel at home there.

- Going back to an even earlier stage, consider that many drugs, such as statin cholesterol-lowering drugs, cause heartburn as a side effect. That obviously leads to a prescription for acid blockers.

- When a drug spoils a person's appetite or causes cravings for bad food that may have a bad effect on the food supply for the GI tract and dictate a change in bacterial communities.

I could go on, but I think it is clear that something that upsets the chemistry of the body is likely to also affect these delicate microorganisms. The website drugs.com is an example of an online resource to learn about drug side effects as well as interactions with other medications and even foods. Unfortunately, neither this type of website nor the fine print on the drug package inserts currently list the effect of medications on our gut bacteria. The FDA does not require that information probably because until now the probiotic role of bacteria was not properly appreciated. Also, the drug manufacturer has a clear *disincentive* to even look for these side effects.

Threats From Conditions And Their Treatments

It may take some getting used to remember that we have to look out for the rest of our team when our attention is understandably focused elsewhere. For example, here are some situations that can create a gut environment not conducive to a thriving microbiota.

- Radiation kills friendly bacteria whether the source is x-rays, medical treatments, or even frequent airline travel.

- Chronic diarrhea is obviously a problem because the probiotics are constantly being flushed away.

- Colon hydrotherapy creates a similar situation on a temporary basis. Some therapists will add probiotics to the flush, but in any case, extra attention should be paid to replacing beneficial strains after a treatment. (Some apparently do survive by clinging to the lining of the intestines perhaps protected in biofilm communities.)

- The reverse problem, constipation, can make the intestinal tract toxic and create an unwholesome neighborhood for good flora.

- Anything that creates a general gut inflammation is not good for the flora conditions and that includes continuing to eat foods to which the person is sensitive (or allergic).

- A newly discovered health threat is sitting too much of the day—it has been called the "new smoking." Based on a study of rugby players, it appears that playing hard leads to a more diverse microbiota.[2] Professor Tim Spector, Director of the Department of Twin Research and Genetic Epidemiology at St Thomas' Hospital, London found from a study of 3,000 twins that the amount they exercised was the strongest determinant of having a rich and diverse microbiome. An animal study showed that rats using the exercise wheel compared to those not exercising created more (almost double) of a substance that promotes colon health. If exercise is good for our probiotics, conversely sitting may be bad for them.

- Chronic stress always appears on the list of risk factors for any disease, and it certainly sends the wrong signals to the digestive system.

The Downside of Herbs

There is a tendency to think that everything natural is healthful. As critics of natural medicine point out, the *hemlock* that was used to poison Socrates was *natural*. However, most natural remedies are safer than their counterpart drugs. Some essential oils and herbs like elderberry extract have anti-viral actions. Many herbs are *antimicrobial* and that means they may be hard on bacterial allies as well as enemies. For example, raw garlic has wonderful health properties and is effective against pathogenic bacteria, but in excess it can apparently kill *bifidobacteria*.[3] The same is true for the adaptogenic (balancing) herb astragalus.[4] When taking these, probiotics should be supplemented but just as with antibiotics, not at the same time of day as probiotic supplements. In Chapter 9 we'll discuss similar problems with some natural remedies used specifically to control yeast.

Vaccines

Immunizations are designed to alert the immune system to be ready to destroy pathogens (bacteria or viruses) if and when they appear. It is beyond the scope of this book to contribute much to the current vaccine debate, except to acknowledge that there is one. In brief, establishment authorities encourage vaccinations and predict that unvaccinated children will spread diseases that were previously under control. The other side questions the actual effectiveness of vaccines; expresses concern that in some cases vaccines might actually *cause* the disease they were to prevent; point to a possible link with the steep rise in neurological conditions, such as autism; and they worry about the unknown long-term effect of the dramatically increased numbers of vaccinations given to newborns and infants over an ever shorter time. Children are already expected to receive over 50 doses of vaccine before they are 5 years old and there are many more vaccines in the pipeline. There is also the concern that many if not most disease-causing bacteria and viruses mutate into slightly different forms that might not be affected by a current vaccine. On page 73 we discussed how the chemicals in vaccines might be more likely to cause damage in the brain if the gut microbiome is not protecting the blood brain barrier as it should.

Maybe it isn't wrong to question the potential for negative effects from at least the so-called "inactive ingredients" that are included in the vaccines. For example, besides live or killed pathogens, vaccines can also contain egg, formaldehyde, ether, aluminum, and mercury. These chemicals may harm probiotics as well as cells. Mercury is a highly toxic metal that is added to many vaccines in the form of Thimerosal, a preservative. It is possible to request a vaccine without this preservative.

The microbiota is vigilant against a vast array of pathogenic threats by identifying them and killing them directly and/or by alerting our own immune cells. Protecting our microscopic warriors seems key. It is very encouraging that scientists are searching for ways to improve vaccines, and in one study they found that probiotics made a Hepatitis vaccine work better—perhaps even better than aluminum which is often added for that same purpose.[5] I'm also encouraged by studies showing that a safe, probiotic-sparing homeopathic alternative to vaccines, homeoprophylaxis, is effective even for curbing epidemics.[6] A good article on that topic can be found on the website nourishedmagazine.com.au. by searching for "homeoprophylaxis."

HOW TO AVOID PATHOGENS

Since medications are not needed if we don't get sick, ideally we would never come in contact with any pathogens. That isn't realistic, but below are some common sense ways to avoid disease-causing microorganisms without becoming a germaphobe like the late Howard Hughes or the very funny Howie Mandel. These are sorted by location and most are logical and relatively easy to implement.

Anywhere

It appears that grandma might have been right about not letting the dog kiss us on the lips. As it turns out they can transmit norovirus to humans. She also was right about us catching a cold from being outside in the winter without a hat.[7] I am disappointed that expert medical advice for avoiding illness during the cold and flu season rarely (if ever) includes information about building immune competence with sufficient sleep, good nutrition, supplements, and probiotics. However, some of the tactics that they do recommend may very well help to dodge whatever misery is going around.

- It is obvious that we should take their advice and steer a wide path around people who appear to be sick. However, that might be harder than it sounds. In response to an anonymous survey taken at a large children's hospital in Philadelphia, Pennsylvania 446 employees (83.1 percent) reported that they had come to work sick at least one time in the past year, and 50 (9.3 percent) reported working while sick at least 5 times.

- Wash hands *frequently* with soap and water for long enough to sing the Happy Birthday song. I admit that for a long time I was pretty casual about the advice to wash hands after visiting the restroom. Then I realized that I am not protecting myself *from me*. Washing my hands is to protect me from all the other people who visit the restroom bringing with them germs from everywhere they have been. That restroom visit is also a convenient time to get rid of the germs I might have picked up all around town. Now I wash my hands at every opportunity. I even go the extra step to use a paper towel to open the door when leaving the restroom because I know not everyone that preceded me did the right thing.

- And/or use an *alcohol-based* sanitizer. I'm now a fan of that too. More about these sanitizers on page 80.

- Sneeze into a tissue or at least a sleeve.

- Stay home when sick. Besides protecting others, rest is a crucial element of getting well. (I list others in the Library on my website.)

At Work, the Gym, Shopping, and Traveling

Pathogenic microorganisms are left behind anywhere people have visited. Some items in the following list may seem surprising, but they are likely just the tip of the iceberg.

- Researchers found that *half* of workplace coffee mugs were contaminated with *fecal* bacteria. Wash them with dish soap and water.

- Researchers at the University of Arizona found that a doorknob coated with viruses could transfer them to as many as 60 percent of the people in the building in just four hours. Brass doorknobs reportedly disinfect themselves in a short time.

- Pathogenic bacteria can survive up to a week on airplane armrests and seatback pockets.

- According to NBC's account of research done on shopping cart handles by Dr. Charles P. Gerba at the University of Arizona: "72 percent turned out to have a marker for *fecal* bacteria."[8]

- Other sources of bacteria and viruses include ATM keypads, elevator buttons, hand rails, exercise equipment, TV remotes, light switches, and phones. The glasses in hotel rooms do not go through a dishwasher to be sanitized. Anticipating that housekeepers have not given them a thorough cleaning, I either wash them with the shampoo provided or use disposable glasses.

- At first thought, tongs on a buffet seem like a good idea. However, consider this. If I grab a roll with my bare fingers, I am the only one that touches the food. But, *everyone* touches the tongs. We probably wouldn't want to grab a Swedish meatball with our fingers, but we could bring a fork from the table.

- A study in the *Journal of Environmental Health* years ago found that bacteria can survive on the chalice rim and on wine-soaked wafers, but those taking communion didn't get sick more often.

- In a study of bacteria found in the New York subway, of the strains isolated, 48 percent were previously *unknown*. Fortunately, just 12 percent turned out to be of the disease-causing variety. Courtesy of subway rats, one is known to cause bubonic plague. The pathogens were present, but not at levels that would be harmful to passengers with normal immune defenses.

In the Kitchen

Paying attention to potential pathogens in food is very important because foodborne illness hospitalizes over 5,000 each year and kills 3,000. It is difficult to know what is going on in the kitchen of restaurants we visit, but we do have control at home. Awareness, not paranoia is the goal.

- Who would have guessed that kitchen sponges are more contaminated than the toilet? Dishcloths that are routinely laundered are much safer. If sponges are used, they should be sterilized in the microwave frequently.

- Shrimp is not well regulated and Consumer's Report found bacterial contamination at alarming rates. We have to remember that the poisons produced by bacteria and molds cannot be cooked away. *When in doubt, throw it out.*

- Consumer Reports also noted in their October 2015 *On Health* that they had found more bacteria and increased amounts of antibiotic resistant varieties in commercial ground beef than in grass fed and other more naturally raised products.

- Follow safe food handling practices, especially with animal products. For example, honor the expiration dates on egg cartons and cook eggs because even the yolk can come contaminated with *Salmonella*. The government website, foodsafety.gov, has many useful ideas—one that surprises many is that we are advised to *not* wash chicken because that spreads bacteria around.

- Speaking of the government, it seems that we are increasingly on our own to protect ourselves. We might rightfully wonder what the FDA is doing to prevent the contamination of the spinach, lettuce, peanuts, melons, caramel apples, hummus, ice cream, green beans and such that we hear about on the news. Lack of water safety in farming is at the root of those problems, but in 2014 the FDA bowed to industry pressure and proposed to *relax* the water safety rules. Under the proposal, farmers will be able to irrigate with water that is less pure and harvest crops sooner after having used raw manure as fertilizer.[9]

- *Campylobacter, Salmonella,* and *Listeria* bacteria have been used in the past as measures of food contamination. Scientists have now discovered that pathogenic *Staphylococcus aureus and E. coli* can also be found in food.

- As mentioned earlier, an antibiotic-resistant *E. coli* strain has been found in grocery store poultry. This bug causes human urinary tract infections and is also associated with meningitis, pneumonia, and sepsis (a potentially fatal whole body infection/inflammation).[10] Regulation and inspection of poultry production is the responsibility of the U.S. Department of Agriculture (USDA). Until now, as many as *4 inspectors* were stationed along a production line to look for birds with problems, such as tumors and obvious contamination with excrement. However, in 2014, the USDA created a new *voluntary* inspection system. Under this system, *only one* inspector would be on a similar line. He or she would be required to inspect at a dizzying 140 or more birds *per minute*. The agency generously allowed that, *at the option of the supplier,* company employees could help. (Apparently another case of foxes guarding hen houses.) And there is no requirement to test for many common disease-causing bacteria.[11]

- When there is an outbreak of food poisoning, authorities require that the product be recalled. Stores will accept returns of those products, but it is easy to miss a recall in the news. The website belltowertech.com/FoodAlert notifies subscribers of recalls. (Of course, by the time consumers hear of a recall, they may have already eaten the food. That is just one of many reasons we need to keep our internal defenses in good repair.)

- Stomach acid is our first line of defense against contamination in food. So, if a person has less stomach acid due to age and/or acid-blocking drugs, they are at greater risk that a pathogen may slip by.[12]

- Our beneficial flora is another important early defense against invading foodborne germs.

Outdoors

Fresh air, nature and sunshine are all well-known health boosters. Unfortunately, invisible threats await us there too. A little advanced preparation can avoid the dangers without interfering with the fun.

Mosquitos carry several serious viral diseases, including West Nile, Chikungunya, and Dengue fever which is similar to West Nile and is also called "breakbone fever." In the tropics mosquitos spread a parasitic disease, malaria. Unfortunately, malathion, the insecticide most commonly sprayed to kill mosquitos was declared a carcinogen by the World Health Organization. We can protect ourselves from mosquito bites with clothing that covers us and with natural insect repellants.

It is also important to eliminate any standing water in the yard where mosquitos might breed—they can lay eggs in as little as the water in the saucers of potted plants. For larger amounts of water, such as rain barrels or ponds, Mosquito Dunks are an effective way to kill the larvae before they become airborne. (Dunks are safe for fish, animals, and plants.) We've had fair results with a garlic powered mosquito-suppressing outdoor system offered by the pest control company Terminix. As an aside, researchers in Brazil, Australia, Vietnam, and Indonesia have used mosquitos as weapons against Dengue fever. They release mosquitos that are infected with a certain strain of bacteria that fights the disease. The infected mosquitos then spread those killer bacteria to other mosquitos.

Ticks spread diseases caused by bacteria, viruses, and protozoa. Among the most well-known are Lyme disease and Rocky Mountain spotted fever. When going into the woods or rural areas, especially in May and June when exposure risk seems greatest, it is important to wear protective clothing and bug repellant that specifically states that it is effective for ticks. Everyone should check for ticks when returning from an excursion where there has been a risk of tick bites. Lyme disease may create a bull's eye rash.

Personal Services

It is tempting to feel that when we are purchasing personal services of various kinds that we have to just go with the flow. However, we can decline the option to take home a disease. It isn't being pushy, it is just being smart and as more of us speak up, the providers will improve.

- We have to watch very carefully in doctors' offices, clinics, and hospitals that workers and even the doctors are following safe hand-washing practices. It is absolutely our right to assure they aren't delivering someone else's bugs to us on their hands, tie, clipboard, or stethoscope. This is serious business because the nastiest, most antibiotic-resistant germs are found where the sick people are. Infections of this type are responsible for about the same number of deaths each year as the combination of AIDS and firearms.

- Tattoo needles and inks can be contaminated and have been linked to hepatitis, staph infections, and even *MRSA*.

- Selecting a nail salon with good sanitation practices helps avoid acquiring fungal and bacterial infections. In some states, the licensing agency may have an online reference rating how well salons comply with regulations.

- It is best to *not* shave legs right before a pedicure. That weakens the skin's protective barrier, and it increases the odds of infection from the scrubbing and massaging of the legs.

HOW TO SANITIZE SAFELY

Knowing how many unsavory microbes lurk in our environment we might be inspired to sanitize everything in sight. However, as seems to be the case with all good things, there is the potential for overdoing it—and not all methods are even safe. Advertisers understandably make their cleaning products sound appealing, but many harbor hidden dangers that they are not required to disclose. We can make better choices among a plethora of options if we know what to look for.

Disinfecting Anti-bacterial Soaps

We were flat out misled about these chemical-laden hand cleansers that are now hard to avoid. At one time such cleansers contained hexachlorophene, but that was replaced with triclosan, a chemical that can also be found in body washes, toothpastes, and some cosmetics. Traces of triclosan have been found in the urine of pregnant women as well as the blood of newborn infants' umbilical cords. Environmental watchdog groups are concerned that triclosan is absorbed into circulation where it potentially interferes with hormones and thyroid function. Triclosan has also been linked to liver cancer in mice, interference with brain development in children, as well as potentially diabetes and other health issues. Researchers also say that, like with antibiotics, they may encourage the development of stronger, more resistant strains of bacteria which would make the next generation of bugs even tougher to combat. All that risk isn't even balanced by a good benefit! According to the FDA, "At this time, FDA does not have evidence that triclosan added to antibacterial soaps and body washes provides extra health benefits over soap and water." When babies are born they are washed with anti-bacterial cleansers that remove a natural protective coating from their skin and remove their friendly bacteria. There are not proven health reasons to sanitize a newborn. A light rubbing with a towel is sufficient to prepare the baby for its photo ops.

Disinfecting Wipes

Many name brand wipes contain questionable ingredients, such as quaternary ammonium compounds and our old friend triclosan. These are not only potentially toxic, but they are also more likely to encourage the growth of resistant species of pathogens. The best choice seems to be alcohol-based sanitizing wipes, such as those by Purell, which are based on the sanitizer discussed next.

Alcohol-based Sanitizer Gels

These products are safe and bacteria cannot become immune to their mode of action. The Centers for Disease Control and the World Health Organization agree that alcohol sanitizers, such as Purell, may be more effective at killing bacteria than even hand washing. (However, they cannot cut through a layer of greasy grime—for that we need soap.) A New Yorker article said of a test of Purell: "After thirteen weeks, the [U.S.] Army found that two test battalions had experienced 40 percent less respiratory illness than the control group, 48 percent less gastrointestinal illness, and 44 percent less lost training time."[13]

I admit that I was always a little suspicious of alcohol sanitizers because I had heard that they were dangerous for toddlers who might lick them off their hands and suffer alcohol poisoning. Mostly, I think I was afraid that they would dry out my skin. However, I became curious enough to look into them when we encountered dozens of Purell dispensers on a cruise ship. I liked what I learned and was surprised that my hands actually became *less* dry and the tips of my nails looked like I had a French manicure. Now I carry some in my purse. (For those looking for a natural alternative, CleanWell sanitizer uses herbs and discloses all ingredients.)

The *New Yorker* article also contained a funny anecdote. "George W. Bush was called a racist and a germaphobe for using a sanitizer after first shaking hands with Barack Obama, but Bush was ahead of the curve: he also gave a squirt to Obama, and recommended it as a cold preventative. (It has been estimated that the President shakes hands with about sixty-five thousand people a year.")[14]

Household Cleaners

The non-profit Environmental Working Group has this to say regarding home cleaning and care products: "Some ingredients are known to cause cancer, blindness, asthma, and other serious conditions." Search their website (ewg.org) for their *Cleaners Hall of Shame.* While efforts to completely sterilize a home might be good for the Lysol stockholders, that would also kill off our protective bacteria and lead to the development of resistance and even more dangerous bacteria. In fact, the collection of family-specific bacteria might just be considered part of the home's "immune system." Natural food stores sell safe cleaners, but it is surprising how much you can do with simple inexpensive options like vinegar, baking soda, and regular soap.

HOW TO AVOID PROBIOTIC KILLERS IN FOOD

There are obviously thousands of food choices, and we all know that some are more healthful than others for our bodies. Until learning of second hand antibiotics in the previous chapter, it is likely that few of us ever consider that substances in the food might damage our good bacteria. In the next chapter we'll talk about what foods the probiotics thrive on, but for now let's look at the chemicals in the food supply and at least try not to send our tiny allies a lethal lunch.

Commercial Produce and Grains

Fruits, vegetables, and whole grains that are intrinsically healthful can become much less so depending on many factors, such as how the seeds are engineered and how the food is grown, stored, transported, processed, and packaged. For example, domestic produce that has not been grown according to *organic standards* likely contains residues of the 1.1 billion pounds of pesticides sprayed annually. Then there are herbicides, fungicides, and antibiotics. Those chemicals are harmful to humans, so how can they *not* hurt probiotics? Check the website of the Environment Working Group (ewg.org) to see how fruits and vegetables currently rate regarding pesticide contamination—the EWG lists of *The Clean 15* and *The Dirty Dozen.* As a reminder, poisonous mycotoxins can contaminate peanuts and grains stored in silos. Grains grown from seeds that are known as Genetically Modified Organisms (GMO's) present another level of risk. Please *see* inset on page 82.

Commercial Meats and Dairy

In the chapter on antibiotics we discussed the problem of the drugs given to commercially raised animals, and the presence of those drug residues in the meat, dairy products, and even produce. But, also note that animals that are not raised according to organic standards are usually fed commercial grains

Concerns About GMO'S

GMO is short for "Genetically Modified Organism"—meaning a living thing whose genetic makeup has been changed by the insertion of genes from some other living thing. I really have no objection if scientists want to transplant genes from various sea creatures in order to engineer gold fish in various neon colors like hot pink, blue, or green. (Yes, they are a real thing, GloFish.) However, when they start doing that sort of thing to the food supply, I am no longer comfortable. It should give us pause that most countries do not consider GMO foods safe.

Part of their concern and mine is that we just don't know the potential for allergic reactions or the long-term health effects of these unnatural "Frankenfoods" created with genes from animals, bacteria, viruses, and so on. As near as I can tell, no one is studying whether or not GMO crops per se are hard on our probiotic organisms. There is an even more alarming concern than the prospect that the foods might be *directly* damaging to the microbiome. GMO's have sometimes been created by inserting genes from bacteria and viruses into the DNA of food plants so that they will generate chemicals poisonous to pests. It is possible that our friendly microorganisms can acquire those genes and turn into little toxin factories. We should know these health factors because 88 percent of the corn and 94 percent of the soy grown in the U.S. are now GMO. Of course, we'd never know that from food labels because there is no requirement to indicate GMO ingredients.

As an example, genes from a bacterium *Bacillus thuringiensis (BT)* are spliced into the DNA of certain food crops. This bacterial species has been used on crops since the 1950's because it releases a toxic insecticide. Animal studies reveal side effects of this BT toxin, including some in the kidney, liver, heart, adrenal glands, spleen, and blood system.[15] There is good reason to believe that it also kills probiotic bacteria. The microorganisms themselves will degrade in sunshine. However, the *toxin* they produce has become incorporated into the genetic makeup of Monsanto seeds so that the only way to escape it is to avoid eating GMO foods. Corn, soy, and even sugar beets are being modified this way.

Another big part of the GMO controversy is indirect because it involves the supposed reason for making most of the genetic modifications. Corn and soy are examples of crop plants genetically engineered mainly to make them "RoundUp Ready," which means that they will not be killed by the potent herbicide (weed killer) RoundUp. Direct exposure to RoundUp, a glyphosate-based herbicide (GBH), is scary business. This sentence from the abstract of an article on the subject in a *cardiovascular journal* is hair-raising: "Millions of farmers suffer poisoning and death in developing countries, and occupational exposures and suicide make GBH toxicity a worldwide concern."[16]

RoundUp creates nutritional deficiencies in plants because it binds up minerals and kills beneficial microorganisms in the soil.[17] That surely diminishes our access to our historical microbial diversity which is so important to agriculture that some farmers transplant soil from wild fields to "inoculate" other fields thereby creating more nutritious food. This chemical apparently is known for disrupting probiotics, interfering with our detoxification pathways and depleting minerals and amino acids.[18] RoundUp is also suspected of being linked to a vast array of health problems, including breast cancer, leukemia, fatal kidney disease, liver damage, autism, reduced fertility, birth defects, Parkinson's, and more. Glyphosate and a by-product were detected in 75 percent of rain and air samples. Worse yet, in the NHANES 2003-04 study 93 percent of children had detectable metabolites of these organophosphates.

Disease connections are difficult to prove because of the power and grandstanding of the vested economic interests. Industry apologists say that glyphosate, the main active ingredient in Roundup is considered "relatively safe" and at least better than the chemicals it replaced. I suspect they may be "cooking the books" by selecting the more flattering studies, and I'm not willing to give them a pass just because they may or may not be killing quite as many of us as they used to.

Digging deeper, we find that glyphosate doesn't act alone in RoundUp. Pesticide and herbicide formulas always contain so-called "inert" or "inactive" ingredients which are akin to those extras I told you about in vaccines. (Chemical products do not even have to put the contents of their inactive ingredients on the label.) For example, surfactants (wetting agents) and adjuvants (activators) used in agricultural products can be 1,000 times more dangerous than the "active" ingredient. They can also increase the toxicity of the main ingredient.

Health advocates are concerned not only about the health of the farmers and the safety of our ground water. But, they also worry that agricultural chemicals like pesticides usually leave residues on the foods that were grown using it. And then we eat them! Should we be comforted that industry always says, " . . . but the exposure is so low." No, not so fast. French scientists found that negative effects (including cell death) on human cells are seen at concentrations of herbicides and pesticides even lower than exposures due to common use on farms or lawns. The researchers also said that "RoundUp was among the most toxic."[19] Most chemicals loose in the environment have not been tested for safety and certainly not in the combinations that we are encountering. When the Environmental Protection Agency or other government agency does require safety studies, they only look at *immediate* toxicity—not the *long-term* effects of chronic low level exposure as might be the case from having a little bit of the chemical in our cereal every day for decades.

Use of these potent killers has spawned new super weeds that are resistant to those poisons and that leads to ever stronger poisons. (Doesn't this vicious cycle sound a lot like the problem of antibiotic-resistant bacteria?) Also, according to the Union of Concerned Scientists, the jury is still out on whether GMO's even deliver the higher crop yields that were promised. This idea may be hard to get our heads around, but some scientists theorize that overuse of pesticides may be a factor in drought because they kill soil bacteria that might otherwise have ended up in clouds to help precipitate rain. Aside from the unknowns, the general health risks and likely adverse effects on our probiotics of GMO's, I am opposed to industry giant Monsanto's heavy-handed bullying of farmers to use their GMO corn. I am also incensed by companies investing big money to defeat consumer initiatives requiring proper GMO labeling of foods.

that carry the contamination risks listed just above. The animals accumulate and *concentrate* residues of those chemicals, including aflatoxin. Grass fed animals produce healthier meat and dairy to begin with, and they are less prone to producing foods contaminated with pathogens.

Food Additives

The rise in consumption of processed foods parallels the rise in chronic degenerative disease. Most attention has been paid to the lack of nutrition in these "foods" and the increased amount of sugars they contain. Those are very important factors, but there are more. Artificial colors and additives of all kind are added for sales appeal, shelf life, manufacturing convenience, or cost reduction with no regard for how they might affect our gut bacteria.

For example, *actual strawberries* supply fiber and a great many vitamins, minerals, and phytonutrients to our own cells, and feed our important gut microorganisms; in contrast, the 51 chemicals that make up *artificial strawberry flavor* do not. I could not find any research asking whether or not the chemical soup that is artificial flavoring hurts our friendly microorganisms. Fortunately, many companies are bowing to public pressure and going with supposedly natural flavors instead of artificial. For example, in 2015 the Taco Bell restaurant chain announced that they were switching to real pepper instead of artificial pepper flavor.

As another illustration, ice cream, salad dressings, non-dairy creamers, pastries, and ever burger patties have emulsifiers added to improve texture and shelf life. Emulsifiers are detergent-like molecules, such as carboxymethylcellulose, polysorbate-80, carrageenan, polyglycerols, and gums such as xanthan and guar. Fortunately, researchers have looked into this category and found that some emulsifiers caused low level inflammation, obesity, metabolic syndrome, and colitis in mice.[20] Lecithin (such as is contained in egg yolks) emulsifies but doesn't seem to have as negative an effect.

Processed foods also contain preservatives to prevent spoilage and some of those chemicals are added *specifically to kill bacteria.* The high fructose corn

What Consumers Can Do About GMO and RoundUp

This problem may sound discouraging, but we are not powerless by a long shot. The following are some helpful steps for the consumer.

- Learn more and find sources of non-GNO foods at JustLabelIt.org and NonGMOProject.org.

- Buy organic foods as much as possible because those will not be GMO and will not contain harsh agricultural chemicals. Buying organic also financially supports the small family-owned farms that are trying to do things the right way and protect the environment. ("Natural" does not mean organic.) Look for a Certified Organic seal or a seal with a butterfly that states "Non GMO Project Verified."

- Lobby for clear labeling of GMO foods and better testing of industrial chemicals. Also, support non-profit groups that do those things.

- Don't use RoundUp or a similar chemical weed killer at home. A friend of mine noted, organic expert landscape architect and horticulturist, Howard Garrett, offers safer and yet still very effective alternatives. Visit DirtDoctor .com/RoundUp-Alternatives_vq5112.htm. (We use his Vinegar Herbicide Formula.)

syrup that is added to a great many processed foods and beverages usually contains mercury.[21] Mercury was sold as a topical antiseptic in the form of Mercurochrome because it killed bacteria, but it is now banned in the U.S. due to mercury's toxicity to nerves.

Artificial Sweeteners

In the beginning it was assumed by the industry, consumers, and even scientists that non-caloric artificial sweeteners (NAS) were kind of a get-out-of-jail-free card in that we could have our cake but not the calories. A recent study published in *Nature* showed that NAS seem to cause an increase in glucose intolerance (a precursor to diabetes). What is new and relevant in that study is that the scientists showed that the harmful effect was due to changes the NAS made *in gut bacteria*.[22]

The sweetener Splenda (sucralose) was shown in one study (sponsored by sugar producers) to harm intestinal bacteria.[23] That is of special interest because this chemical is often used to reduce the sugar content of yogurt marketed as a source of probiotics. Later reviews of that study (possibly a counter attack by the makers of Splenda) found that study unreliable and challenged the findings. One study showed that the herbal sweetener Stevia was okay.[24] Another said that Stevia was not so good for probiotics.[25] In another study using pigs, an artificial sweetener containing saccharin seemed to *promote* lactic acid bacteria.

Studies are under way to determine why aspartame (known commercially as NutraSweet is associated with increasing insulin insensitivity and weight gain. Most recent studies of artificial sweeteners show that they reduce the diversity of our microbes and disproportionately harm the beneficial strains. Take what you like from all that. Many artificial sweeteners do reduce diversity of microbes. For those reasons and a variety of others I just think we should reduce our collective sweet tooth and that real food is better than chemical substitutes.

Salt

We are told by the "authorities" to reduce sodium intake. But, just as was the case with their prior pronouncements about fat, the advice turns out to be an oversimplification. Reducing sodium seems to help a small percentage of persons with elevated blood pressure, but lowering salt intake across the board to a very low level is actually problematic for most of the rest of us. Potassium salt substitutes may be useful for persons who are salt-sensitive, but it seems that *extremely high* levels of either potassium or sodium are bad for our probiotics.[26]

MORE EVERYDAY THREATS TO PROBIOTICS

It is no wonder that our friendly bacteria are in decline. As we will see in the next chapter we may not be getting a good start from having them passed on from one generation to the next as we have in the past. Besides the items above that kill them, modern life hides many more hazards for our probiotics in plain sight. Take cookware as just one example of a threat that most people would never even remotely consider. Acidic foods cooked in aluminum or copper pans will acquire a small amount of the metals which are antibacterial. Non-stick Teflon which coats pans and the insides of many toaster ovens contain off-gas chemicals (PTFE or PFOA's) that have been known to kill pet birds. Those chemicals are not good for our gut and are a likely negative for our flora. Also, any toxin we breathe, we swallow. Being aware of these threats will make it easier to take precautions.

Drinking Water

Unfiltered tap water contains chlorine which is put there specifically to kill bacteria. Chlorine (the same chemical that is in bleach) is an equal opportunity poison, killing good and bad bacteria with equal ease. The U.S. manufactures over 70,000 different chemicals of which only 1,500 have been studies for toxicity to humans. Ground water can contain pesticides, herbicides, industrial solvents, petrochemicals, heavy metals, antibiotics, and other medications which municipal water treatment plants are simply not set up to remove. On the shop/recommended products page of my website (HBNShow.com) I provide a link to whatever home and kitchen filtration systems I currently find to be the best value.

Alkaline Water

The body works hard to maintain a normal acid/alkaline balance in blood and tissues. In the face of an excess of acid-producing foods and sodas, it may have to pull alkaline minerals out of storage to buffer that acid. It is on that basis that water alkalinized by either ionizing water filters or the addition of alkaline drops has become popular in some circles. Vegetables contain minerals that can also help maintain balance as can mineral supplements. The colon maintains a relatively acidic pH between 5.2 and 6.5 (neutral is 7) which is appropriate for the colonization and proliferation of probiotic strains. Therefore, there is the potential for overdoing a good thing. For reasons similar to those I've mentioned in regard to the use of acid-blocking drugs, I'm a little concerned about overly aggressive attempts to alkalinize the body with water. Drinking alkaline water continually may tend to disturb that gut pH. I also have to wonder if a reduction of the acidity of the stomach might interfere with the absorption of B12 and other nutrients. At the least it would seem that alkaline water would be best consumed away from meal time when we need strong stomach acid.

CONCLUSION

The principles for protection of our beneficial microbiome are all relatively *simple*. However, that doesn't make the steps *easy* because changing habits rarely is. I doubt that any reader is going to throw out everything in their cupboards and start over. But, hopefully, we can give our friendly bacteria a break by at least making some gradual improvements in our choices of medications, sanitizers, yard care, foods, drinking water, and health practices. After seeing the variety of threats they face we should now have more motivation to learn how to acquire an ample, robust, diverse army of protective probiotics and to support them with appropriate food and supplements. We will discuss that positive side of the story in the next chapter.

7.

Recruit and Support the Troops

Bacteria contribute in a major way to our digestion, our immune competence, our general metabolic operation, and even our genetic memory. So, clearly we will be healthier and have greater vitality if our gut is host to a large, complex, and well-balanced community of microorganisms—but where do we get these good bacteria to begin with? And what should we eat to attract more and do to maintain them? Those questions seem basic enough, but surprisingly scientists are just beginning to figure out the answers.

ACQUIRING THE BACTERIA WE DEPEND UPON

So far in this book we've learned that there are perhaps up to 10 thousand subspecies of probiotics. There are similarities in the blend of microorganisms according to geographic area, to family association, and even to the type of diet (for example, vegetarian or omnivore). But, men and women differ and, in fact, each individual has his or her own unique assortment. The answer to how our microbiome develops begins even before we are born.

In the Beginning

Long held assumptions are being challenged about the role and origins of our natural complement of probiotic strains. Now that scientists are cataloging the serious negative effects suffered when infants and children have inadequate protection of friendly bacteria, they are asking all kinds of interesting questions and making sometimes shocking observations.

- Recent research has shown that far from being sterile as previously assumed, the placenta (that temporary organ lining the uterus which supports the fetus' needs) is a rich depository of bacteria. It not only contains a variety of bacteria but a combination not found elsewhere in the body.[1]. It can't be a mistake, but we don't really know yet exactly what the bacteria are doing, but surely they must be preparing the fetus for life on the outside. It has recently been discovered that mothers with lower levels of *lactobacillus* are more at risk for having preterm babies.

- Many things mom does during pregnancy are very important in part because microbes are already communicating with the baby while it is in the womb. Alcohol consumption during pregnancy is known to disrupt the infant's immune system. Is that in part because it kills some of the mother's beneficial microbes which would otherwise have helped the infant? Also, at least with mice, when the mom is stressed she passes on lower amounts of the bacteria known to create calming compounds. Incidentally, the mom's microbiome balance changes with each phase of the pregnancy. The bacteria respond to and perhaps even participate in changes. At some points the blend looks a bit like that of someone with metabolic syndrome.

- It seems that the original plan was that babies would gestate for nine months and then pass through the birth canal being naturally inoculated with their mother's friendly bacteria along the way.[2] It turns out that even premature birth alters the baby's microbiome as does simply being born in a hospital. And now that about one-third of children are delivered surgically by Caesarian Section (C-section), there are concerns that in those cases, the starter set is not being supplied as effectively. For example with C-section, the baby usually acquires a microbiota that looks more like mom's skin than gut. Maybe it does make a difference. It is at least interesting that babies born by C-section have twice the risk of being obese by age 3 compared to those delivered normally.[3]

- And that omitted trip down the birth canal might not be the only factor with C-sections. I have to wonder if part of the problem isn't that mothers who deliver surgically are routinely given antibiotics to prevent infection from the incision. That may help the moms, but it is perhaps not in the best interest of the infant if it lessens the availability of probiotic strains even in the placenta.[4]

- Breast feeding is the next opportunity for newborns to acquire a healthful microbiome. However, consider that the mother is given antibiotics before and after the C-section. The antibiotics surely reduce the microbes that mom has available to contribute via breast milk, and there is evidence that antibiotics taken by the mother also transfer into breast milk. Therefore, that infant is effectively also taking antibiotics.[5] Children are more likely to be overweight if given antibiotics as babies.[6]

- I found it fascinating that breast milk is quite rich in complex carbohydrates (oligosaccharides) which infants cannot digest. What would be the evolutionary point of a mom's chemistry spending precious energy to create something that baby couldn't use? It turns out that these oligosaccharides are food (a prebiotic) for at least one of the baby's probiotic bacteria (*B. infantis*). That is a strain that protects the baby's delicate digestive tract which is as yet not fully functional.[7] Interestingly, the bacterial balance in breast milk is similar to that in the stool of a healthy baby.

- It has been shown that supplementing with probiotics before delivery changes the probiotic composition of breast milk.[8] Commercial infant formulas now add prebiotics, but they cannot duplicate the natural bacterial assortment. Breast feeding will always be the ideal because it offers so many other advantages, such as protection from obesity, inflammation, cardiovascular disease, diabetes, asthma, and celiac disease at the least.

- A small study (of 10 children) showed that the blend and ratio of various beneficial bacterial strains in babies change substantially between age 6 months and 12 months. At that point things were relatively stable on to age 13 (and likely into adulthood). Researchers also noted that supplementing probiotics very early in life did not have a long lasting effect on the strains present later.[9] However, the study was small and it isn't clear that the ideal supplement of strains was given. In any case, it is less important exactly how the blend of strains was affected over time. What I would want to know is whether the supplemented children were healthier than those not given probiotics.

Environmental Sources

Humans have apparently acquired much of their basic microbiome from contact with the environment. Children who are in contact with farm animals, the animals' surroundings, and drank raw milk have been shown to be much better protected from allergy and asthma. The improvement is apparently due to a combination of new probiotic species acquired and a training of the immune system about what is a threat and what is not. Germ free mice raised in a sterile environment do not have the degenerative diseases with which we are all too familiar. But, neither do their nervous systems develop naturally. For example, they may not recognize mice they are raised with which brings to mind some traits of autism. These germ free mice also do not become tolerant to environmental allergens. That may be in part because we know that much of the training of our own immune cells is provided by the microbiome.

There is scientific concern that young children in a modern sanitized society lack exposure to normal environmental bacteria, thereby preventing their immune systems from learning to properly differentiate between "friend" and "foe." That theory is called the "hygiene hypothesis" and was advanced by David Strachan in 1989. It is also referred to as the "biome depletion theory" and the "lost friends theory." Scientists have recently given us a fresh wakeup call. They somehow managed to secure stool specimens from a remote hunter/gatherer tribe on the border of Venezuela and Brazil. These villagers had lived separated from modern society for perhaps eleven thousand years with no antibiotics, no Lysol, no pesticides, no chlorinated water, or any of the other bacteria-killers so common to us. These so-called primitive people were found to have microbiomes that are up to 50 percent more diverse than ours. Many sub-species to which they are host are unknown here.[10]

We have been trained to sterilize everything that baby might touch and to reach for Lysol if we even *think about* bacteria. Modern life also offers fewer opportunities for children to play in the dirt outside. In what may be a related finding, children exposed to pets during the first year and who have more siblings are less likely to have allergies and asthma.[11]

We hear complaints of kids bringing home diseases from school. However, parents (over age 24) were shown to be 52 percent *less* likely to develop a cold than non-parents.[12] So, even as we age, our immune systems continue to be educated by microorganisms encountered. I'm not suggesting that we should all adopt a school-age child. Or that we should go out of our way to be exposed to pathogens or stop washing our hands.[13] It just seems a cautionary tale that we best not get carried away sanitizing our environment and overprotecting our children from normal exposures.

Our Diet

We will soon cover fermented foods which seem an obvious source of good bacteria, but there is a more direct and important source. We seem to understand the need for a pregnant woman to get good nutrition because she is "eating for two." To nurture our probiotics, we should remember that we are eating for *trillions*! It stands to reason that our armies of protective bacteria will perform better if they have a nutritious food supply. But, beyond that, the *type of food* we eat actually dictates the *type of microorganisms* that we will cultivate. Learning this factor was an "aha" moment for me. Surely, one reason that certain foods and diets (for example, the Mediterranean diet) that have earned a reputation for supporting good health is that they encourage a better class of microbes! Our microorganisms have developed right along with humans over millennia and continue to adapt to our changing diet. In fact, the proportion of various strains in the gut can change in a day depending on what we eat, but apparently it is our long term food intake that largely determines the composition of our microbiota.

We have much less diversity of probiotics in our systems than in centuries past. That makes me wonder if we haven't caused some species to become extinct because giant industrial farms have depleted them at the source with chemicals. And they no longer use microbe friendly practices, such as crop rotation, allowing soils a rest with cover crops, and avoiding soil compaction by making fewer passes with equipment. Also, our "civilized" processed diet doesn't help. We've already touched on some problems with modern processed foods. For example, they have fewer vitamins and minerals that our bacteria need. Fiber is important for our flora and the substances our bacteria make.

Our hunter/gatherer ancestors are said to have consumed 135 grams of fiber where today we are lucky if folks get into double digits. Sugary and starchy foods are the favorite fuel of yeasts and encourage them to overgrow into a problem. Food additives harm our microbiome. Professor Tim Spector who studies human twins found that junk food diets support pathogens and drive down the diversity and quantity of healthful bacteria. But, there is more. Variety in food leads to variety in species of microbes. Dr. Spector says that fifteen thousand years ago man regularly consumed 150 separate food ingredients in a week but now eats a mere 20 per week. Now the same few ingredients are typically just rearranged into forms that look and taste different. That is possible in part due to the artificial flavors that we discussed earlier. In his book, *The Dorito Effect*, Mark Schatzker explains how to serve economic interests flavor that has been bred out of our food. As he points out that there may be 14 flavors of Doritos, but they are all still corn chips. The food for bacteria conversation is really just getting into full swing.

- The Hadza tribe of Tanzania, Africa, one of the world's last remaining hunting and gathering tribes, is the most comparable to our Paleolithic era ancestors. Researchers found a richer microbial diversity and stability of strains in the Hadza than among urban Italians eating a Mediterranean diet or even other African tribes. Women of the tribe had slightly different assortments of bacteria because they tend to eat more of what they gather, and the men eat more of what they hunt. Specific strains (*Prevotella*, *Treponema*, and *Bacteroidetes*) are much more prominent in these hunter/gatherer people than in groups that consume a Western diet. These bacteria help digest the very fibrous Hadza diet and make human fuel from it—something their hosts could not do on their own.[14] It is interesting that when hunters bring home their kill, the intestines are eaten, likely greatly expanding the diversity of microbes to which the Hadza are exposed. While this practice may be distasteful by our modern hygienic standards, we should remember that the tribe also does not share our modern degenerative diseases.

- An elegant study compared changes in microbes when subjects ate a plant-based diet or a diet based on meat and fat. The results provide some insight into how we might adjust our diet to promote the growth of bacterial strains that in turn promote our health. *See* the inset on page 95.

- Recent research comparing vegans and omnivores living in the same area and eating controlled diets showed less difference in the proportion of strains than was expected. However, there was a significant difference between the two groups in regard to substances *found in the blood.* Apparently similar bacteria produce different output based on what they are fed. The scientists found the influence of geography to be quite strong and suggest that we may acquire our balance of microorganisms from the community early in life. That might explain why vegans in this trial were less able to process soy than their counterparts in Asia.[15]

- Researchers have found that when elderly persons enter residential institutions, changes in their diet create changes in their intestinal bacteria (rarely, if ever, an improvement on either count). That means a loss of diversity which in turn correlates to an increase in fragility, inflammation, and disease.[16] There are other factors too, such as lack of contact with diverse persons and reduced activity. Perhaps we can help by visiting and bringing real food instead of candy and cookies.

- Some gut bacteria like to eat mucilage. (That is a substance in plants that holds water. You might have noticed it as a slimy layer surrounding a soaked flax or chia seed.) If those types don't have fiber available from for example, plants in the diet, they can erode the mucous lining of the gut.

- Eating disorders are hard on our microbiota simply because the microbes can be left with little to eat.

- Consumption of high amounts of alcohol is a cause of an imbalanced microbiome and disturbing changes in the substances that are produced—protective substances are reduced and harmful ones increased. Interestingly, one metabolite that is reduced, caryophyllene, is one that would help suppress the inclination to drink more.[17]

What Is a Perfect Diet
for a Healthy Microbiome?

We know for sure that both what we eat and our microorganisms affect our health. What is a whole lot less clear is how those affect each other.

A very ambitious human intervention study published in Nature January 2014 focused on that question.[18] Researchers assigned 10 subjects to eat two radically different diets—one vegan and the other high in animal fat and protein and then to alternate. For five days on each plan the subjects' food intake was tightly controlled and the resulting alterations in the balance of microorganism types were meticulously measured using genetic analysis. One finding was that concentrations of species changed markedly and in as little as *single day* on the animal-based diet. (That there was a bigger change is not too surprising in that in their normal lives all participants had been eating at least some plant-based foods.) We know that substances (metabolites) made by bacteria differ among species. This study documented that effect, but also showed that a given strain may make different substances in response to a change in diet. That happens because the bacterium activates or quiets certain of its genes. Interestingly, subjects on both diets showed increases in live fungi carried in on the foods. Subjects' microbiota acquired similarities due to the food provided, but their personal characteristics were still detectable and the community structure returned to normal two days after the diet ended. In the notes below about the study, strain names are included mainly for health professionals who might be interested. Then we discuss the implications of the findings and attempt to reconcile this input with other information in this book.

Plant-based Diet

"Subjects on the plant-based diet ate cereal for breakfast and precooked meals made of vegetables, rice, and lentils for lunch and dinner. Fresh and dried fruits were provided as snacks on this diet." Not surprisingly, the types of bacteria that digest carbohydrates (for example, *Prevotella*) increased. The subjects' body weight remained stable. Viruses that affect plants appeared in the stool of subjects on this diet.

Animal-based Diet

"Subjects on the animal-based diet ate eggs and bacon for breakfast, and cooked pork and beef for lunch. Dinner consisted of cured meats and a selection of four cheeses. Snacks on this diet included pork rinds, cheese, and salami." Subjects began to lose weight by day three even though they *did not eat fewer calories* than those on the plant based diet. (Let that sink in a minute. We are often told weight gain or loss is only about calories, here is one of many indications that it is not the whole story.) This diet created a greater and faster change in species balance than the plant-based diet. It also "increased the abundance of bile-tolerant microorganisms (*Alistipes, Bilophila,* and *Bacteroides*) and decreased the levels of Firmicutes that metabolize dietary plant polysaccharides (*Roseburia, Eubacterium rectal,* and *Ruminococcus bromii*)." This high fat and protein food supply increased the expression bacterial genes that make vitamins and those that break down cancer-causing substances produced when meat is charred. There was also more activity among genes that degrade antibiotics. Bacteria used in the making of fermented foods, such as cheese and sausage, found their way to the intestine.

Of major interest to the researchers was that the animal-based diet significantly increased the fecal levels of the strain *B. wadsworthia* which, in response to the fat in milk, makes a bile acid that in animal studies is linked to intestinal inflammation.

Nutritionist's Questions About the Study

I'm in awe of the prodigious amount of work, great care, excruciatingly fine detail and overall brilliance of this study. However, as a nutrition professional, I must ask some big picture application-related questions.

- Processed and cured meats, such as those provided (lunch meats, bacon, and salami), are well-known as risks for a number of diseases. Isn't it possible that one reason for that increased risk is their effect on the microbiome? Might their content of preservatives or emulsifiers, such as carrageenan, have introduced confounding factors that might not have been seen with fresh meat? I'd love to see a similar study using a more healthful selection of animal products. Grass-fed meats with their improved fatty acids and other benefits might offer useful insight. Likewise, organic dairy products might produce different outcomes than commercial cheeses because organic dairy does not contain antibiotics, pesticides, and added hormones that affect gut bacteria.

- Fish is also an animal-based food. A study of mice showed that inflammation and insulin sensitivity were improved on a diet containing fish oil compared to one with the same calories as lard. The researchers attributed the difference to changes in the signals sent by bacteria.[19]

- Fresh garlic and onions were used at lunch and dinner in the plant-based diet but not in the animal-based diet. Since they are both known to reduce pathogenic bacteria and boost certain strains, did that possibly introduce a confounding factor that affected the data?

Discussion

The study used *extreme* diets to isolate specific research endpoints. But, real life is not nearly as tidy. For example, even many consumers who describe themselves as being vegetarian consume some eggs and dairy—for example, a little milk on their cereal, an egg in their muffin, or cheese on their gluten-free veggie pizza. Therefore, they are getting some animal protein and saturated fat and would be expected to have bacteria to process those and gain the benefits. Likewise, most people on what they consider a healthful low-carb or paleo diet would eat vegetables, nuts, seeds, and at least berries. They certainly do not consume *zero* plant nutrients and fiber as was the case in the study. It just seems unwise to make radical behavior changes based on *this or any other single study.*

There is a risk for error in human studies called the "healthy user bias." That acknowledges that folks who have one good behavior might have others which were not measured in that research. Apparently there is also a research risk in the opposite situation. For example, when we hear about a study that casts doubt on red meat, we should remember that the average red meat eater *also* consumes more processed foods, more pro-inflammatory omega-6 oils, fewer fruits, vegetables, and less fiber than the average person who shuns red meat. Fiber alone can make a big difference. In mouse studies showing weight gain on high fat diets, it has been found that the presence of the fat was not as much of a problem as the absence of soluble fiber in the experimental chow.[20]

So, we have to ask, is the problem due to the *inclusion* of the animal products *per se* or other factors such as the absence of fiber?

Variety and balance are important. High fat intake generates bile acids to help digest the fat. The working theory is that bile acids sometimes cause intestinal inflammation because they generate free radicals. However, when a person eating fat also eats fruits and vegetables they are eating the antidote—antioxidant nutrients. Plant foods contain up to 4,000 flavonoids which are just one class of antioxidants. Spices also contain antioxidants. At least in lab studies, extracts of fruits, vegetables, and spices, such as garlic, ginger, and pepper, enhanced the growth of beneficial bacteria and/or inhibited pathogenic strains.[21] Even red pepper improved the growth of lactic acid bacteria in a Japanese fermentation project.[22]

Plant foods in general offer a great variety of health benefits. Adults are advised by the U.S. government to eat $1^1/_2$ to 2 cups of fruit and 2 to 3 cups of vegetables daily. However, an extremely large national survey released by the CDC revealed that only 13 percent of Americans eat the recommended amount of fruits and vegetables and only 9 percent ate sufficient vegetables. Telephone surveys are notoriously inaccurate, so I have to hope many respondents weren't fooled into reporting errors, calling artificially strawberry-flavored foods fruit.

I'm not saying that we all need to become vegan. On the other hand, although the protein and other nutrients in non-processed animal foods are valuable, I'm also not saying that we should all eat red meat constantly. Red meats add to our stores of iron—good for the young or anemic. However, as we age we can accumulate *excess* stored iron to the point it becomes an aging factor. We shouldn't neglect fish, of course, because it is a good source of anti-inflammatory omega-3's. (Incidentally, useful probiotics have been found in the gizzards of chickens.)

The Probiotic Diet Takeaway

Our microbiome composition is dictated by our long term diet, but due to our genetic differences there may *not* be one *perfect* diet. However, I can't image that any amount of supplemental probiotics will compensate for a consistently unhealthy food intake that is the Standard American Diet or SAD. (I like to quote Dr. David Kolbaba's thought "just because you can chew and swallow it doesn't make it food.") In addition to macronutrients (fat, protein, and carbohydrate) as the above research aimed to study, our bacteria also need micronutrients (vitamins, minerals, and plant antioxidants) and fiber. Each food substance comes with pros and cons. Therefore a variety of foods leads to a variety of bacteria and the beneficial substances they make. For example, the fiber in plant foods encourages species that create butyrate which protects the gut. Those species wane on an extreme low carb diet. As noted, fat intake causes more bile acids to be secreted, so we want to avoid extreme fat intake. Friendly bacteria do not need and are harmed by the chemical additives in processed foods.

So, it seems to be, the bottom line is to do what our ancestors did: Eat a wide variety of real whole foods, such as clean fresh animal foods (preferably wild and grass fed), vegetables, fruits, nuts, seeds, spices, and for those that tolerate them beans and whole grains. Raw honey has a reputation for helping with many health conditions perhaps in part because it is a source of beneficial microbes—some of them ancient varieties now rare elsewhere.[23] *Avoid ganging up on any single type of food and especially avoid refined foods, such as those made with white flour, sugar, and chemicals.*

Fermented Foods

Fermented foods are a major source of probiotic strains and their beneficial metabolites. Archeological evidence indicates that fermented foods have been around about as long as humans—perhaps predating the discovery of fire. Fermented foods still provide important health benefits for us today because they make foods more digestible, more nutrient-dense, and less allergenic. Fermenting reduces the impact food sugars on the body's blood sugar. The fermenting process also creates lactate (a helpful signaling molecule) and reduces what are known as anti-nutrients, such as phytic acid, a substance that binds up minerals making them less accessible. Fermenting can increase the potency of beneficial substances. An example is the fermented mushroom supplement Immpower. It supports the vigorous function of immune cells, such as natural killer cells, T-cells, and macrophages, and is therefore popular with those who have severe immune challenges. Fermented foods have been shown to reduce social anxiety symptoms, but the mechanism has not yet been proven.[24] Fermentation can even totally change the nature of the starting material (think grapes into wine) and add flavors (some of which are definitely an acquired taste).

For our early ancestors, the food supply was unpredictable and seasonal at best. The fact that fermentation makes food too acidic to support the growth of spoilage bacteria and preserves it for an uncertain future was surely critical to survival. It is likely that primitive populations also noticed that fermented foods helped them stay healthy. Now we know several reasons why—not the least of which is their content of good bacteria and the biochemical substances they create.

In Japan, the incidence of Irritable Bowel Disease (IBD) has increased 100-fold over the last thirty years which scientists blame on loss of microbiome diversity. Japanese experts explain that Tokyo has basically the same hygienic conditions as New York City, the same processed foods with excess sugars and reduced fiber, as well as the same overuse of antibiotics. They add as a major factor the reluctance of the younger generation to eat the historic fermented foods.[25]

It is said that there are several thousand fermented foods in existence. Below, I list just a few examples of types that are popular around the world grouped according to the base food used. Looking at that starting material may give us an idea what type of food our own intestinal bacteria might like to have for lunch.

Fish

In Barcelona, Spain we viewed some fascinating Roman ruins discovered under layers of buildings from the city's more recent inhabitants. I was surprised to learn that large kettles were dedicated to fermenting a sauce (*Garum*) made from fish parts. That was an idea they apparently borrowed from the Greeks. This sampling from around the globe shows how popular the fermenting of seafood is:

- *Bagoong* (Philippines)
- *Fesikh* (Egypt)
- *Hákarl* (Iceland)
- *Hongeohoe* (Korea)
- *Igunaq* (Inuit)
- *Jeotgal* (Korea)
- *Kusaya* (Japan)
- *Pla ra* (Thailand)
- *Prahok* (Cambodia)
- *Rakish* (Norway)
- *Surströmming* (Sweden)

Another, *Ngari*, from Manipur, India has been studied because of its reputation for health benefits, such as healing stomach ulcers. It was discovered to have potent antioxidant effect associated especially with its bacterium, *Enterococcus faecium*.[26]

There is a fine line between fermenting and rotting. Some of these fish preparations have an "aroma" so putrid that it makes one wonder if they are on the wrong side of that line. Since Americans were typically not brought up eating them, the whole idea of fermented fish isn't appealing to the average person.

Dairy

High intake of milk has been linked to unpleasant health outcomes for many. However, consumption of fermented dairy is better tolerated and has been shown to reduce the risk of many diseases, including bladder cancer.[27] One fermented dairy product, yogurt, is enthusiastically embraced by Americans. By law, commercial yogurt must be made with milk heated to kill potentially pathogenic bacteria (pasteurized), but that also kills the probiotics. Except for raw yogurt purchased directly from a farm, yogurt brands that claim to have live cultures would have added them back after heating. The label usually indicates which strains were added, but there is no assurance they are still alive.

Yogurt has proven benefits, especially for digestion. However, we are aiming for great diversity of strains and there is only one or two in each brand of yogurt, most of which are transient. So, it is best to not rely solely on that source. Then there is the puzzling problem of what to buy. One example on the healthier end of the spectrum is from Maple Hill Creamery. It uses milk from grass fed cows and organic ingredients. It also contains the natural fat, less sugar, and live cultures.

The most advertised yogurt is Activia by Dannon. I'm guessing that most consumers have not noticed the fine print in the instructions. It says that the product helps relieve slow intestinal transit time (constipation) *when consumed 3 times a day*. Each 4 ounce cup contains 120 calories. If nothing else in the diet changes, that means adding 360 calories a day which could lead to a weight gain of one pound every ten days or so. A serving of their flavored yogurt contains 5 teaspoons of sugar. The roughly two dollar cost per day of their recommended intake might better be invested in a good probiotic supplement.

Even unsweetened yogurt contains 2 teaspoons of sugar because of the sugar that naturally occurs in milk. (When a label says a product contains 4 grams of sugar; that equals one teaspoon.) When bacteria ferment milk, the process makes the yogurt sour, and in the U.S. we like things sweet. Therefore, grocery yogurts are typically loaded with sugars and jams sweetened with high fructose corn syrup (remember that this is a source of mercury). Yogurt shops also add sugar, making that yogurt's taste (and nutritional value) virtually distinguishable from ice cream. Kefir is a less well-known dairy product made by bacterial fermentation that shares the same good and bad attributes as yogurt.

There is understandably a negative effect on our blood glucose from all those sugars. But, sugar also feeds intestinal yeasts and slows down the immune cells that our probiotics are busy trying to speed up. (Even if you buy them in a health food store, yogurt-covered pretzels are not actually a health food.) As discussed in the previous chapter, the artificial sweeteners often used as an alternative in dairy products are controversial.

Americans love cheese! Dairy becomes cheese through fermentation. However, all the processing required by law (adding rennet, salt, and aging) kills the probiotics. Products described as "processed cheese food" or that are squirted out of a can are even further removed from the real thing. Raw milk cheese is a source of probiotics, but we typically have to buy that as imported cheese or directly from the farmer.

Soy

Except for edamame (the immature bean and pod eaten as a vegetable), the consumption of soy by humans is controversial. We have a substantial exposure to soy via protein powders, soy milk, soy protein bars, and soy additives in every imaginable food. Basically, nutritionists worry that large quantities of soy interfere with thyroid function and upset hormones. A new worry is that most soy used in the U.S. is GMO which we discussed previously as problematic. None the less, the producers of soy products have convinced most consumers that soy is hot stuff, and for marketing reasons they often quote benefits found in studies that aren't quite applicable. For example, they may use data on isolated extracts of soy. More commonly, they point to Asian health statistics.

That is not really fair because in Asia, soy is typical eaten as a condiment in small quantities. Also, the forms, such as miso, tempeh, soy sauce, and natto in the Asian diet, are *fermented* and that changes the basic nature of soy. In traditional Asian fermentation, friendly bacteria reduce the soy liabilities and they add assets in the form of substances that we will discuss in the next chapter. With the unnatural process of commercial U.S. tempeh, the bacterial element and its benefits may be missing altogether. Commercial soy sauce may also be a chemical-laden pasteurized mixture that bears little resemblance to naturally-brewed Asian soy sauce. Geography does affect our microbiota. It is interesting that U.S. vegans seem less able to process soy the same way as their counterparts in Asia.[28]

I had to try natto when I was in Japan, but once was enough because I thought the smell, gooey consistency, and taste was very unpleasant. It has a well-deserved reputation for supporting cardiovascular health, but I believe most people would find it easier to benefit from that enzyme in natto (nattokinase) in the form of a blood pressure supplement from Kyolic, a Japanese maker of aged garlic products that are available in the U.S.

Almased is a soy-based meal replacement weight loss product that uses *fermented* soy. That doesn't make it a source of probiotics, but the fermentation would at least improve the healthfulness of the soy.

A novel home remedy for burns recommends immediately splashing on soy sauce. Why does it help, because of the saltiness or because soy sauce contains some mysterious bacterial metabolite?

Vegetables

In their natural state, plants have their own probiotic systems and many of those would be helpful to us.[29] One reason for the dwindling diversity of our microbiome is the use of pesticides and weed killers, but probably also that we just don't eat enough plant foods. Plants also protect themselves with some antimicrobial properties, so those who eat a lot of *raw* produce should probably take care to include some fermented foods and/or probiotic supplements. Canned vegetables and vegetable juices have been pasteurized (heated) to kill microbes. Canned vegetables and vegetable soup are pasteurized and then cooked again at home so we cannot get any of the plant probiotics. All things considered, we fare better if we eat vegetables in fermented form. In discussing viruses in Chapter 3, I mentioned that Kimchi, the Korean dish of fermented cabbage, cruciferous vegetables, and healthful spices was found to have benefit against a flu virus.[30] Other researchers describe Kimchi with its probiotic and nutrient content as having antiaging, antioxidative, and fibrolytic (fiber digesting) properties as promoting the health of the brain, colorectal tract, immune system, and skin. It is believed to reduce cholesterol and to be helpful against cancer, obesity, and constipation.[31] Perhaps doctors should consider writing prescriptions for Kimchi.

Pickles used to be a familiar American fermented vegetable food. However, please note that there is a very important difference between foods that have been made tart by fermentation and common "pickled" foods. For example, cucumbers are marketed as "pickles" after simply being brined with salt and vinegar. Vegetables pickled in this way do not provide the benefits of microbial fermentation and, worse yet, seem to increase the risk for certain cancers, such as breast cancer and multiple myeloma. Similarly, old world cabbage becomes sauerkraut via fermentation in contrast to the bottled varieties on store shelves which may have simply been brined, of course, been pasteurized. To enjoy probiotic benefits, look for krauts in the refrigerated section of natural food stores.

Fruit

In addition to the alcoholic beverages below and a few chutneys, there is Tempoyak. It is an interesting fermented fruit dish made from the foul-smelling Southeast Asian fruit, durian. It will not likely be popular in the U.S. because besides liking our foods to be sterile, sweet, pretty, and non-bitter, we also like them to smell good. What treasures are we missing by being so finicky?

New-Fangled Ideas

Probiotics are being added to everything from salami to peanut butter. These are not fermented foods in the true sense, but they are an alternate way of delivering probiotics in food. Olives would naturally contain probiotics, but because of their loss in commercial processing researchers are looking to add some back. The addition of probiotics to sausage is under study. I don't have an objection to the idea of adding probiotics to foods, but I do question how they are going to decide which microorganism to use. I also have to hope that the products will not be full of sugars, preservatives, and other artificial ingredients. Most of those microorganisms will not colonize the gut, and I doubt that people will consume them consistently enough to keep the right balance in their intestinal tracts. But, I guess that every little bit helps.

Fermented beverages

Some fermented beverages are a source of probiotics; most are a source of alcohol. Although newer studies challenge the notion, moderate alcohol intake seems to keep popping up as a factor associated with a lowered risk of various diseases. I've often wondered the reason. Is it the relaxation factor? Or maybe people who can be moderate about alcohol are moderate in other areas of their lives? Now I have a new wondering. Are there traces of goodness (Postbiotics) left behind by the microorganisms used to make the beverage? The following are some common examples of fermented beverages.

Beer. This may be one of the original fermented foods because it provided a convenient low-tech way to preserve food and provide nourishment for a long period of time. (The feel-good factor surely had something to do with its sustained popularity.) Fermentation is done mainly through the use of "brewer's yeast." (Incidentally that was one of the earliest dietary supplements in health food stores and was appreciated for its content of B vitamins.) Both fermenting the mash to the point of creating a buzzworthy alcohol level and pasteurizing it *inactivates* any microorganisms. Draft beer is often less pasteurized because it does not need to be stored as long. In any case, beer is not a good source of probiotics. It is also typically made with grains, and although most of the proteins in the source material have been digested during fermentation, persons who are extremely sensitive to grains should ask about the source. (I find that I am more likely to get a headache from Weisse beer because it is made from wheat.)

Wine. Grapes, oranges, apples, elderberries, prunes, or anything with substantial sugar content can be turned into wine. Although bacteria are also present, the fermentation is created mainly by friendly yeasts. One reason for pasteurizing wine is to stop the process of fermentation before the vat blows up or the brew turns to vinegar. In Asia, coconut wine and rice wine are known to deliver several probiotic bacteria strains. However, commercial domestic wine is not considered a source of probiotics. Even so, as we'll see in the next chapter when we cover prebiotics, it may somehow stimulate our good bacteria. "Pruno" is the name of "wine" created in prison cells—in plastic bags or even the toilets, from whatever the inmates can get. That might include fruit cocktail, catsup, or candy. Due to the lack of pasteurization, it may well have the highest probiotic content, but besides being unappetizing, it can also be the source of dangerous botulism.

Kombucha. This is a fermented sweetened tea (green or black) concoction with roots in Asia. The very slight amount of alcohol contained is not the aim, but rather the probiotic content of yeasts and bacteria used in the fermentation. The many testimonials for health effects were previously discounted by mainstream medicine. Now that scientists are starting to appreciate the power of probiotics, a recent review of studies indicates an apparent benefit for kombucha for detoxification, increase of antioxidants, improving energy, and supporting immune function.[32] Now my fantasy prescription pad would list Kimchi and Kombucha.

Homemade versions of this lightly carbonated drink are a bit shocking to see with its "scoby" (symbiotic colony of bacteria and yeast) or "mother" that looks like a gross floating mushroom top. Care must be taken in making Kombucha to avoid contamination with microorganisms that we don't want to grow. (A book noted in the Resources, page 207, tells how to do it safely.) Natural markets in the U.S. carry beautifully labeled bottles of flavored and nutrient-enhanced Kombucha by GT. The probiotics *Lactobacillus* and the friendly yeast *S. Boulardii* are used to ferment their brew. Their products are organic, raw, and unpasteurized. Interestingly, they are not even flash-pasteurized because the FDA does not require pasteurization of products that are not grown in soil and do not contain any animal byproducts.

Meat. Fermentation of meat (for example, into sausage) is an ancient way of improving its nutritional value and extending its shelf life. For safety's sake, the practice logically requires more attention to details of the quality of raw material and selection of strains.

CONCLUSION

They say "it is never too late to have a happy childhood." That, of course, refers to adopting a better attitude about whatever transpired when we were young. We can't go back now to be born and reared with the original lineup of probiotics that we were supposed to have, but we can certainly fill in some of the blanks. We do that in part by consuming fermented food and drink.

We will acquire a greater *variety* of probiotic cultures if we don't camp out on one source, such as yogurt, but rather eat a variety of fermented foods. Obviously, they need to be naturally fermented types rather than vinegar flavored imitations. They should also be products where the beneficial microorganisms have not been killed by pasteurizing and processing. Homemade is a budget-friendly approach. These days most of us were not taught about fermentation at our mother's side, but it isn't too late to learn. The internet abounds with recipes, and in Resources, page 207, I list a useful book on the topic.

You will remember from above that we also attract and foster bacteria based on the foods we eat. As a refresher, bacteria need a variety of carbohydrates, protein, fats, salts, vitamins, minerals, and more.[33] That probably means that the most healthful probiotic strains wouldn't thrive on Cheetos because they are nutrient depleted, and it is unlikely that probiotics crave orange food coloring. If we have been dieting or have had no appetite due to illness, we may have to make a point of feeding our microbiome its favorite foods and prebiotics. Prebiotics are special bacteria food discussed in the next chapter where we'll see how to jumpstart our new and improved microbiome with supplements.

8.

Restoring Order

We are about to dig into the potential value of supplements in assuring a robust, diverse, and well-balanced population of microorganisms in our intestinal systems. But, since that means making a modest financial investment, it might not hurt to reinforce our motivation with a quick reminder of why we care so much about our friendly bacteria. Lest we forget, at a very fundamental level they supply some of our genetic memory and support our cellular power source, the mitochondria. That gives them a big say in how well the body does virtually *everything*. Our human chemistry is unbelievably complex. Now we know that our friendly bacteria are responsible for a great deal of it. They are miniature biochemical manufacturing facilities busily producing a large number of essential substances discussed below under Postbiotics. Bacteria improve our systems that deal with detoxification, digestion, energy, hormone balance, immune function, inflammation, insulin sensitivity, nutrient absorption, and oxygen uptake. They also communicate with our brains to improve our mood and help us decide important things such as if we are hungry or full. They are even involved in sending signals that maintain our circadian rhythms and changing hormones that affect sleep cycles.[1] As further evidence of that, mice without bacteria do not respond to changes from light to dark. In Chapter 2 we saw how all of those functions relate to some specific health conditions, and we'll cover more concerns in the next three chapters. Each time I review what our bacteria do for us I am even more inspired to make sure that they are well taken care of. I hope the reader is as well.

Our goal is to build a substantial microbiota (weighing several pounds) that contains a great diversity of strains consisting of at least 85 percent *beneficial* microbes. When the probiotics no longer have the upper hand, the imbalanced situation is called "dysbiosis." Dysbiosis can be so slight that we experience only minor symptoms which we don't even associate with the gut. Or it can be so severe that it sends us to the emergency room. In previous chapters we examined a wide range of factors that can easily damage probiotics and allow dysbiosis to occur. However, the good news is that dysbiosis can be corrected and internal order restored, with probiotic supplements being a powerful tool. As with any investment, there are a range of choices, and this chapter establishes criteria for evaluating products so that real value is received. We'll also discuss how to use them for best results.

WHAT TO LOOK FOR IN A PROBIOITC SUPPLEMENT

Obviously, supplementing may be less successful at achieving an ideal probiotic balance if we continue to kill them off as fast as we add new ones. So, for the sake of moving on, let's assume that the positive steps covered in earlier chapters have already been implemented to the extent possible.

There are hundreds of commercial products claiming to have probiotic benefits. It is likely that they all do at least some good, but how do we know what is really a good investment? The answers to the fundamental questions below point the way. My recommendations in the Shopping Guide at the end of this chapter and in Resources on page 207 are based on these factors.

Numbers May Not Be Crucial

Is the greatest number of microorganisms per dose contained in a product the best way to judge a probiotic? I am starting with this question not because it is the most important, but rather because we've been told that it is. Even though it is so often the American way, more is *not* always better. I'm reminded of what happens when a consumer magazine renowned for guiding us to the best values among brands of laundry soap and lawnmowers discusses nutritional supplements. The magazine staff actually *tests* toasters, but they don't conduct clinical health outcome *studies* on dietary supplements. Rather they rely on *opinions* from their go-to mainstream health experts—experts who tend to cling to conventional and often outdated ideas. If the magazine were to rate probiotics, I'm afraid it would be only on the basis of which brand offers the most billions per buck—apparently without realizing that their advice is woefully oversimplified.

Many health opinion leaders make the same mistake. (Many also say to only buy probiotics that need to be refrigerated which is advice that also doesn't always apply.) A popular TV medical host advised his viewers to ask for 25 billion per capsule. I wondered why not ask for 23, 27, or 100 billion? The real problem is not so much that this number is arbitrary and as far as I can see not supported with studies, but that there is so much more to the story. For example, if we swallowed just 100 probiotic cells, given that they can double their numbers twice per hour we could have over 25 billion in about fourteen hours. Through special communications methods using a chemical language and special sensors (called "quorum sensing") microorganisms can decide that they are now in control and change their behavior as a group. Curiously, when we supplement one strain, others may multiply as well. Therefore, it seems to me that we need to be just as concerned to make sure the gut environment is conducive to normal multiplication, and of course that the strains are what we need.

For sure, taking a whopping big dose of probiotics does usually generate a reaction. However, sometimes that reaction is an uncomfortable flushing of the bowels caused by the system ridding itself of what it senses is an abnormal influx of one species. In contrast, a slow and steady supplementation with a lower dose may allow the digestive system to accommodate and restore order more naturally. Cautious scientists in Japan, understanding how the immune system can react to a sudden huge load of bacteria, *purposely* allowed the quantity of bacteria in their supplement to be reduced from mega-billions by implementing a multi-year fermentation process. In spite of a lower cell count, they actually improved potency and effectiveness because that process puts the emphasis on the other factors explained below.

Postbiotics—A Unique Component

We are repeatedly told to look for giant numbers of microorganisms in a supplement and maybe a variety of strains, but we never hear about what is perhaps the most important benefit we should look for in a supplement. Probiotics serve us by actively competing with pathogens for space and nourishment, but their main power may come from the substances they manufacture and from messages contained in their cell walls and DNA. "Postbiotics" is a term that I coined in 2007 to describe that collective output of substances and remnants of cultured probiotic microorganisms (such as the cell walls and DNA of even dead cells). Because there was (and to my knowledge still is) only one commercial probiotic supplement capsule that contained them, I encouraged that company to trademark the term. Starting in 2012, I began to see the term appear in a few studies. (The terms "metabolites," "biogenic substances" and "pharmabiotics" are also used, but those are applied in many diverse ways elsewhere and do not seem specifically descriptive.) I'm sure scientists will find more constituents, but so far we know *at least* the following are contained in rich full Postbiotics. Even if we don't buy a product that specifically contains Postbiotics, just knowing what the bacteria produce should encourage us to work harder to nourish and protect our diverse flora. Just remember that different strains specialize in creating different metabolites.

Amino acids. Amino acids are the building blocks of proteins and are used in the body not only for muscles, but also they are used for making hormones, neurotransmitters, and so on.

DNA and cell walls of bacteria that are no longer alive. Curiously, even dead bacteria can have a positive effect on reducing gut inflammation and stimulation of the immune system.[2] It is also believed that the DNA from the bacteria may send immune-boosting signals.[3] Dead cells also seem to somehow bind up toxins.[4] That said, scientists are beginning to appreciate the increased benefit of live bacteria and, as we will see, they are a key component of an important medical procedure (FMT described in the inset on page 112) that saves lives and is being suggested for many other issues, even obesity.

Some forward-looking scientists think that the probiotics of the future may focus less on the bacteria themselves and more on the beneficial cell components and byproducts—in other words, the Postbiotic.[5] Fermented foods have accumulated Postbiotics during fermentation. Since each fermented food may have only one or two bacterial strains and the metabolic substance those make, we would need to eat a variety of foods to acquire the most beneficial diversity.

Likewise, fermented dairy liquids would contain the substances that their one or two cultures make, but as noted, I'm only aware of one domestically available probiotic supplement *pill* that contains significant Postbiotics. It is made in the same way as fermented foods, but with many more strains and over a period of years rather than days or weeks as might be the case with sauerkraut, for example. During that extended time, billions of bacteria have reproduced and lived out their lives leaving behind the multi-generational accumulation of their Postbiotics and even the spent, but still beneficial, cells of their ancestors. Therefore the longer the fermentation continues, the more potent the mixture becomes. This supplement type is discussed under "cultured food probiotic complex."

Enzymes. Some enzymes aid digestion and others serve as antioxidants or catalysts for a variety of metabolic processes. Digestive enzymes can be extremely specific for types of foods and even species of plants. While humans make a handful of enzymes for processing carbohydrates, our bacteria make thousands, including some to digest the cell walls of yeasts. The bacteria can monitor food intake and adapt their secretions accordingly.

Neurotransmitters. Serotonin and melatonin are examples of neurotransmitters made in the gut. In some cases they may be made by the bacteria and in other cases the bacteria create substances that influence how the neurotransmitters are produced and managed by the body. The most immediate effect of these nerve-communicating substances may be that they improve gut function. For example, roughly 90 percent of the body's serotonin is made in the gut where it regulates movement of feces.

Organic acids. These acids are substances such as acetic acid, formic acid, fumaric acid, and lactic acid. They likely have many yet to be discovered benefits, but they are already known to aid in the adhesion and colonization of lactic acid bacteria perhaps in part by maintaining an appropriate pH in their environment. Organic acids may provide another exciting area of research. For example, formic acid seems useful in treating warts. Acetic acid is the acid in vinegar which is praised in many folk remedies.

Selective antimicrobials (bacteriocins). In Chapter 5 we saw the devastating effect of pharmaceutical antibiotics that kill both good and bad bacteria. Because probiotics work in teams, they have evolved the ability to create "antibiotics" that kill only enemies, not friends. These substances are called "bacteriocins," but some are also effective against fungi. (Probiotics help fight viral infections, but as we'll see, that effect may not be direct so much as it is the bacteria sending messages to our immune system.) It is less likely that pathogens can become resistant to these natural antibiotics because they are produced by living organisms that can adapt to changing challenges. There are commercial applications for bacteriocins, such as use as a substitute for antibiotics in chicken feed.[6] Even washings of cells (called "supernatant") can help fight pathogens and candida yeast.[7]

Short chain fatty acids. Among these short chain fatty acids (SCFA's) is butyric acid which feeds cells that line the intestines and is considered cancer-protective. SCFA's produce energy for our cells and have an important role in boosting immune function, reducing inflammation, and quieting allergies. They may help keep yeast from turning into a more invasive form where they developing hyphae (a bit like roots). Most SCFA's are in the colon, but some make their way to the bone marrow where they can have wide effect. Because the SCFA's offer so much health benefit, medicine has tried supplementing them, but that turned out to not have as positive an effect as having them produced internally by bacteria who eat fiber.

Signaling molecules. For example, some molecules inform our immune cells of threats and apparently coordinate with other probiotics. I suspect that we will soon see a lot more research into this fascinating area.

Vitamins. One of the most interesting we've discussed is vitamin K2.

Fecal Transplant

I imagine that many of you may be thinking "surely this isn't what it sounds like." But, that is exactly what it is. This procedure which is now often called "Fecal Microbiota Transplantation (FMT)" is a medical procedure (please don't try this at home) whereby the entire microbiological content (feces, and the Postbiotics discussed previously) of a healthy person's GI tract is inserted into the GI tract of a very ill person. That may sound shocking or even disturbing.

While this unusual measure seems beneficial for tough cases of Irritable Bowel Syndrome and other chronic GI conditions, it is typically reserved for patients in serious trouble with *Clostridium difficile (C. difficile or C-diff)*. This pathogenic bacterium may reside harmlessly in a person's system for years. However, when antibiotics clear out its competition, *C-diff* cells can multiply wildly to the point that they cause intractable and potentially fatal diarrhea. *C. diff* can reoccur because it leaves behind spores. FMT is a life-saving treatment for up to 90 percent of even elderly *C-diff* patients who are the most affected, and it usually works almost instantly.[8,9] FMT seems to be much more effective than the antibiotics which curiously doctors are still more comfortable using.[10]

Fecal donors are carefully screened to make sure their "contribution" doesn't harbor any known diseases. The material is then delivered to the patient via enema, colonoscopy, or a tube through the nose. The practice had been to use feces within just hours of donation, but it was found that frozen material also works and is more convenient. That discovery led to the founding of something on the order of a blood bank. (Read more at openbiome.org.) The newest idea is to offer a custom made concentrate

Single Strain vs Multistrain

In the early days of natural food stores, the only probiotic supplement available was known generically as *"Acidophilus."* It was of the 128 species in the genus *Lactobacillus*. The strain, *Lactobacillus Acidophilus*, was sold as a liquid and then in capsule form. Those traditional *acidophilus* products were a single strain and did not contain anywhere near 25 billion microorganisms per dose, and yet, they still managed to develop a great testimony-based reputation for improving digestion and vaginal infections. (A 1924 Yale paper suggested that even benefits that had previously been attributed to *Bulgaricus* in yogurt might actually have been due to *acidophilus* colonies stimulated to grow by the lac-

that has been processed into odorless oral capsules (roughly 2 dozen of them) containing just the bacteria. Oral delivery harkens back to the origins of fecal transplant in China where a medication called "yellow soup" was used.

Back in the 1950's when FMT first appeared in the U.S., the establishment thought it to be a crazy dangerous idea. Now the practice is broadly accepted for GI diseases and perhaps Medicare may soon cover screening of the donor. The FDA regulates the procedure as an "experimental new drug." Well, good luck with that since the FDA system likes a one molecule/one effect approach and the contents of each person's gut is vastly complex and unique to the individual.

Scientists are now asking why the benefits should be limited to just gut diseases. Virtually any condition that has been shown to have a microbiota connection might theoretically benefit.[11] (Are there actually any conditions that do **not** in some way relate to our gut bacteria?) The early chapters of this book covered prospects such as asthma, autoimmune diseases, cancer, cardiovascular disease, diabetes, kidney disease, obesity, autism, multiple sclerosis, and Parkinson's disease. FMT is being investigated for possible benefits for many of these conditions and more.

Other scientists think that FMT is simply a stepping stone practice whose time is limited.[12] Surely, there are supplements that are as effective, less distasteful in concept, and less prone to accidentally transferring a pathogen. The scientists think that the particular microorganisms in FMT that seem to have the most impact will be identified and isolated. That's a start, but I believe that might be an oversimplified approach because it doesn't account for the importance of the Postbiotics and the prebiotics or diet that will support the helpful bacteria.

tose in yogurt.[13]) Because *acidophilus* was discovered so long ago, it is one of the best researched. Recently, it has been shown to offer benefits for lowering cholesterol, protection from pathogens, lactose intolerance, inflammation, and more. *Acidophilus* provides a good example of how a single species can indeed perform a variety of tasks, and it is quite likely that this old standby performs many more that just haven't been discovered yet.

The study discussed in the inset on page 95 showed that supplementing one strain results in increases in allied strains. However, because the gut community contains hundreds of strains and thousands of sub-strains, pumping in a large load of a single strain doesn't seem the most logical way to restore a normal diverse balance. If one strain is forced to predominate, then we would miss out on the benefits of the other probiotic strains that it crowded out. The single strain method also increases the pressure to make sure that the single strain is the best and safest choice. Earlier we discussed the slight risk of creating an *opportunistic* infection when supplementing bazillions of cells of a *single* probiotic strain to an immune-compromised patient. But, even when the immune function is healthy, a large influx of one single strain of bacteria could *theoretically* trigger an unnatural response.

Enterprising companies are beginning to ride the wave of interest in probiotics and market new strains that lack the long-established track record of stability enjoyed by *acidophilus*. Because bacteria can multiply so very quickly, it is obviously important to deliver a beneficial variety and some experts express concern about very new strains because it isn't so easy to tell the good guys from those that have morphed into harmful ones.[14] In contrast, *ME-3* that I discussed in Chapter 4 has been studied for more than twenty years and has shown itself to be very stable and to offer its benefit by boosting the master antioxidant, glutathione. I called attention to it because glutathione is so fundamental to our general good health and improves such a wide range of conditions. That doesn't mean that some combination of other strains wouldn't also have a positive, if perhaps less dramatic effect on glutathione. I wouldn't want consumers to feel they must treat bacterial strains like drugs and buy a different one for each symptom because they could spend a lot of money and end up with a fridge full of bottles. These special purpose single strains should be used as a *complement to* a general purpose probiotic, *not a replacement.*

From what I've seen in hundreds of studies, those that compare multiple strains to single strains find more benefit with multi-strain supplements.[15] Even in probiotics created for use with *plants* the trend is to supplement diverse communities of bacteria, not just single strains.[16] The multi-strain trend is showing up in the marketplace sometimes in subtle ways. I was amused to see that a long time popular brand still labels a liquid product as simply "*Acidophilus*" even though it now contains three strains of *acidophilus plus six other strains.*

There Is a Logical Limit

Could we supplement every strain? I pose this question to hold down the other extreme end of the continuum from using just one strain. Only FMT can deliver an entire balanced microbiota with its thousands of sub-strains. FMT saves lives because it honors the diversity and synergy of a *typical* healthy person's microbiota and supplies a lot of healing Postbiotics. Even so, FMT does not accomplish the *ideal* which would be to replace one's own *personal unique blend*.

A Rational Number of Strains to Use

Generally speaking, more strains are better as long as each one has a legitimate unique purpose, and is not just added for window dressing. Except in the special purpose cases listed above. I would rather use more than two or three strains. A combination of six to twelve seems better. Including a couple dozen strains may be useful or it might be a marketing gimmick and compensation for lack of thoughtful formulating. (Perhaps it is sometimes a "let's throw in any strain we ever heard of and see what happens" sort of philosophy.) I suspect that there is not much scientific support for a few of the strains included in such a potpourri, and there is no evidence of how these freeze-dried strains react when they wake up together in the gut and begin competing for resources. There is no magic number of strains, so I recommend selecting a blend of several strains in a product supplied by responsible, well-established manufacturer who bases its formula on science not hype.

Sources—Human, Animal, Plant, or Soil

Dirt from the garden contains a huge number of bacteria, including *Tetanus* (lock jaw), *C. difficile,* and deadly *Anthrax*. It just seems safest and most logical not to simply pull potential probiotics out of soil, but rather to supplement with bacteria isolated from either healthy humans or at least from our normal food supply. In my counseling practice I had many clients who suffered lingering problems after taking a soil-based microorganism supplement that was trendy at the time. They felt good for a short time (perhaps due to relief from chronic constipation), but later they could not seem to restore a comfortable balance. That doesn't mean there are no beneficial soil-based products; just that it is important to be assured of a *long* record of stability and safety.

Bacteria that originated in the soil seem safer to use if a mammal has eaten it and survived. For example, one strain commonly found in soil, *Mycobacterium vaccae,* was isolated from cow droppings. Killed cells of that strain are being studied for use in stimulating mood hormones and for use in vaccines for treating drug-resistant tuberculosis and metastatic melanoma.[17] Deciding if strains are appropriate is hard enough without their names being manipulated for advertising purposes. For example, the popular yogurt Activia uses *Bifidobacterium animalis*. We could research that and learn that it is found in the gut of most mammals. However, the yogurt brand calls it a made up marketing name, *Bifidus regularis*.

Permanent Residents and Visitor Strains

Some probiotics adhere (implant, multiply, or colonize), meaning that they become permanent residents. Others just pass through offering benefits along the way, such as latching onto a pathogen and taking it away. Both permanent and temporary types are useful. There may be a difference from one person to the next in which strains are able to adhere. *Lactobacillus acidophilus* is an example of a species that is native to the intestinal tract and therefore adheres. However, a cousin, *Lactobacillus rhamnosus* DR20 apparently does not. It was administered in milk to human subjects daily for six months. The study was only able to detect that probiotic strain in the stool *during the supplementation period,* but not after supplementation stopped.[18] *Bifidobacterium longum* occupies a middle ground. It is prevalent in the gut of babies, but less prevalent in adults. Ultimately, the regular intestinal residents will competitively eliminate any strains that are not well suited to staking out their own territory. Again, supplementing a variety gives the gut community more options from which to choose.

Spore-Formers

A relatively new idea is to create probiotic products from spores, a form that some types of bacteria (mostly bacillus) can retreat into if they are stressed. Spores are something like bacterial seeds and have even been found in archeological digs and reanimated. You may recall that one reason C-diff infections are very hard to treat is that they form spores. Spores apparently make it past the acidic stomach and some adhere in the colon. That may be a reason spores are being studied as a means of delivering vaccines. However, as potential probiotics, I did not find studies comparing the effectiveness of spore delivery with the more familiar forms of probiotics. There are fewer species from which to choose and those seem to have largely been studied in animals. The fact that some pathogenic spore-forming species are closely-related to those proposed as supplements would seem to make it imperative to select a high quality manufacturer and a product with a history of safety.

Freeze-Dried Bacteria

Most probiotic pills and powders fall in this category. In making a selection for the blend, the producer must consider the ability of each bacterial strain to tolerate this extremely challenging manufacturing process because some shapes, sizes, and strains of bacteria seem to better tolerate such handling.[19] In brief, here is how the process works. First, a probiotic strain is cultured on a medium of some kind (usually dairy or soy) for a short time (hours to days). Then the microorganisms are cleansed of their food supply. During that centrifuging process, colonies become disconnected. Freeze-drying can kill substantial numbers of lactic acid bacteria because ice forms in the cells and/or the stress of the sub-zero temperatures damages their cell membranes.[20]

Researchers are still looking for high tech methods to protect bacteria from these manufacturing stresses. That includes ideas, such as encasing them in nano particles made from components of shellfish and algae. (Those methods are also being researched as a drug delivery system.) It seems quite counterintuitive, but in one study, researchers found that the probiotics were more stable and more likely to arrive at their target in viable shape when processed into *tablets* rather than in powders or powder capsules.[21]

The fragility of frozen cells is likely one source of the idea that a supplement should contain huge numbers of organisms. Large quantities may be needed to compensate for the percentage that will not awaken or reproduce in the intestinal tract because of the accumulated damage.[22] Because some manufacturers create less damage than others makes it hard to generalize about how many organisms make for the ideal CFU (colony-forming unit) count.

To make a multi-strain probiotic product from freeze-dried organisms, the various strains are generally mixed together *after they are dried*. The bacteria that do wake up after surviving the manufacturing process and the perilous journey to the intestines, must then establish their territory—perhaps at the expense of their fellow freeze-dried travelers. That competition further reduces their numbers. For those reasons and because the culture medium has been washed away in processing, it is hard to see how there can be a Postbiotic benefit until after those bacteria wake up, find a food supply, secure their territory from competing strains, and begin multiplying and generating metabolites.

With all these risk factors for bacteria, how can there be so many consumer testimonials and significant research success with freeze-dried combinations? The fact is that many do survive the journey, and if conditions are acceptable in the intestinal tract (for example, sufficient amounts of the food that they like) they can proliferate sufficiently to have a noticeably positive effect. It is also likely that other bacteria and even human immune cells pick up information from substances on the cell membranes and from the DNA of even the bacterial casualties. Freeze-dried probiotics are a better option when the supplier of raw material to the brand has extensively studied the science and maintains the highest quality assurance, such as one I've listed in Resources on page 207.

Inactive Versus Active Bacteria

Although *inactive* bacteria (those in freeze-dried suspended animation) as noted above certainly have value, bacteria that are *active* may provide even more powerful benefits. Fermented foods (those that have not been pasteurized or cooked) show remarkable benefits in part because they contain live, active cultures. Incidentally, just sixty years ago it was thought that most of the bacteria in the intestines were dead because they didn't move under the microscope. It turned out that they just didn't like the high-oxygen environment of the laboratory.

How To Choose A Culture Medium

As mentioned, most commercial probiotics are cultured on either dairy or soy. Since these are 2 of the top 6 allergens, people with allergies need to read the fine print. In most cases processing washes away the bulk of the culture medium (and Postbiotics), but remnants of the food material might be an issue for those who are extremely sensitive.

What we eat determines which bacteria thrive and therefore what metabolite substances they are likely to produce. The same bacteria make different substances in response to different foods. Therefore, when shopping for a base probiotic, it may be important to know what their diet has been.

A scientist studied 189 strains of lactic acid bacteria that were found in 16 traditional fermented foods and beverages in Southeast Asia. From those he selected a dozen strains for their diverse health benefits and matched them with the foods that they preferred. He created a culture medium consisting of more than 90 food fruits, vegetables, herbs, and seaweeds. The components of this medium are unlikely causes of allergic reactions to begin with and enzymes developed during fermentation digest them making them even better tolerated.

Prebiotics

A substance added to a probiotic supplement to feed the bacteria on its arrival in the gut is known as a "prebiotic." A supplement containing both prebiotics and probiotics is called a "symbiont." Since a bacterium's most important job upon landing in its new home is to find lunch, it is not surprising that these combinations seem to offer much more benefit than microorganisms used alone. The food is such an important factor that in some studies simply giving the prebiotic alone had a similar effect to supplementing the bacteria itself. That stands to reason given that bacteria can multiply meteorically when the fuel they need is present. Foods may stimulate bacteria in surprising ways that we don't yet fully understand. For example, although most wine does not contain actual bacteria, a study found that wine (with or without alcohol) increased fecal levels of 3 probiotic strains. Apparently, even after fermentation into wine, something remains to feed the wine drinker's bacteria or to at least signal them.

Studies comparing food as a delivery system for probiotics to supplements of isolated probiotics show that the food approach may work better.[23] According to one researcher, the probiotics "*Lactobacillus* and *Bifidobacterium* species are generally fastidious bacteria, and they require rich media for propagation."[24] To that point, research shows that adding trace minerals to a culture medium increases the growth, diversity, and output of lactic acid bacteria.[25] We consume our own prebiotics when we eat a broad range of fruits, vegetables, and whole grains.

Many natural foods, such as prunes, potatoes, nuts, and seeds like chia, have benefits as prebiotics. Studies show that there is some prebiotic type benefit in everything from bamboo and coffee to quinoa and squid ink. However, it doesn't seem that the ingredients typically added as prebiotics to symbiont products are that "rich media" the scientist described. What I've listed here are the prebiotics more commonly added to commercial probiotic supplements.

Inulin

This is the prebiotic that seems to appear most frequently in studies and in products. Inulin is a rather broad term used to describe a type of indigestible fiber, fructan. (Fructans are fructose polymers—for example, long chains of simple sugars called polysaccharides.) They can be found in many plants, especially in the roots. However, in the products of commerce, inulin usually refers to polysaccharides derived from chicory or perhaps artichoke. Inulin is known as a "full-spectrum" prebiotic because it can feed bacteria all along the GI tract. However, it appears that this somewhat unnatural approach to feeding bacteria increases the *quantity* of probiotics but not the *diversity*.[26] Since *Bifidobacteria* seem to especially like this type of prebiotic, the amount of that strain in our gut can be increased simply by ingesting inulin. Fructans may also have a direct beneficial effect on immune function. On the other hand, for many people this kind of indigestible fiber cultivates varieties of bacteria that produce methane gas.

FOS

Although its main use is to add sweetness to food, FOS is listed on some product labels as a prebiotic. FOS stands for fructooligosaccharides which are indigestible fibers similar to fructans. FOS can be made by extraction from a variety of plant materials; by processing inulin; or by having a type of fungus convert sugar into it. FOS, especially in amounts greater than 10 grams a day, is also known to cause gas and bloating in some people, and consumption of an *excess* of it (or inulin in some instances) can feed the wrong type of bacteria. FOS is a bit less likely to cause distress when it naturally occurs in foods, such as bananas, garlic, onions, asparagus, and artichoke.

Whole Real Foods

I do believe that a symbiont is a step in the right direction, but there is concern about attempting to maintain our intestinal flora based on whatever manufactured prebiotic is convenient and economical for industry. Blueberries have been shown to act as prebiotics. In Resources on page 207, I list a source of an organic prebiotic based on them. The closer we can come to a *variety* of fermented foods as a prebiotic, the better. For example, the Japanese approach discussed that uses a rich array of fruits, vegetables, herbs, and seaweeds puts that culture medium into the capsule as a prebiotic. There is also another reason this approach might be preferable. There is some evidence that for the immune system-stimulating DNA of probiotics to be most effective, the probiotic should be consumed in the same medium in which the lactic acid bacteria were originally cultured. (My guess is that reveals the importance of the Postbiotics created during fermentation.)

Importance Of Acid/Bile Tolerance

The vast majority of probiotics are "lactic acid bacteria" meaning that they tolerate and even need an acidic environment. We acquired our innate microbiome by swallowing the bacteria, and so those microbes somehow made it past the stomach. The probiotic bacteria must also survive another acidic digestive fluid, bile.[27] Interestingly, a type of *bifidobacteria (B. Longum)* isolated from a person who was over 100 years old was found to have adapted to be bile resistant.[28] The instructions for most probiotics say to take them on an empty stomach to avoid *peak* stomach acid levels and there is no harm in that.

Going a step further, some probiotics are "enteric coated" meaning that the capsules (or even the microorganisms themselves) are coated with one of a number of materials to keep the pill from dissolving until it is past the stomach and into the more alkaline environment of the upper small intestine. Coating the bacteria with a seaweed extract and forming tiny beads does seem to improve acid resistance *in the laboratory*. But, some of those tests don't sound much like how our systems work, and I did not find studies comparing what actually happens in the body with enteric coated probiotics versus uncoated.

Coating adds questions about the additional materials themselves and the slight risk that a consumer might react to them.

It seems prudent to at least investigate how enteric coating and micro encapsulation is done. One animal study showed that the material itself used for microencapsulating probiotics (in that case sodium caseinate or rennet gel microcapsules) altered the gut microbiome and increased intestinal inflammation.[29]

I'm not opposed to enteric coating, but I'm also not enthusiastic about it. I have had clients whose digestive systems did not work well enough to allow pills with enteric coatings to even dissolve. Perhaps we want to encourage the bacteria that are the most adaptable to various conditions rather than fragile ones that must be smuggled by the normal system. And, if the benefits of the probiotics are needed in the mouth, the esophagus, or stomach, it is sometimes best to chew a soft gel probiotic. In that case an enteric coating would be useless.

Testing Probiotics

We obviously want probiotic products that have been tested for safety and evidence of benefits, but it is rare that an actual probiotic *product* is studied for either. I feel comfortable with the strains commonly seen in multi-strain products because they have individually stood the test of time for safety. Where I start being concerned is with supplementation of newly-isolated single strains. There may be no immediate risk evidenced in a short-term test, but how might it behave over a longer term or under different circumstances or with a different type of individual than was used in the test?

It can be difficult for consumers to know what benefits may have been shown in research because according to FDA regulations, probiotics can only make the most general of claims—for example, they support digestive health.

Antibiotic Resistance

Stay far, *far* away from a probiotic product that claims to contain antibiotic resistant bacteria. If indeed it does have that ability, the good bug could donate its genetic coding for antibiotic resistance to a bad bug. Some probiotic bacteria even without such a claim have been shown to be resistant to common antibiotics.[30] Perhaps we should require assurance of antibiotic sensitivity before ingesting products with exceptionally high CFU counts. The probiotic yeast, *S. Boulardii* is safe because it is not targeted by antibiotics.

SHOPPING GUIDE

Although I've done my best to make a strong case for consistently eating a probiotic supportive diet and a variety of fermented foods, I expect that the average person will not have time to make their own and may not even buy a variety of these cultured foods because tastes and habits are so hard to change. So, how can we find supplements that come close to this ideal? I can't imagine that there will ever be a single ideal probiotic product because we are all so very different. Consumers see benefit (especially for obvious digestive difficulties like constipation) with a wide variety of probiotic products, so perhaps there are no outright bad choices. However, there is definitely a continuum of quality and effectiveness. Budget is a factor for most people, so I want to give suggestions that provide *good value*. That is a much different thing than a *low price* because what we really want are *results*. The following are some good examples in the different categories.

Probiotic Shots

These are fermented food—cultured dairy products similar to yogurt but in a more liquid form and with a greater concentration of probiotic content. Bio-K+ is a popular shot-sized bottle preparation containing three strains (*L. acidophilus*, *L. casei*, and *L. rhamnosus*). It is produced in a base of milk, soy, or rice and in flavors.

Although these shots have developed a good reputation and as mentioned in Chapter 2 was the product given for ten years with good results in the Quebec hospital, I am not very impressed with their new capsules. It seems a fairly ordinary freeze-dried product which doesn't appear to contain the culture medium. That would miss out on the power of the Postbiotics the liquid likely contains. Also, capsules come with ingredients added for the convenience of the manufacture. In this case those include cellulose, hypromellose, ethylcellulose, medium chain triglycerides, sodium alginate, ascorbic acid, magnesium stearate, silicon dioxide, and titanium dioxide.

Advantage: Bio-K+ liquid is known for helping with diarrhea and, under Canadian regulations, its use in connection with *C. difficile*. Bio-K+ can be found in the refrigerated case in natural food stores and some supermarkets.

Liquid Drops

An unusual approach used in Probimune is further proof that enormous numbers of CFU's are not necessarily the only route to success. Cells from a number of strains are contained in a liquid packaged dropper bottle. The bacterial cells are not freeze-dried but rather microencapsulated. That puts them into a state of suspended animation until they arrive at their final destination. The strains are individually well researched and one that is referred to as a "toxin-

How to Use Probiotics

Since there is such variety in products, it is a little hard to make generalizations about dosage and timing. Of course, the label on product bottle or box should be the main guide. Sometimes people are surprised to find by looking at the Facts Panel that a single dose may require two capsules to obtain the quantity of organisms noted on the front. Label cautions might include warnings for those with allergies or certain health conditions. Here are some other common questions about taking probiotics.

Q. When do I take probiotic supplements?

A. Instructions to take with or without food vary based on the way the product was made. Nutritionists usually recommend taking probiotic supplements on an empty stomach, first thing in the morning or the last thing at night. Time of day matters less with the liquid probiotics because those are more food-like.

Q. Should I start slowly?

A. Each person is a case of one. My general recommendation is to take the dose recommended on the label. However, for those in a hurry to restore order, it sometimes works well to take a "loading dose" of double or more the usual amount. I recommend to those who are extremely sensitive that they start slowly to avoid the effects noted below.

Q. How long does it take to restore balance?

A. That is a good question but a tough one to answer. People are told to wait up to eight weeks for an anti-depressant to be fully functional but may expect *instant* results from a probiotic. A person might actually see a quick benefit from a probiotic taken for something like diarrhea or constipation. However, the time needed to fully rebuild a healthy microbiota will vary based on how long things have been out of hand and how many of my positive diet and lifestlye recommendations the person implements. In the worst cases the process may take months. On the bright side, it is certainly encouraging that the body repairs itself so handily.

Q. What does it mean if probiotics cause discomfort?

A. Usually this is what is called a "Herxheimer reaction" or a "healing crisis." If gas, nausea, or a change in stool occurs, that may mean that the person is moving too swiftly to change over the gut balance—at least too swiftly for his or her comfort. In a positive view, Sherry Rogers, MD uses these reactions as a measure of how active and powerful a probiotic is.

Q. Will probiotics interfere with my other medications?

A. In general, the answer would be "no." Probiotics are *supposed to be in our systems,* and typically they are already working to heal the same issues that the drugs are addressing. The only *theoretical* exception I can imagine is that right after an organ transplant, the doctor may wish to suppress the immune system and would not appreciate having probiotics improve its function.

Q. Is my mother/father/aunt too old and too frail for probiotics?

A. The elderly are consistently shown to benefit from probiotics. As for being too sick, it seems the only caution is to be sure to use a multi-strain (not a single strain) probiotic with severely immune-compromised patients. Another exception might be that the jury is still out on whether probiotics are a help or a problem with acute pancreatitis. But, otherwise, often those that are the most ill will see the most benefit.

Q. Is my child too young for probiotics?

A. Probiotics are supposed to be onboard *in utero,* and they seem quite helpful in preventing problems even with the tiniest preterm babies. Again, a multi-strain probiotic is safest. Ideally, if a high count dry powder is used, use one that is formulated specifically for infants. The nursing mother should also supplement herself. Some moms spread the paste from a cultured food probiotic complex capsule on the nipple of the bottle (or her own) as an easy way of administering probiotics to babies.

Q. How long should I supplement probiotics?

A. I think that people can stop supplementing probiotics as soon as they live on a relatively toxin-free mountain top; have no stress; take no medications; grow their own organic food; and eat lots of fermented foods to continually get a booster shot of beneficial bacteria.

scavenger." The testimonials are impressive, but I'd like to see a clinical study on the finished product.

Advantage: This is a conveniently small bottle with a dose being just 4 drops, 2 times per day (before meals). That makes a 0.5 oz bottle a 30-day supply. Probimune is available by mail order from Young Health which is listed in Resources.

Freeze-Dried Blend

As successful as Bio-K+ is, they still felt the need to add capsules. That speaks to reasons for the popularity of this type of supplement. Not only is there a convenience factor, but also the fact that often people don't want to *taste* their supplements. VSL#3 (from the pharmaceutical company Sigma Tau) seems to be the probiotic combination most often identified in research. It is a "medical food" and as such is supposed to be used under medical supervision. However, it can be found on the internet. The product contains 8 common strains and a high cell count. Although there may be hundreds of freeze-dried probiotic products, I probably have enough fingers on one hand to count the laboratories that actually culture the bacteria contained in them. That is a good thing because the big suppliers are culturing facilities that have been long-established and are sophisticated enough to assure control of the strain identities and quality. The product brands order whatever custom blend of strains they plan to market (hopefully from a top notch supplier, such as the one I've listed in Resources.) I'm starting to see a little competitive one-upmanship, not only in the quantities of CFU's but also in the numbers of strains.

Jarrow Formulas is a fine company that has been marketing probiotics for decades. For those that subscribe to the more-is-better idea, they have new products with many strains and up to 50 billion microorganisms per capsule. They also have a product specifically for vaginal health that we will discuss in Part Two. I've had good reports over the years on their original simpler product, Jarro-Dophilus.

Advantage: It has a blend of 6 popular strains (*B. longum, L. acidophilus, B. Lactis, L. Rhamnosus, L. casei, and L. plantarum*) each of which are extremely well researched. The product has CFU's in reasonable quantities (3.4 billion); is not enteric coated; is reasonably priced; and has a very modest list of encapsulating ingredients. Find it in the refrigerated case of natural food stores.

Cultured Food Probiotic Complex

I confess that I had to create this category because it seemed to be needed to describe a product type that is so different from all the others. To meet the criteria for this new category, a product must contain the fermented food culture medium, not just a fiber added as a prebiotic. The probiotics must be alive and active, not freeze-dried. Perhaps most importantly, the capsules must also contain the Postbiotics made by the bacteria during fermentation.

It was not hard to pick the specific brand for this category because, as far as I can tell, there is only one in the U.S. that qualifies. I've used Dr. Ohhira's Probiotics (or OM-X internationally) successfully myself and with clients for nearly fifteen years. Respected Japanese scientist Dr. Ohhira ferments 12 probiotic strains that he selected from fermented foods for their range of special abilities (*B. breve, B. infantis, B. longum, E. faecalis, L. acidophilus, L. brevis, L. bulgaricus, L. casei, L. fermentum, L. helveticus, L. plantarum, and S. thermophilus*). You will recognize these as strains cited in many studies throughout this book. The strains are fermented together from the beginning rather than being combined at the time of encapsulation. That allows them to sort out their territorial issues before arriving in the gut. The culture medium is that unique blend of dozens of fruits, vegetables, herbs, soy, and seaweeds. The still active bacteria are put in vegetarian capsules along with the culture medium and the Postbiotics.

The content of Postbiotics (probiotic-produced substances and spent cells) is quite substantial because the bacteria have had years of fermentation time to create it. The younger paste (three years) is encapsulated and sold to consumers. It goes to prove my point about the power of what the bacteria create, that a version fermented for an additional two years has fewer active organisms but more Postbiotics. It is sold to doctors as a *Professional* Formula.

One of the strains, *E. faecalis TH10*, is proprietary and is noteworthy because it is particularly potent. It is what is known as a keystone strain in that a small amount can have a big effect. In the laboratory, it eradicates several of the most worrisome causes of food borne illness and antibiotic resistant infections. In an animal study, even when killed by heat, *TH10* improved immune function and markedly increased nitric oxide (NO).[31] (NO plays an important role in stimulating natural killer cells and in promoting cardiovascular health.) On the flip side, unlike antibiotics, it is not aggressive against friendly bacteria. Dr. Ohhira's is one of the very few probiotics extensively studied for both safety and effectiveness *as a completed combination product.*

Advantage: This supplement is closest in form and effect to eating a variety of live cultured (fermented) foods. I sometimes recommend it be taken as support for individual strain probiotics because Dr. Ohhira's seems to improve conditions in the intestinal tract so that the consumer's own unique assortment of thousands of sub-strains bacteria can thrive. (That may be due to its unusual Postbiotic content.) Because it does not contain huge quantities of any one strain, it will not create an imbalance in the gut. This product is created at room temperature, and so it is quite stable without refrigeration in its blister packaging. It can be found on shelves in natural food stores and natural pharmacies, but sometimes retailers like to put it with their other brands in the cooler.

Lookalike. There may not be another cultured food probiotic complex any time soon at least in the U.S.. I believe that is because domestic corporations are unlikely to have the patience to wait through *years* of fermentation. I did find a product promoting itself as a "whole food," "live" probiotic. However, on closer inspection, the prebiotic is just inulin (apparently added not during culturing but rather at the time of encapsulation). I am puzzled at the intended value of the "whole food" component because that is just .016 of a teaspoon of organic apple added to each capsule. The strains are cultured on soy and then freeze-dried. That does not meet my definition of "live." The company did not answer my question about whether the fermentation process is long enough to create any meaningful amount of Postbiotics. This may be a useful product, but it doesn't meet my definition of a "cultured food probiotic complex."

Probiotics for Children

Children resist taking pills, but fortunately there are many other ways to sneak the friendly bacteria in. Some will chew a soft gel pill. Powdered capsules can be pulled apart and the contents stirred into foods or beverages. Probiotics themselves are flavorless and will not distract from whatever they are added to. For a candy-like product that will motivate children, Nature's Bounty makes Probiotic Gummies containing *Bacillus coagulans*. That strain apparently resists damage from the high temperatures it takes to make a gummy chew. The flavor and colors are natural. I'm not keen on the 6 grams (one and one-half teaspoon) of sugar a dose contains, but depending on the health issue, it might be worth that to get a child to eagerly comply.

Probiotic Yeast

Saccharomyces boulardii is tropical yeast found on the skin of the fruits lychee and mangosteen. You may recall that this strain has come up a few times previously in this book, especially in connection with protecting us from some side effects of antibiotics and it will come up again in regard to control of fungus overgrowth. Florastor is a very well-studied brand. They list the *weight* of the effective dose rather than microorganism count. (Those with allergies should note that the product does contain a small amount of milk, sugar, and soy.)

Advantage: *S. boulardii* it is not killed by antibiotics and can be taken along with one's regular probiotic while on the medication. The product does not need to be refrigerated, but natural food stores and pharmacies often put it in the cooler with the other probiotics anyway.

Pet Probiotics

Yes, pets benefit from probiotics. Our vet sold us some expensive tablets that are supposed to be chewable, but they do not appeal to our persnickety rescues. When the need arises, our dogs do just fine with Purina FortiFlora that we sprinkle on their food. It is available from websites, such as Amazon and 1800petmeds.com. The label claims among other things to stop the dog's gas.

CONCLUSION

Each of the strategies and tactics for resolving various health problems covered in the balance of the book depends on a diverse balanced robust microbiota. It is reassuring to know that no matter what kind of shape we are in, we can help by restoring normal gut function. When we take supplemental probiotics, we are not replacing our own personal assortment. In the most desperate cases restoring order might require the rather extreme FMT. The rest of us can make major improvements with a healthier basic diet, a wide variety of fermented foods, and the addition of high quality probiotic supplements.

9.

Strategies and Tactics—
Basic Digestive Challenges

The amount of shelf space that drug stores devote to medicines for indigestion, heartburn, constipation, gas, and diarrhea (which we'll get to in Part Two) is ample evidence that *observable* digestive complaints are a big problem and therefore big business.

Those painful symptoms are an obvious warning of digestive trouble, but we can also tell a lot from the *appearance* of the stool. For example, a very dark stool might hint at internal bleeding (or a harmless sign that you've recently eaten deeply-colored foods, such as beets, blueberries, or pasta colored with squid ink). If, on the other hand, the stool is very pale, the gallbladder may be struggling to release the normal amount of bile. Visible bits of undigested food are a clue that there may not be sufficient digestive enzymes. A bowel movement that floats or the appearance of fat droplets on the water may indicate poor absorption of fat and/or a lack of pancreatic enzymes. If that is a frequent occurrence and assuming that the person is not taking a diet product such as Alli designed to block fat absorption, it would be best to see a doctor and rule out problems with the pancreas or celiac disease.

None of the drugs offered for relief of digestive distresses actually solve what is so often their underlying cause—dysbiosis. Dysbiosis, an imbalance of gut microorganisms, is also behind a massive number of health problems that are not usually thought of as even distantly related to digestion.

The reason for this disconnect will become clearer after a close-up look at two fundamental digestive challenges—leaky gut and fungus overgrowth. Solving these often closely linked digestive issues usually offers fast and widespread health benefits throughout the body. Addressing them also lays an important foundation for the strategies and tactics for dealing with specific health complaints which will be laid out in Part Two of the book.

It is difficult to effectively address leaky gut and fungus if we are not taking appropriate steps to build and protect our probiotic colonies. Because we've covered so much, a quick review of key positive actions seems in order:

- **Avoid unnecessary chemicals.** In Chapter 6 we talked about using safer natural products for yard care, home cleaning, and body care; filtering tap water; and choosing whole natural foods (if possible organic) without chemical residues and additives.

- **Drink in moderation.** Excess alcohol consumption tends to sterilize the gut.

- **Feed the team well.** A wide variety of foods provides a greater variety of nutrients and fosters a wider variety of microorganisms. We foster better microorganisms with a diet of unprocessed foods that are rich in nutrients and high in plant fibers—even spices. In contrast, sugary and starchy foods feed unfriendly yeasts.

- **Maximize life style effects.** Exercise is good and sitting too many hours is bad. Stress seems to have a damaging effect on probiotics.

- **Recruit new team members.** Fermented foods supply beneficial microorganisms as well as the Postbiotics they have made. Again, variety is important to create diversity in the microbiome. The natural loss of probiotics caused by modern life can be offset by taking probiotic supplements.

- **Reduce exposure to antibiotics.** We discussed strategies for that in Chapter 5.

- **Research all medications.** Most medications are hard on our friendly bacteria. Natural remedies or even watchful waiting are safer choices for many conditions.

With those health-building factors for background, let's look deeper into two particular effects of ending up with a microbiome that is out of balance.

LEAKY GUT SYNDROME

In terms that may be more medically acceptable this condition is known as "increased gastrointestinal permeability" or "hyper-permeability." Leaky gut is just easier to say and to visualize. In short, leaky gut is a breakdown of the lining of the gastrointestinal that allows toxic substances and even microorganisms to escape into the blood stream. Functional medicine has recognized and treated this condition for decades, but the conventional wisdom has been that the lining of the intestines prevents such large molecules from being absorbed. At a Harvard symposium on the microbiota I had the unique opportunity to meet a researcher whose work I had referenced in this book. W. Allan Walker, MD published work in the 1970's showing that larger molecules were absorbed from the intestines than could be explained by the then prevailing theory.[1] There are now many thousands of scientific articles and studies on the subject. This is a good example of the common forty-year lag between a discovery and general acceptance. In addition to the unwelcome absorption of substances, leaky gut also reduces the uptake of nutrients. This double whammy contributes to a wide variety of health complaints, such as those in the following list.

- Abdominal pain, diarrhea, fatigue, fevers of unknown origin, food intolerances, joint pain, muscle pain, poor exercise tolerance, shortness of breath, skin rashes, as well as problems with thinking and memory are listed on gastrointestinal guru Leo Galland, MD's website (mdheal.org/leakygut.htm).

- According to a submission to the *Journal of Clinical Gastroenterology*, problems such as Crohn's disease, celiac disease, food allergy, acute pancreatitis, non-alcoholic fatty liver disease, alcoholic liver disease immune dysfunction, chronic diseases, and even multiple organ failure are also related to leaky gut.[2]

- An apparent link between dysbiosis, leaky gut, and Type 1 diabetes has been the subject of research for several years.[3]

- Research is under way into a suspected connection between increased intestinal permeability and multiple sclerosis (another autoimmune disease).[4]

- Leaky gut is even suspected as a culprit in schizophrenia.[5]

- At least part of the reason for depression might be a dysfunctional gut lining.[6] Fixing the cause seems more likely to provide a lasting cure than simply diagnosing "depression" and prescribing an anti-depressant medication.

- Mice develop negative changes in the intestinal barrier (and non-alcoholic fatty liver disease) over time when their diets are high in fructose, fat, or fructose and fat.

The list of diseases linked to leaky gut will likely continue to become longer because this dysfunction is so widespread and can affect every part of the body. Actually, leaky gut is not quite the most fundamental problem because we still have to find and fix whatever has *caused* that increased permeability. Toxins, medications like NSAIDS (even low-dose aspirin), an inflammatory diet (including eating foods to which we are allergic), and most significantly, dysbiosis and *Candida* (which we will cover later in this chapter) can all cause leaky gut. The simplified drawings below illustrate the situation.

Figure 9.1 shows a greatly enlarged caricature of healthy cells lining the small intestine. Food passes across the top and blood flows below. Normally, only when food is digested into its most fundamental nutrients is it then absorbed by the gut cells and sent into blood circulation. Wastes and pathogens should continue across the top of the cells along with gut contents ultimately into the toilet. Note these details.

- The little finger-like projections are called villi, Latin for "shaggy hair."

- Each of those tiny fingers is covered with kind of a fuzzy layer comprised of even smaller projections called "microvilli." These textures function to increase the surface area for the absorption of nutrients. To put that in perspective, if the entire surface area of the intestinal tract lining (including the surfaces of the villi and microvilli) were ironed out flat, the square footage would be only a little less than the footprint of an average U.S. home—3,000 square feet.

- The crossed lines are like little rubber bands and represent an exaggerated depiction of the mechanism that holds the cells closely together. Those, for obvious reasons, are called "tight junctions."

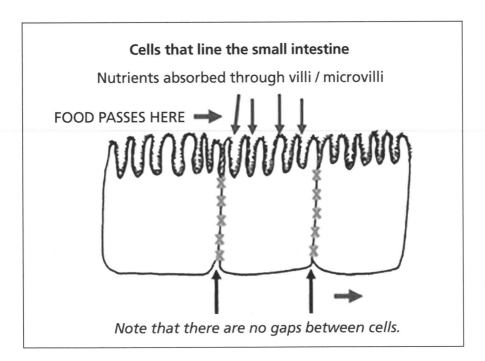

Figure 9.1. A Greatly Magnified View of Three *Healthy Cells* in the Intestines

Figure 9.2 illustrates the same cells but as they would appear in a leaky gut lining. Note the details.

- The villi have been mowed down.

- The microvilli are missing. The surface area for absorption of nutrients has obviously been dramatically diminished.

- The *tight* junctions are now *sloppy* junctions, as though the rubber bands had become old and stretched out. All bets are now off about what particles of incompletely digested food, microorganisms, wastes, and other toxins can escape the interior of the intestine into blood circulation.

Conventional Treatment

Hyper-permeability condition is not observed and is not diagnosed during a colonoscopy or with tests done during routine office visits. Therefore, mainstream medicine is much more likely to simply treat the resulting symptoms and use drugs to manage diseases caused by leaky gut than it is to look for and address the intestinal breakdown. The condition can be identified with a biopsy or specialized testing, but the doctor has to be knowledgeable about the condition and suspect it.

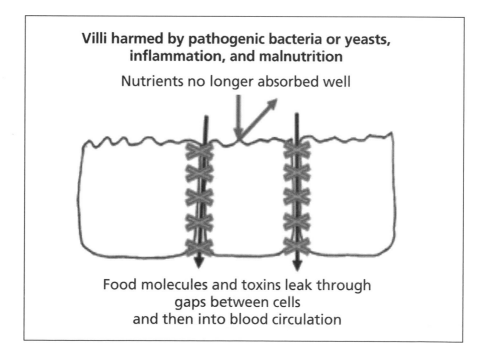

Figure 9.2. A Greatly Magnified View of Three *Damaged Cells* in the Intestines

It is hard to blame physicians for treating symptoms as they have been taught in medical school. Moreover, even if physicians do go to the trouble to independently acquire training in leaky gut and fungus, it is difficult to do the in-depth analysis and patient education required in the average six to ten minute office visit. (Even that average visit is interrupted by computer entries and others entering the room). The prescription pad is just too convenient—especially when third party payers do not usually reimburse for long office visits or the required testing. (Consumers who suspect they have leaky gut may have to look for a functional medicine practitioner.)

A Functional View

Without addressing leaky gut, a vicious cycle is unleashed. The condition itself makes it increasingly hard for the body to correct its problem since it cannot absorb needed nutrients and will be slowed down by toxins and inflammation. Unfortunately, medications given to suppress symptoms can make the underlying dysbiosis worse. Functional medicine physicians often perform a double sugar test that relies on these two factors. First, a healthy intestinal barrier should only absorb small amounts of one sugar (lactulose). Secondly, conversely, another sugar (mannitol) should be well absorbed by the villi.[7] If the test shows the reverse happening, leaky gut is suspected. Food sensitivity may alter the results, and other fine points of how to better utilize this test can be found on Dr. Galland's website (mdheal.org/leakygut.htm).

How Probiotics Relate

Clinicians have long found that probiotics were crucial to healing leaky gut. Researchers are now busy validating that concept and trying to better understand the mechanisms at work.[8] For example, the small intestine permeability of Irritable Bowel Syndrome (IBS) patients improved significantly when they were given milk that was fermented with multiple strains of probiotics in comparison to subjects on plain milk.[9] Another human study showed that a multi-strain probiotic reduced leaky gut and complications from surgery.[10] Unpublished animal research showed that the strain *Lactobacillus fermentum ME-3* helped resolve leaky gut. (*See* Resources for how it is sold.) Yeast overgrowth (*see* page 136) is a major cause of leaky gut and probiotics are essential to rectifying that problem.

Suggested Steps

Each functional medicine practitioner has a remedy preference and that may be further individualized to each patient. However, the use of probiotics and implementation of the basic *Candida* protocol steps, page 138, is typical. After stopping whatever process has degraded the gut lining, it is necessary to heal the damage that has been done. Fortunately, the digestive tract is constantly remodeling itself. For example, the small intestine sheds up to fifty million cells per minute and the colon up to five million.[11,12] The mucous lining totally regenerates itself every three to eight days, but we have to assure that the body has adequate amounts of the nutrients required to replace the shed cells with better ones.

Consumers find Aloe Vera a reliable remedy not only for improving digestion but for also healing the intestinal lining from top to bottom—canker sores in the mouth to stomach ulcers and on to anal fissures. I studied Aloe Vera for a small book on the subject and learned that while there is scientific research to back up these claims, there should be more.[13] Hopefully, when those studies are conducted, they will use the brand (Lily of the Desert) that I found to contain far and away the richest amount and highest molecular weight of the active properties, polysaccharides. Unfortunately, some aloe processors accidentally break those polysaccharide chains down into simple sugars. I mentioned earlier that polysaccharides also act as prebiotics.

A number of studies have demonstrated that zinc L-carnosine (or polaprezinc as a drug) helps to heal the mucosal lining. One study looked at it in regard to repair of injury from long-term low-dose aspirin therapy.[14] That same form of zinc was shown to prevent leaky gut in humans challenged with an anti-inflammatory drug known to damage intestinal lining.[15] GastricSoothe by Source Naturals is a good choice. Other supplements may be added to the leaky gut protocol to reduce inflammation and provide antioxidant protection. For example, the amino acid l-glutamine may help heal the lining.[16]

Other Considerations

Zonulin is a molecule that loosens those tight gap junctions that we depend on to keep the intestinal cells close together. It is thought by some researchers that proteins found in wheat, rye, and barley (gluten and gliaden) may increase zonulin and lead, for example, to depression symptoms.[17] In fact, overuse of products made from these grains and the hybridizing of the grains to contain ever more gluten may be a significant cause of leaky gut even among those who do not have documented sensitivity to gluten.[18] Recent research by Dr. Ken Fine, MD at EnteroLab indicates that immune sensitivity to gluten is exceedingly common, present in perhaps 30 to 40 percent of all Americans. Probiotics may reduce that effect.[19] In addition, vitamin D deficiency can apparently worsen leaky gut.[20]

FUNGUS OVERGROWTH

Yeast loves to colonize the gut! Years ago there was a lot of attention paid to a type of fungus or yeast, *Candida albicans.* (Incidentally there are many, perhaps hundreds, of types of potentially pathogenic yeast in the human body, but *Candida* is the most common group and will be used here as representative.) These days *Candida* seems no longer "fashionable," but not because the problem has gone away! In fact, incidence may have increased substantially. It is a little hard to be precise about that because, in contrast to other diseases, fungal infections do not need to be reported to the Centers for Disease Control, the official keeper of such stats. It is quite likely that a great number of fungus infections are reported as other diseases. For example, in 2013 the medical journal *Lung* reported on 27 patients who, based on x-rays and other clinical evidence were assumed to have *lung cancer,* but who were eventually diagnosed with fungal disease.[21] It is anyone's guess how many such cases receive surgery, chemo, and radiation instead of antifungal meds.

Yeasts (in part due to their creation of leaky gut) are associated with a wide range of problems:

- digestive difficulties
- food sensitivity
- gum issues
- headaches
- joint pain

- mood and focus problems
- rectal itch
- sinus congestion
- skin rashes
- weight gain

Candida can also cause such trouble because it may imbalance hormones, overload detoxification systems, suppress immune function, and cause general inflammation which can in turn aggravate virtually any health condition. Fungal infections can be very serious business indeed, and they are of special concern in intensive care units where according to one study they are known to be "associated with significantly increased mortality."[22] Fungus can even form cysts that resemble tumors, but beyond that some experts believe that candida is the real culprit behind cancer and diabetes. My friends, Doug Kaufmann and Kyle Drew from the television program, *Know the Cause,* often say to think "FUPO"—Fungus Until Proven Otherwise. I think they might be right. The quiz in the back of the book (*see* page 211) shows how likely it is that any problems the reader is experiencing might be yeast-related.

In Chapter 3 we covered a few fungus basics, but a quick recap here might be warranted. Women often notice an irritating vaginal yeast infection after having taken an antibiotic. What they don't know is that they are likely experiencing the same overgrowth in their intestines. Candida can overgrow in other parts of the body, including ears, eyes, eyelids, nose, lungs, and of course, the intestinal tract. Most of the factors (such as drugs, second hand antibiotics, chemicals, and sugars and starches in the diet) that diminish our beneficial microbes make conditions in our bodies more favorable for yeasts. Unchecked, yeasts can become aggressive and change their form going from being a minor factor to a major player in the gut environment and as noted a common cause of leaky gut.

Fungi make mycotoxins which are poisons. They are like the *evil twins* of the beneficial Postbiotics created by probiotics. Mycotoxins can be extremely toxic to every cell and organ in our bodies, but their ability to damage genes and cause cancer is one of the most serious threats that they pose. Mycotoxins can be acquired externally from foods, such as grains (especially corn) and peanuts stored in silos. But, fungus can also generate mycotoxins right inside us. Mycotoxins are toxic to nerve cells and *Candida* has been shown to slow recovery from mental illness in part because they interfere with nutrient absorption.[23] Yeast overgrowths can persist for decades!

Conventional Treatment

If a patient shows up in a medical office with a fuzzy white tongue and a vaginal yeast infection, he or she might be given an antifungal drug. Unfortunately, most of the effects of yeast infections are *subclinical* (not easily observed or evident on standard tests), and so they are not treated *at all*. Antifungal drugs are relatively safe. (But, surely they should be combined with changes in diet and support for probiotics or the condition is likely to return.)

A Functional View

Candida can be shared back and forth with sexual partners, so it is probably best if both parties do at least the non-drug treatments. External yeast problems like athlete's foot, jock itch, and nail fungus can be treated topically, but it is wise to consider that the immune system may have been unable to fend off those conditions because it was also fighting yeast *internally*.

How Probiotics Relate

Candida gets a foothold when probiotic strains are not robust (most often after antibiotic use). With reduction of probiotics and the overgrowth of yeast, we experience a double whammy. We not only suffer the yeast harms, but we also miss out on all the benefits of the good bacteria. Any bacterium is going to be competitive with the yeast and therefore provide some inhibitory effect.

One probiotic strain (*E. faecalis TH10* proprietary to that cultured food probiotic complex discussed in the last chapter) has been shown to be as effective an antifungal as some medications. Even killing *TH10* microorganisms with heat did not keep them from working.[24]

Suggested Steps

There is more than one cause of a yeast overgrowth and so a multi-front approach seems to work best to tame *Candida*. The natural tendency is to jump right into trying to *kill* the fungus, but I think that steps 1 and 2 below are at least as crucial and are practices to continue for a lifetime.

1. **Deprive them of the foods they like.** Chief among those foods are starches and sweet foods and drinks. It just makes no sense to try to kill the pathogen while delivering gourmet meals that give them strength. Happily, fresh vegetables and fruits are *antifungal*. If we get cravings for carbohydrates like bread, pasta, cookies, cereal, and sugar, we should remember that the craving might just be the yeast ordering its lunch. Chemicals they release give them the power to do that!

2. **Restore probiotics.** This step includes supplementing varieties of probiotic bacterial strains, but also all the ways we can improve the environment in which they live, some of which were reviewed at the beginning of this chapter. Adding friendly yeast (*S. Boulardii* such as Florastor) to the probiotic program gives the pathogenic yeast competition from its own kind. In a study of low birth weight babies, the *S. boulardii* was been shown to be just as effective at preventing yeast overgrowth as a common antifungal medication, Nystatin.[25] More about this yeast in step 4 below.

3. **Kill yeasts.** There are many natural products (such as colloidal silver, elderberry extract, garlic, Gymnema sylvestre, olive extract, oregano oil, and Pau D'Arco) that kill yeast or slow its transformation to pathogenic form. However, the trick is to find one that doesn't also damage our good bacteria because those just listed do. They can still be used but with a bit of caution—like antibiotics, at different times of the day from probiotic supplements. And we may have to increase the dosage of supplemental probiotics when using such remedies.

   Certain enzymes can digest the cell wall and interior of yeasts without damaging our bacteria. Candidase by Enzymedica is a product that contains these. However, it would make sense to take Candidase and *S. boulardii* at different times of the day to avoid having the enzymes digest the friendly yeast. One way that *S. boulardii* helps is by creating a substance, capric acid, which inhibits *Candida*.[26] That hints at additional help. We can also get capric acid from monolaurin capsules, Lauridin pellets, or in certain saturated fats like coconut oil. Macadamia nut oil contains similarly beneficial fats.

Honey bees are quite remarkable. It has been shown that bee hives have a microbiota and that the more diverse the beneficial microbes in the hive are, the healthier the hive.[27] It appears that as a survival instinct, bees make propolis as a very selective antibiotic to protect their hives from pathogens. As you will recall, that is also the case with bacteriocins created by our human beneficial bacteria. In both cases, pathogens are targeted, not beneficial strains. The substance containing the selective antimicrobial is *propolis*. It is being researched for benefit with cancer and is mentioned here because it has been found to be a very good defense against yeast. Brazilian green propolis seems to be the most effective because of the particular plants the bees visit to gather their raw material. In the Resources guide, page 207, I recommend a source.

Rotating compatible fungus-killing approaches is not a bad idea. In severe or persistent cases of *Candida,* antifungal medications may be required.

4. **Retrain the immune system:** It stands to reason that if the immune system has been encountering *Candida* for decades, as is often the case, it may have come to assume that this is the "new normal" and just give up. Added strains of probiotics can help retrain the immune system. Also, the homeopathic Aquaflora Candida by King Bio is worthy of a try. It only claims to alleviate *symptoms* of *Candida,* but I think it does that by signaling messages that re-educate the immune system. That product is available in most natural food stores.

Other Considerations

Many natural antifungal remedies, such as tea tree oil may be effective for topical yeast problems. (It should not be swallowed.) The helpful site, Dirtdoctor.com lists a popular home remedy for toenail fungus using cornmeal. Efforts at such topical solutions will be much more effective if combined with a plan to fight internal fungus.

CONCLUSION

Dysbiosis, yeast, and leaky gut are behind a huge number of symptoms. So, no matter what health issue may be bothering us, it surely wouldn't hurt to *at least ask* if one of those three might be a part of the cause. Unlike the *side effects* that often accompany a pharmaceutical drug taken to quiet a symptom, taking positive steps to repair balance in the microbiome, fix a leaky gut, and/or reduce fungus will most likely also offer *fringe benefits*. However, sometimes the situation is so far out of balance that a person can't even tolerate the yeast remedies mentioned. In that case I might suggest trying Aloe Vera to first calm things down and then building up the others very slowly.

Please keep these digestive fundamentals in mind as we move on next to specific health issues in Part Two of this book.

PART TWO

Strategies and Tactics for Common Complaints

Exciting research into the use of probiotics to benefit serious and chronic diseases was reviewed in Chapter 2. Of course, the stage of those studies doesn't yet permit writing a specific probiotic-only protocol for any one of those conditions. Perhaps that may be a blessing in disguise because the trends seem to show that matching a *specific bacterial strain* with a *specific disease* may not be necessary or even the most desirable approach. We already know without question that a healthy gut flora is fundamental to the functioning of a healthy body, and there is absolutely no harm in establishing one. In the process we might well resolve systemic imbalances that have led to disease symptoms.

Virtually *any condition* will likely be helped either directly or indirectly by an abundant, diversified, and well-balanced microbiome. However, I had to narrow the list down, so for this section of the book I simply chose to focus on health complaints that are very common. In addition to a bit of basic information about each topic, I hope to open up a new way of looking at each issue; describing the conventional treatment; providing a functional view; showing how probiotics relate; and, providing other helpful suggestions; as well as including other important considerations. For convenience in referencing, the items are listed in alphabetical order.

ACID REFLUX

This condition goes by many names, including heartburn and GERD (Gastroesophageal reflux disease). It is an inflammation or irritation of delicate tissues that occurs when digestive acids (hydrochloric and bile) back up from the stomach where they belong into the esophagus which is not prepared to handle acids. Barrett's Esophagus is a premalignant condition which arises from chronic acid reflux. It leads to cancer of the esophagus in about 1 out of 1,000 patients annually.

Conventional Treatment

The typical treatment is to shut down production of stomach acid with acid-blocking medications, such as those in the proton pump inhibitor class (for example, purple pills). Even though these medications have only been approved as safe for use for just two weeks every few months, it has become common practice for patients to stay on them for years. PPI's may stop stomach acid production and relieve pain, but they do not actually prevent reflux of stomach content into the esophagus. (That is controlled by the mechanical action of a muscular ring.) They are also not known to help with problems due to bile acid. Because PPI's as intended reduce stomach acid, they reduce the absorption of critical nutrients, such as minerals and vitamin B12. That can account for many of the extremely worrisome long term side effects. For example, persons on PPI's have been shown to be roughly 20 percent more likely to have a heart attack. In addition to reduced absorption of magnesium, that increased risk is in part due to the fact that the drugs reduce nitric oxide which help keep the arteries healthy and flexible. New research warns that PPI's contribute to kidney serious kidney damage.[1] They also cause dysbiosis and worsen the damaging GI effects of NSAIDS.[2]

A Functional View

The problem is almost *never* an *excess* of stomach acid. Acid is critical to digestion, to the absorption of nutrients, and to our defense against pathogens, such as those that cause foodborne illness and pneumonia.

The real problem is inadequate functioning of the muscular ring, the lower esophageal sphincter (LES) that is supposed to keep stomach acid in the stomach. Acid blocking drugs do not address that problem, and the extensive list of side effects resulting from long-term use of these medicines includes hip fracture, dementia, and many other frightening possibilities. I'm especially concerned about the trend to give these medications to infants. It makes more sense to correct the *cause* of the problem by fixing digestion rather than to essentially shut it down. One surprising cause of acid reflux is medication side effects. For example, heartburn is one of many side effects of most statin cholesterol-lowering drugs.

How Probiotics Relate

Researchers have found that probiotics reduce the disease markers of Barrett's esophagus.[3] Probiotics help assure absorption of nutrients needed to strengthen the LES and to repair tissues. In addition to many other indirect benefits of probiotics, they speed the emptying of the stomach. That in turn reduces the opportunity for the stomach contents to splash into the esophagus. Sometimes we just don't know *why* they work, but a recent study found a reduction in reflux symptoms when patients consumed yogurt containing small amounts *Lactobacillus gasseri OLL2716 (LG21)*.[4] I've received similar reports for other probiotic strains and mixtures. When a meal doesn't seem to be sitting well, I get nearly instant relief by chewing one or two soft gel probiotics that I always have with me. (The one that I use may work quickly because it contains the Postbiotic enzymes and organic acids made by the bacteria. I can't say if other brands would be as effective.)

Suggested Steps

It is important for reflux sufferers to understand what is causing their problem. If for example, the cause is hiatal hernia, that would dictate a different natural remedy than if the problem is insufficient stomach acid. This is too complex a subject to explain in detail here, but I should at least point out that a great many people see their heartburn or acid reflux subside when they reduce the amount of refined carbohydrates in their diet. There is no cost to trying that approach and it offers additional health bonuses.

Other Considerations

Chewing gum stimulates saliva which helps keep the esophagus clear. A natural heartburn remedy has recently been introduced. It is an unusual formulation in that it addresses various root causes of reflux rather than interfering with digestion. Garligest has natural ingredients to improve bile flow, normalize stomach acid, absorb air and gas, and to help control *H. Pylori* which is another cause. It also contains an enzyme to reduce dairy intolerance. *See* Resources for where it is available.

ALLERGY

We throw the term "allergy" around pretty loosely. Here are some examples of how we use that term and a more accurate translation of each.

- When a person says, "I'm allergic to Mondays," we get the message that the speaker has a negative *emotional reaction* to going back to work. But, of course, that isn't an allergy in the medical sense. Probiotics do help level emotions, but the person might also be advised to look for a job that he or she loves.

- When a person gets gas or other GI distress from milk, they may refer to it as an allergy. That usually isn't an allergy either, but rather *intolerance* because the person lacks an enzyme (lactase) to fully digest milk. Probiotics help with intolerance.

- A very observant person (or one keeping a food/symptom diary) may notice a connection between eating a food and a reaction (such as a headache) that occurs many hours or even a day or two later. While there are some similarities to allergy, that is called an *acquired* or *delayed food sensitivity*. The most common cause for this condition is leaky gut which we covered in Chapter 9. The sensitivity can be unacquired by eliminating the food for a period of time, healing the gut, and reintroducing the food slowly. (My website Library offers suggestions for using an elimination diet and a pulse test to help track down which food *ingredient* is the cause of the symptoms as well as ideas for reintroducing it after a clearing period.)

- When a person gets dizzy from being around the formaldehyde fumes in a fabric store or coughs because of the mold in a basement, those are not allergies, but rather *overreactions to toxins* that at some higher dosage would bother anyone. Improving gut health boosts the body's ability to deal with such toxins. As we discussed in Chapter 4, probiotics improve detoxification. The strain *ME-3* has been shown to be especially useful.

- A true allergy is an overreaction by various immune system mechanisms to something (usually the protein component) that is not realistically a threat. The damage is caused by our own defense mechanisms' excessively enthusiastic response to killing what it senses is an invader. True allergic reactions can range in severity from mere annoyance, such as a red bump (hive), to *chronic* reactions, such as an embarrassing skin rash, to life-threatening *acute* conditions as is the case with difficulty breathing. Sneezes and itchy eyes from exposure to pollen or freshly cut grass are expressions of seasonal or environmental allergy. Allergic reactions to insect stings can be quite severe as can those from food allergies. According to the support group, Food Allergy Research & Education (foodallergy.org), although an individual can be allergic to *any* food, these foods represent 90 percent of allergic reactions: peanut, tree nuts, milk, egg, wheat, soy, fish, and shellfish.

Conventional Treatment

Management of severe allergies is a serious and complicated medical matter that is not appropriate for a do-it-yourself manual. So, in this section, I'll stick with the less dangerous expressions of allergy. Avoidance of the offending substance is the first line treatment in both conventional and functional treatment. However, drugs that reduce the impact of an allergic exposure are also used. Desensitizing injections (allergen immunotherapy) have been a staple of allergy treatment for seasonal allergies and for allergy to dust mites for a long time. The idea is to reeducate the immune system in a way similar to the principle of vaccines. Drops and even tablets are an alternative to shots. In the past there was a division among major camps of allergists over the utility and the method for dealing with food allergies. Of late, they seem to be coming to agreement that gradually making the immune system comfortable with a reaction-producing food is indeed possible.

A Functional View

It is likely that, as is the case with autoimmune conditions, a leaky gut at some point might have put the immune system on heightened alert. And, then because of constant overexposure to some of the ingredients in our food supply, it never stands down. Although there is certainly a genetic component to allergies, as we are finding with most genetic traits, our diet and lifestyle can determine whether or not those traits stay dormant. Air filtration may be very helpful for inhalant allergies.

How Probiotics Relate

A search of PubMed for "probiotic and allergy" returns many hundreds of listings. A number of them show beneficial effects in double-blind placebo-controlled clinical trials of allergic rhinitis or seasonal allergy.

British scientists supplemented a probiotic to expectant mothers whose babies were at increased risk to develop allergies because of a family history of atopic eczema, allergic rhinitis (nasal irritation), or asthma. They then continued supplementation in the babies for six months. The rate of eczema was one-half of that experienced by the control group. (Eczema is an important issue in its own right as we'll see below under Skin, but it is also an indicator of increased risk to asthma and other problems.) The probiotic used was *Lactobacillus GG,* chosen because they reasoned it to be not only safe for newborns, but also "effective in treatment of allergic inflammation and food allergy."[5]

In another study, researchers showed that supplementing two common probiotic strains (*Bifidobacterium breve M-16V* and *Bifidobacterium longum BB536)* to the mother beginning one month before delivery and to their infants for the first six months significantly reduced skin allergies and eczema during the first eighteen months of life.[6]

Australian researchers studied children who were allergic to peanuts. They gave them peanut protein in an increasing amount along with the probiotic *Lactobacillus rhamnosus* for eighteen months. At the end of the trial, 80 percent were no longer sensitive.[7] Aside from the probiotic I would guess that a major factor in the success was the gradual buildup which itself has been shown to be somewhat effective.

Consumption of dietary fiber helps prevent asthma perhaps because that feeds our beneficial bacteria. It is likely that fiber would also help other allergic conditions.

I didn't find that any particular strains were routinely the most beneficial. In fact, not all studies even show benefit with allergies. That may be due in part to the fact that there are endless options for using single or multiple strains and a great many methods for conducting studies. I find many people become congested from eating dairy products (I'm one) and so it seems odd that some studies of allergic nasal congestion use probiotics delivered *in dairy products.* Consumer feedback for the use of probiotics for allergies is overwhelmingly positive, and following the guidelines in this book to rebalance gut microorganisms is very likely to help.

Suggested Steps

For seasonal allergies, pollen counts are highest from 5 to 10 AM. Staying indoors with the windows closed and not wearing outdoor shoes indoors will help during peak pollen weeks. It is counterproductive to dry out the nose too often with sprays. Not only does that risk rebound reactions, mucus is a first line defense against pathogens, and it is supposed to wash them into the stomach to be dissolved by stomach acid. Cleaning the sinus area using a Neti pot or the equivalent might be a better approach.

Other Considerations

Whatever we breathe we swallow! For typical seasonal reactions to airborne pollen I've often had success with a trick I learned long ago from lay healers.

Persons prone to extremely serious reactions (for example, anaphylaxis) to *anything* should *not* try this. The remedy uses local bee pollen in the form of loose granules found in health food stores and farmers' markets. (Local pollen is best.) The process begins with one single tiny granule. Assuming that the person does not react to the single granule, the second day dose is doubled to 2 granules. The amount eaten continues to double each day up to a teaspoonful. Besides imitating the gradual buildup of tolerance that we gain from allergy shots, pollen is quite nutritious. Other home remedies include the herb stinging nettles, Vitamin C (it has anti-histamine properties), and the plant pigment quercetin.

See also **CELIAC DISEASE.**

BLOATING

See **GAS and BLOATING.**

BRONCHITIS

See **INFECTIONS.**

CELIAC DISEASE

In addition to a variety of gastrointestinal issues (GI) such as very smelly stools and abdominal bloating, symptoms of celiac disease can include chronic fatigue, aches and pains, anemia, arthritis, headaches, and neurological problems. One less common manifestation of the disease can be itchy bumps or blisters on both sides of the body (can be on forearms near the elbows, knees, or rear) often with no GI symptoms. I certainly cannot improve upon the definition given by the Celiac Disease Foundation (celiac.org): "Celiac disease is an autoimmune disorder that can occur in genetically predisposed people where the ingestion of gluten leads to damage in the small intestine. It is estimated to affect 1 in 100 people worldwide. Two and one-half million Americans are undiagnosed and are at risk for long-term health complications." Gluten is a protein found in wheat, rye, and barley. There are also genetic factors, associations with leaky gut and environmental triggers. One of the main effects of celiac is that the damage to the intestines reduces nutrient absorption. The reader may remember that gluten is suspected of contributing to leaky gut, but celiac is an even more serious problem.

The incidence of celiac has greatly increased. A chart showing the rise mirrors the increase in C-section deliveries, corn syrup intake, and probably a host of other changes that are not supportive of our microbiota.

Conventional Treatment

Celiac disease (CD) is often misdiagnosed as any number of other conditions in part because the symptoms vary so much from one person to the next. For example, if a woman presented with osteoporosis, celiac disease might not be considered as a cause. Of course, there are medications for the inflammation and complications of Celiac disease, but with conventional and alternative doctors alike, the first and main treatment is to have the patient *totally* abstain from gluten. Even a small hidden amount can wreak havoc. That makes avoiding gluten quite challenging because of the wide use of those grains and their byproducts. (There is a quick reference article and a page of gluten sources on my website.) Scientists are looking for an alternative treatment, such as a vaccine that will improve tolerance to gluten.[8]

A Functional View

Functional medicine seems to have a much greater appreciation for the impact that digestion can have on health and for that reason might be more likely to suspect Celiac and test for it. Because they are always looking for a deeper level of cause, functional medicine doctors would be less likely to treat a Celiac rash with a steroid cream, and to try to instead identify the cause, probably starting with the gut.

How Probiotics Relate

Leaky gut seems to worsen CD.[9] In Chapter 9 we discussed the important role probiotics plays in solving leaky gut. Some bacterial strains help digest gluten, but they are not a substitute for avoidance.[10] It appears that some probiotics may help keep gluten from entering cells.[11] Probiotics are apparently needed even for those CD patients on a gluten free diet.[12] Supplementing with two strains of *Bifidobacterium breve* reduced inflammatory markers in children with Celiac disease.[13] Incidentally, some researchers have blamed the increase in CD and gluten intolerance on the increased use of glyphosate herbicides like RoundUp that we discussed earlier as having a nutrient-depleting effect and being hard on our probiotics.

Suggested Steps

Anyone with long-term GI problems, osteoporosis, symptoms listed at the beginning of this section, or a family history of Celiac disease should be tested.

To make the test more accurate, it is best for people to get tested by a Celiac specialist *before* attempting to eliminate gluten from their diet. A properly designed stool test may be much more accurate than the typical blood tests and can detect Celiac even in persons who have no obvious symptoms. Enterolab's patented test (*see* Resources) is more convenient than the common but more cumbersome seventy-two-hour tests and has an exceptionally good record of sensitivity.

Other Considerations

Those with CD have to be careful of even medications and dietary supplements because many of them contain gluten. It is best to look for language that clearly says the item is "gluten free." I believe that routinely taking a gluten-specific enzyme (GlutenEase by Enzymedica is an example) may be a useful backup plan for dealing with the gluten that sneaks into the diet in spite of the patient's best efforts.

See also **Gas and Bloating.**

CROHN'S DISEASE

See **INFLAMMATORY BOWEL ISSUES.**

COLDS

See **INFECTIONS.**

COLITIS

See **INFLAMMATORY BOWEL ISSUES.**

CONSTIPATION

For roughly forty-two million Americans, nature doesn't call—or at least doesn't do so regularly enough. Something is amiss given that Americans are buying over 300 different brands of laxatives to the tune of $400 million a year! Some readers will be surprised at the actual definition. The official mainstream medical reference (the Rome III Diagnostic Criteria), defines "constipation" as when a person (has not met the definition of Irritable Bowel and) has *two or more* of the following which occur at least 25 percent of the time:

- lumpy, hard, or very small stools
- sensation of incomplete evacuation
- feeling of an obstruction/blockage
- loose stools are rare without the use of laxatives
- fewer than three bowel movements per week

I've talked to people whose doctors said something along the lines of "once a week is normal for you." That may be *usual*, but it is certainly not *normal* even by the strictest definition. Nutrition-oriented practitioners usually recommend at least one fully formed bowel movement a day and often prefer one for each meal.

Functional medicine doctors are less concerned with avoiding the *minimum* criteria for a diagnosis than in obtaining *optimum* function such as a healthy transit time—that's the time it takes for a meal to be digested and excreted. If material goes too fast (diarrhea) there is insufficient time to absorb nutrients. If it lingers too long, we begin to absorb into blood circulation noxious waste breakdown products, such as two with worrisome names, putrescine and cadaverine. (It is easy enough to measure transit time by swallowing an indicator like a spoonful of sesame seeds or a charcoal capsule, and then to see how long it takes to appear in the stool.) Opinions seem to vary widely on what is normal transit time. In the 1980's the Mayo Clinic found the average to be fifty-three hours which seems too slow. Functional medicine seems to aim for a transit time of something more on the order of twenty-four hours or less as is typical in Asia and Africa.

Conventional Treatment

Given the importance, it would be great if more doctors asked about digestion and bowel habits. At least when asked by patients about constipation, most no longer suggest habit-forming stimulant laxatives. They may recommend stool softeners which are relatively safe, but as you will see below, magnesium also serves that purpose, and we get so much more benefit from that mineral.

Fiber is a common prescription. One reason that fiber helps both constipation and diarrhea is that it not only adds bulk, but it also provides food for our good bacteria. That is probably constructive since the standard American diet does not come close in fiber content to the recommended daily intake of 38 grams for men and 25 grams for women. (By the way, only plant-based foods contain fiber.) Psyllium fiber has been the medical go-to fiber for some time. It is considered relatively safe, but according to the National Institutes of Health Medline reference, potential side effects can include difficulty breathing, stomach pain, difficulty swallowing, skin rash, itching, nausea, and vomiting.[14] MiraLAX (polyethylene glycol) is another frequent choice, but it should not be given to children because it seems to be absorbed to some extent and has side effects. I like Super Seed Fiber by Garden of Life. It uses sprouted seeds and uncommon grains (for less risk of allergy), and it is low in carbs. Although it has no wheat, rye, or barley, because it is not specifically labeled "gluten free," it may not be safe for those with celiac disease.

There is another fiber choice I want to mention because it illustrates the principle of picking products that multi-task and therefore offers fringe benefits instead of side effects. Organic oat fiber has been shown to not only absorb toxins, but to also speed their elimination (especially when combined with the amino acid taurine).[15] It is low in starch and contains antioxidant substances (avenanthramides) which seem to be anti-inflammatory for at least post-menopausal women.[16] In the laboratory, it suppresses cancer cells.[17] Oat fiber may help lower cholesterol two ways—one, by absorbing cholesterol before it can get back into circulation, and perhaps secondly, by providing food for the friendly bacteria that are known to lower cholesterol.[18] I don't think common flavored instant oatmeal products are an ideal source of this fiber because of their high sugar content. NuNaturals packages an organic oat fiber and Bob's Red Mill brand makes oat bran in the form of a hot cereal. If your natural food store doesn't carry these, they would likely be happy to order your choice.

A Functional View

Without sufficient fluid, fiber can make constipation worse. Since 90 percent of the water that arrives in the large intestine is absorbed, there needs to be enough left to keep the stool from becoming hard. Eating fibrous fruits and vegetables adds fiber and water at the same time along with nutrients. A water intake formula that seems to work for most people is to daily drink one ounce of water for every two pounds of body weight. For example, a 150 lb. person would drink 75 ounces.

How Probiotics Relate

Thanks to yogurt advertising, it is becoming common knowledge that probiotics help regularity. Researchers selected 14 studies from a field of 660 to form a meta-analysis regarding probiotics for constipation. They found that probiotics improved stool consistency, reduced transit time, and increased frequency of bowel movements.[19] That is logical because probiotic bacteria stimulate peristalsis (the muscular action keeps things moving along). Also, a major portion of the feces is bacterial. Looking for a citation to be more specific, I ran across a listing in the online Encyclopædia Britannica. They say, "Normally, feces are made up of 75 percent water and 25 percent solid matter. About 30 percent of the solid matter consists of dead bacteria."

As discussed previously, 90 percent of the neurotransmitter, serotonin, is made in the gut where it stimulates movement. We know some beneficial bacteria are involved in making neurotransmitters.

Insufficient probiotics contributes to a toxic environment that can kill whatever beneficial microorganisms are present, creating a vicious cycle. *Bifidobacterium* strains are so far among the most researched in regard to constipation. Most multi-strain probiotics contain that type—including some that I recommended in the Shopping Guide on page 121.

Suggested Steps

Building digestive competence is the plan, but sometimes people want to get quick results with a "loading dose" (more than the recommended daily amount) of probiotics. By having stirred things up so quickly, a person might experience gas or a loose stool. Those are inconvenient, but not harmful if temporary.

Other Considerations

There are other constipation causes. In all the following cases, the natural remedies noted are also supportive of general health.

- The mineral magnesium pulls water into the colon, explaining why Phillips' Milk of Magnesia is used as a laxative. It seems smarter to take a nutritional form of magnesium routinely rather than waiting for constipation. That is because the body uses magnesium in over 300 enzyme systems, and there are so many additional benefits—improved mood, relief of cramping, reduced blood pressure, heart rhythm support, and many more.

- An under-functioning thyroid is a common cause of constipation and many other health issues. It should be checked. (The thyroid quiz on HBNShow.com is a good first step.)

- Exercise helps relieve constipation (and most every other problem).

- It pays to have a good chiropractor assure that a spinal subluxation isn't slowing things down by impinging on the nerve supply to the digestive tract.

- Stress reduction helps constipation.

See also **INFLAMMATORY BOWEL ISSUES.**

DIARRHEA, OCCASIONAL

Traveler's diarrhea may affect more than half of travelers. Temporary or frequent, a runny stool, especially with excessive urgency to go, is a bit frightening. Food going through the digestive system should follow a timetable something along these lines:

- in the mouth = one minute (hopefully being chewed)

- in the esophagus = three to twelve seconds

- in the stomach (where breakdown starts) = two to three hours

- in the small intestine (where nutrients are absorbed) = five to six hours

- in the colon, *see* next paragraph

Transit time faster than that does not allow our system to absorb needed nutrients or remove excess fluid. The next stage of digestion is where the most confusion on timing seems to exist. In the large intestine (where water and electrolyte minerals are to be absorbed), the minimum may be about twelve hours. That Mayo Clinic study referenced above under Constipation found that this stage took an average of forty hours.

If the digestive system contains something the body doesn't like, such as a pathogen, toxin, or allergenic food, it can greatly speed up emptying time on a temporary basis. However, if a runny stool is experienced more than once in a while, we may be talking about one of the inflammatory bowel conditions outlined in later sections.

Conventional Treatment

If diarrhea lasts long enough for people to see a doctor (in the absence of clues to a more chronic disease), they may just be prescribed one of the many over-the-counter anti-diarrhea medications, such as Imodium, Kaopectate, or Pepto-Bismol. If the "runs" are experienced in connection with something like the flu, most attention will be directed to that condition. For any type of practitioner, rehydration is always important along with the replacement of lost electrolyte minerals.

A Functional View

Although eating tainted food is a common cause of diarrhea (see Chapter 6 for prevention ideas), so is exposure to antibiotics. When an antibiotic is necessary, probiotics should accompany it to head off that effect. Package instructions on other medications should be checked to see if diarrhea is a side effect.

How Probiotics Relate

It seems that a *majority* of the thousands of studies in the government database about probiotics are about their use for prevention and treatment of chronic or frequent diarrhea. My clients, friends, and family have always gotten fast help from probiotics in the event of a spell of the runs. A fellow radio host quickly shut down a raging case of food poisoning with a large dose of my favorite probiotic. During a bout of diarrhea, probiotic supplements may need to be taken every two hours.

Suggested Steps

Fiber also helps diarrhea. At first that might seem counterintuitive since fiber was also recommended under the opposite condition, constipation. Fiber helps achieve normalcy because it absorbs toxins and fluid—*and as noted, it feeds probiotics.*

Other Considerations

Large doses of vitamin C and magnesium can cause loose or pasty stools because they increase fluid in the colon. If that is an issue, it may help to switch to a better tolerated form or a reduced dose of the supplements. Coconut (even as macaroons) is a home remedy for diarrhea, perhaps because of its antimicrobial fatty acids. Zinc was found to help reduce diarrhea in children, but that was in poor countries where the children may be deficient in the mineral.[20]

See also INFLAMMATORY BOWEL ISSUES.

DIVERTICULOSIS / DIVERTICULITIS

When depressions or pockets develop in the intestinal tract their presence is called *diverticulosis*. They are sort of the opposite of polyps which are outgrowths. These pockets usually occur in the large intestine and less frequently in the small. They can collect food and worsen other digestive upsets, but they often produce no symptoms. According to the Harvard Health Letter (Aug 2010), by age 60 one-third of all Americans will develop the condition and by age 85, two-thirds will. In up to 25 percent of cases, the pockets become inflamed and/or infected and are then called *diverticulitis*. Obesity is a risk factor as is straining at stool due to constipation.

Conventional Treatment

At the diverticulitis stage, a clear liquid diet and antibiotics may be recommended until the situation calms down. In emergency cases (like when an infected pocket bursts), surgery may be necessary.

A Functional View

In the past patients were told to avoid nuts, seeds, popcorn, and foods with peelings, but as it turns out there seems to be no evidence that those are harmful and they may in fact help prevent the condition. Apparently, the more whole, wholesome, and fiber-rich the diet, the less likely it is that these conditions will develop.

How Probiotics Relate

Some researchers say there is growing evidence that antibiotics are not indicated in uncomplicated diverticular disease, and they point to interest in probiotics and fiber.[21] While there are a lot of studies showing that probiotics benefit the conditions preceding and associated with diverticular disease, only a few look at probiotics specifically for relieving established diverticulitis. One study found that *Lactobacillus casei* subspecies *DG* was effective (along with an anti-inflammatory medication) at maintaining remission of symptoms.[22] Unfortunately, although a blend might be useful, research is often done on a single probiotic strain because first of all, that makes a more specific scientific point, and secondly, sometimes the motive is to find a strain that can be patented.

Suggested Steps

Patients certainly have the option of using what might be more effective—a multi-strain probiotic and a fiber-rich, healthier, and less inflammatory diet that will strengthen the colon wall (as well as their overall health). When the diet is rich in insoluble fiber, the risk of diverticular disease is reduced 40 percent.

Other Considerations

Although I have heard experienced colon hydrotherapy professionals claim that they have *reversed* diverticular pockets by removing toxic material and "exercising" the colon wall with colonics, it seems potentially a bit risky to the have pressurized water pushing against the relatively frail intestinal walls in severe cases. With any colonics, replacement of the probiotics flushed away seems logical.

See also **CONSTIPATION.**

ECZEMA

See **SKIN TROUBLES.**

FATIGUE

Fatigue may be the most common complaint in the doctor's office (or at the water cooler for that matter). Fatigue can result from most diseases, but even if there is not a diagnosis, clearly *something* is sapping a person's energy because fatigue is not the natural human state.

Conventional Treatment

Physicians would usually check for clues to serious diseases and eliminate that possibility. If a patient mentions that sleep issues may be a part of the problem, a prescription for a sleep drug is likely the outcome of the office visit. If the patient reports sleeping a normal amount, but he/she wakes tired and is tired all the time, an anti-depressant may be the prescription. In some countries it is actually official policy that chronic fatigue is psychosomatic—basically all in a person's head. Consumers often self-medicate with an energy shot or a Venti Caramel Macchiato. (Venti, from the Italian for twenty, is a 20-ounce Starbucks coffee beverage. It is loaded with 10 teaspoons of sugar.) Those approaches give relief in the short term but grief in the long run.

A Functional View

Those sleep and depression medications can have very serious side effects, and they do not address the question of *why* the person isn't sleeping or is tired. Chronic fatigue syndrome (CFS) is a real *physical* thing, and at least one psychiatric journal finally acknowledged the fact.[46] CFS is hard for doctors to treat, and not just because they lack the special training, but also because third party payers do not reimburse for the amount of time these complex cases require. Functional medicine doctors are much more likely to deal effectively with CFS because they are accustomed to considering hormones (including thyroid) and health of the gut, cells, and mitochondrial health as at least a part of the solution to puzzling problems.

How Probiotics Relate

As has been the case with every disease condition that I've checked, with CFS the blend of gut bacteria in patients turns out to be different than that of the healthy controls.[47] There are also other connections.

- Repairing leaky gut has been shown to achieve clinical energy improvement even in cases of CFS.[48]

- A study of fatigue among athletes undergoing intense training showed that their levels of a latent virus (*Epstein Barr*) increased. The burden of the virus was likely adding to fatigue. Administration of *Lactobacillus acidophilus* for one month normalized immune function.[49]

- I have quite often been told that my clients' fatigue started after a round of antibiotics which surely depleted beneficial bacteria. Typically, I find that reducing fungus overgrowth greatly boosts energy.

- Overcoming constipation boosts energy as well.

- Diarrhea causes fatigue from loss of nutrients and hydration until the process is stopped. As discussed, probiotics are fundamental to solving diarrhea.

- Virtually all the functions of probiotic bacteria listed in Chapter 4 provide direct or indirect help for fatigue. Those include improved nutrition, detoxification, oxygen uptake, and more.

Suggested Steps

Many people are tired because they do not get sufficient protein, and partly as a consequence of that they have unstable blood sugar. (The HBNShow.com Library offers some basic information about managing blood sugar with diet.) Proper hydration is also important for energy production. Vitamins and minerals do not technically *create* energy, but they do help us extract it from food, store it, and help our bodies utilize it. Therefore, it is important that insufficiencies be corrected. Vitamin B12 is the nutrient perhaps most closely associated with energy, and I have had good success with NoShot B12 micro-lingual lozenges from Superior Source. Magnesium often makes people feel better too, for any one of 300 reasons.

Other Considerations

Energy is made in components of our cells called mitochondria. Keeping them humming will not only maintain energy, but also protect against the diseases of aging. Probiotics seem to help the mitochondria. In addition, D-Ribose is a special sugar used by the mitochondria. It is made in the body, but sometimes not in sufficient quantities and so supplementing with it seems to improve energy. (Jarrow Formulas offers D-Ribose in powders and chewables.) Other natural supplements, such as L-carnitine, alpha-lipoic acid, and coenzyme Q10 have been shown to help restore mitochondrial function.[50] Since few in the public are aware of the role of the mitochondria, formulations combining those nutrients and more are usually available mainly from companies that supply health professionals.

FLU

See **INFECTIONS.**

GAS AND BLOATING

Anyone who has suffered with one these unpleasant conditions does not need a definition. I'm guessing that is *everyone* because we all generate gas in our stomachs and intestinal tracts as result of swallowing air and the normal breakdown of food. It is only a real problem if gases get trapped inside the stomach or GI tract and cause pain; or there is an excess of noisy flatulence; or the gas has an embarrassing odor. (I can't resist noting that a Frenchman has invented a pill that makes users' flatulence smell like chocolate.)

Conventional Treatment

If flatulence occurs along with another digestive condition, such as acid reflux or irritable bowel, medical attention is usually focused on that. Medications containing simethicone do not address what has *caused* the gas, but they do help small bubbles organize into larger ones that may be easier to expel. Di-gel is a well-known over-the-counter remedy containing that ingredient along with antacids which may or may not be needed.

A Functional View

The gas that is produced depends mainly on the combination of foodstuffs and microorganisms. Probably any food can cause gas if a person doesn't digest it due to insufficient enzymes. That deficiency could be caused by a genetic lack of enzymes and/or overindulgence in that food which over-whelms available enzymes. Beans are the poster child of gassy foods. The Mayo Clinic website lists these other foods as common gas culprits:

- broccoli
- Brussels sprouts
- cabbage
- carbonated drinks
- cauliflower
- chewing gum
- fruits (such as apples, peaches, and pears)
- hard candy
- lettuce
- milk and milk products
- onions
- sugar alcohols found in sugar-free foods (sorbitol, mannitol, and xylitol)
- whole-grain foods

Increased yeast in the system can ferment starches and sugars into gas. Some gut bacteria like *Methanobrevibacter smithii* cause us to produce more hydrogen and methane gas. Increased amounts of those gases were linked to greater weight gain and increased body fat presumably because the gut bacteria were not the slimming kind.[23]

How Probiotics Relate

We've covered a great number of ways that probiotics help the underlying digestive issues that might cause gas. For example, the worst smells come from foods that have not been digested and some probiotics create enzymes that help digest them. Lactose intolerant folks for instance get gas because they cannot digest lactose in milk, and they are helped by probiotics that can.

Suggested Steps

Pain in the upper midsection can feel like a heart attack. If forcing a belch doesn't relieve the pain, prudence dictates taking emergency action because, especially for women, what seems like stomach gas sometimes *is a heart problem.*

Other Considerations

Gaseous emissions may be reaching a new level of respectability because scientists believe that a substance emanating in flatulence with the odor of rotten eggs may actually have a number of protective effects against degenerative diseases. The reason is likely that the smell is liberated by our good bacteria from healthful sulfur-containing foods like eggs, broccoli, and garlic. Researchers also think that our personal "smellprint" may lead to new ways of early detection of colon cancer and other diseases.[24] On a tangentially related note, there are indications that loss of the ability to identify odors might be an early indicator of future Alzheimer's disease.[25]

See also **INFLAMMATORY BOWEL ISSUES.**

GERD

See **ACID REFLUX.**

GUM DISEASE AND TOOTH DECAY

Our mouths are the site of a constant battle among billions of microorganisms representing as many as 700 bacterial species. Although *H. Pylori* is a strain that can cause cavities, *Streptococcus mutans* is the number one suspect in causing decay and gum disease. These bacteria also pose a threat to cardiovascular health, and the gum inflammation caused by bacteria has even been linked to increased risk of Alzheimer's disease. Infection of the gingiva (gums) and consequent receding of bone in the jaw is the major cause of tooth loss in adults. Although gums renew their cells every one to two weeks, bacterial toxins interfere with that process. The bacteria hide from our mouthwash in colonies under protective coatings (biofilms) that we know as plaque. "Dry mouth" (a lack of saliva) degrades the health of the mouth, and it leads to trouble with both teeth and gums.

Conventional Treatment

Cavities are drilled and filled up until decay reaches the nerve when root canal is often recommended. Regular scaling and deep cleaning of the plaque from the roots of the teeth removes a burden on the gum tissue. In serious cases, periodontists may resort to antibiotics, gum surgery, and bone reconstruction. Failing those, tooth extraction and replacement with, for example, an implant or bridge may follow.

A Functional View

Holistic dentists (and most functional medicine doctors) believe that root canal and improper extraction lead to chronic low level infections. They also believe it is smart to be exceptionally cautious when removing amalgam fillings because they are composed of more than half mercury. The *Dental Resources* page of my website lists links to learn more and find holistic practitioners.

Dry mouth can result from diseases, dehydration, and medication side effects. According to the Mayo Clinic, antihistamines, decongestants, muscle relaxants, and pain medications are common culprits. The functional approach is to solve the underlying problems, and to eliminate the need for those medications.

That reminds me of one of my earliest clients who came to me with a mouth filled with canker sores. (If you have ever suffered just one you can imagine her distress.) It seemed the problem was caused by a particular medication. However, as I unraveled her story layer by layer, it was apparent the process had started years ago when she was given an anti-depressant for grief after her mother died. The side effect of that drug led to another drug with another side effect. Long story short, she was then on 7 drugs. Fresh cabbage juice and aloe helped heal the ulcerations, but the real answer was in getting off the drugs one by one. I didn't know at the time to consider probiotics, but now I would because of their benefit to other mucous membranes. Although canker sores are considered a relatively minor problem that may not often justify grant money, there is some research evidence that probiotics help, and that those with recurrent ulcers of this type lack a healthy diverse microbiome.

How Probiotics Relate

There are good microbes in that teeming population of bacteria in the mouth. Dozens of studies show that various probiotic varieties (*lactobacilli*) work directly to keep the troublemakers from multiplying. Probiotics also produce selective antibiotics (bacteriocins) as well as immune-signaling compounds. Probiotics help reduce the inflammation caused by gum disease, and I found these other interesting connections in the research.

- Probiotics slow the formation of biofilm plaque hideouts.[26]

- Certain organic acids, including those contained in probiotics and Postbiotics, are important to the protective effect.[27]

- Judicious application of fluoride directly to teeth seems protective against decay. However, one study found that kefir (similar to yogurt) was just as effective.[28] (The idea of medicating the entire population with potentially toxic fluoride in drinking water is quite controversial and banned in some areas.)

- Well respected nutritionist, Dr. Nan Fuchs, PhD said this in her September 2007 *Women's Health Newsletter*: "My gums no longer bleed and the inflammation is gone. What's more, I have almost no plaque—it took less than two weeks to get these amazing results." She was speaking of a practice she and her dentist had just devised which involved squeezing the paste from one or two cultured food probiotic complex capsules (Dr. Ohhira's) and spreading it around the gum line. I've had two reports of people eliminating a toothache the same way. Probiotics can make vitamin K2 which is thought to repair tooth structure, but that seems like a stretch. Surely someone with a toothache should see his or her dentist.

- Although bad breath can originate much further down the digestive tract, it often results when bacteria in the mouth digest sulfur containing food particles. One test tube type study showed that a probiotic (*Streptococcus thermophilus*) reduced numbers of the offending bacteria and their odor-producing output.

- Adding probiotics to ice cream reduces levels in children of the bacteria that cause decay.[29]

Suggested Steps

There is no substitute for brushing and flossing because those actions break up the bacterial biofilms. Several dentists have told me that in that role it is the abrasion not the toothpaste that is critical. Makers of various static and moving types of toothbrushes spend a lot of money trying to convince us of the superiority of their brand. But, oddly enough, a study showed that a traditional Arabic chewing stick (Miswak) may be just as good.

As we've been told since childhood, sugar feeds decay-causing bacteria and encourages them to release acid that breaks down tooth structure. Those are reasons for chewing sugar-free gum sweetened with xylitol. This low-calorie sweetener also prevents harmful bacteria from adhering to the teeth, and it reduces their acid output while seeming to spare the probiotic bacteria. Even more surprising, xylitol also helps rebuild tooth enamel. I use Vita-Myr natural toothpaste, which not only contains xylitol but also nutrients with known benefits for oral health, such as zinc, CoQ10, and myrrh.

Probiotic gum was bound to appear and it has. That supports the credibility of probiotics for oral health, but I prefer another plan. I chew xylitol gum (sometimes it is dessert) and at bed time follow Dr. Fuchs' plan.

Other Considerations

I am also impressed with an ancient Ayurveda (Indian) oral health practice called "oil pulling" which is finding new fans and even some validation from scientific studies. Tradition has it that the practice also improves many systemic diseases. We may not know for some time if that is true, but it certainly points again to the connection of oral health to whole body health. Basically, a teaspoon of oil is swished around the mouth for ten to twenty minutes. Then it is spit out because it contains bacteria, perhaps from having disrupted biofilms. (To save your plumbing, spit into the trash rather than the sink.) The first thing in the morning before eating seems to be the best time, and it is then followed by brushing. Sesame oil was used in India, but today many use coconut oil.

Dentist Weston A. Price was the author of *Nutrition and Physical Degeneration*. Written in 1939, it is still highly regarded for the insights he gained from investigation of the relationship of dental health to the diets of various populations around the world. He found that many diverse cultures still eating their traditional diets did not have decay, and they did not need orthodontists. *See* Resources, page 207, for a book I recommend that includes a summary of this work.

HEARTBURN

See **ACID REFLUX.**

INFECTIONS (Colds, Flu, Bronchitis, and Sinusitis)

We are routinely attacked by a slew of pathogens, such as bacteria, viruses, and fungi, some of which we discussed in Chapter 3. Usually our immune systems fight them off before we are even aware of any symptoms—we might feel just a little tired or slightly "off" one day while the battle is going on, but then feel normal the next. We experience symptoms when the pathogen gets the upper hand over our immune response. This section covers mainly infections known as "Upper Respiratory Tract Infections" (URTI's).

Conventional Treatment

For URTI's, most health care practitioners will recommend rest and fluids, but they will also prescribe various medications, including antibiotics, antivirals, and drugs for relief of symptoms, such as cough, sore throat, sinus congestion, and fever. Each of the symptom-relief medications (even the over-the-counter variety) come with side effects that should be considered. But, at least it is no longer common to put radioactive material (radium) up noses for chronic sinus infections as was done in the 1950's and 60's. (Not surprisingly cancer, thyroid trouble, brittle teeth, and other problems appeared years later.)

A Functional View

Sinus congestion can serve as a good example of the issues. It is rarely caused by bacteria but rather by allergy, viruses, toxic exposure, and most often yeasts. A Mayo Clinic study found that 96 percent of chronic sinusitis patients had infections with one of a wide variety of fungi and were suffering allergic reactions to them.[51] Their findings were later confirmed by a sinus center in Austria. (In the preface I mentioned that in my twenties I had sinus congestion and that a doctor wanted to operate. That would *not* have solved what I now know was a fungus problem.) Mayo wisely recommends against the use of antibiotics in these cases because that would likely lead to a worsening of the condition (and long term gut issues). In another study it was found that the antibiotic amoxicillin and a nasal steroid were not effective for treating acute sinusitis.[52] The functional viewpoint would be to use antibiotics reluctantly, and if possible to avoid drug-based nasal sprays since they can cause dependence and rebound problems. A more natural approach is reviewed below.

How Probiotics Relate

I've presented ample evidence that probiotics improve immune function in general, but here are some examples that apply specifically to these upper respiratory type infections.

- A probiotic given to children attending daycare significantly reduced episodes of both diarrhea and URTI's.[53]

- Children aged 3 to 5 years who were supplemented twice daily for six months with a combination probiotic experienced much less severe fever and upper respiratory symptoms and almost 30 percent fewer days absent from daycare.[54]

- College students receiving a supplement of two probiotic strains experienced 34 percent less severe symptoms of URTI's, and they missed two fewer days of school.[55]

- An animal study showed that pretreating with probiotics protected the subjects from influenza.[56]

- A review of 10 studies showed that probiotics were better than placebo for incidence and severity of URTI's and reduced the incidence of antibiotic use.[57]

- Probiotics can improve a senior's response to flu vaccines.[58]

Suggested Steps

Functional doctors would typically use non-toxic natural remedies for immediate relief (such as those in the immune section of the HBNShow.com Library) while working to identify and fix the root cause and build immune strength. To speed recovery from illness, they might emphasize good nutrition, sleep, hydration, and immune-boosting supplements. As with allergies, they might suggest flushing nasal cavities with a natural saline solution, possibly using a neti pot or spraying with a xylitol spray such the Xlear brand.

They may also be in less of a rush to medicate symptoms. For example, fever is an immune system weapon. Likewise, coughing may perform a useful function in expelling mucus from the lungs.

Other Considerations

Vitamin D plays a very important role in immune system functions, and that applies to preventing and curing URTI's. (See the nonprofit VitaminDCouncil.org for more information.) Olive leaf extract is helpful against viruses, but if not used with caution may negatively affect probiotics.[59]

IRRITABLE BOWEL ISSUES

Irritable Bowel Syndrome (IBS), Irritable Bowel Disease (IBD), Colitis (including collagenous colitis, lymphocytic colitis, and microscopic colitis), Crohn's Disease, and Ulcerative Colitis are in a spectrum of digestive dysfunctions with fine and overlapping distinctions among them. It is estimated that in the U.S. perhaps 10 percent to 15 percent of the population suffers with IBS which is the most general of these terms. However, 70 percent of those do not think that their condition is serious enough to seek medical help.[30] Symptoms can include constipation, diarrhea, cramping, pain, or even vomiting, as well as various combinations thereof. (Sometimes acid reflux and even bowel incontinence are lumped into this category.) The names are applied according to severity and the ability to identify inflammation upon physical examination. The secondary symptoms in the rest of the body can include everything from fever to rashes. In the case of Ulcerative Colitis (UC), there is also damage to the intestinal lining apparently caused by some type of attack by the immune system.

A single cause has not been confirmed, but it is generally accepted that there is some combination of genetics, immune dysregulation, dysbiosis, an environmental trigger, and/or a sensitivity to a food, such as gluten. There are probably prevention clues in the fact that the incidence of IBS in the U.S. is massively greater than in other parts of the world. We are big consumers of dairy products, milk fat, pro-inflammatory omega-6 from vegetable oils, wheat, and processed foods that seem to increase risk. We are also more likely to consume medications and chemicals that kill our friendly bacteria.

Conventional Treatment

Generally, medicines to control the symptoms of IBS (such as constipation or diarrhea) are prescribed. Alosetron (Lotronex) was the first drug to be FDA approved specifically for IBS. It slows movement in the intestines by blocking the action of serotonin (that "happy hormone" neurotransmitter we have discussed). It was taken off the market just months after its approval in 2000 due to life-threatening gastrointestinal side effects. In 2002, FDA allowed it to be sold again but only as a part of a tightly managed drug company-sponsored program.

Antibiotics are also sometimes given. Typically, if there is an indication of inflammation on testing, anti-inflammatory drugs, including corticosteroids, are prescribed. Although the steroids soothe, they are not believed to contribute to solving the underlying problem. When an autoimmune component is suspected (for example, as would be likely with Ulcerative Colitis or Crohn's) doctors may give medication that suppresses the immune system. For example, Remicade (infliximab) is frequently used. (Those carry predictable risks including increased incidence of lymphoma.) More medications may be given for the secondary effects such as joint pain, which can accompany one of these bowel dysfunctions. Many docs traditionally recommended a "bland" diet (for example, steamed fish and white bread) which is surely a short term solution.

There has recently been a lot of interest in positive results from diet changes, such as eliminating the intake of wheat even among those without celiac disease or even proven sensitivity. There is also research into improvements from sharply limiting other sources of the fructans that ironically were discussed in Chapter 8 as helpful prebiotics. These substances which are contained in grains, fruits, and vegetables are collectively called FODMAPs (fermentable oligo-di-mono-saccharides and polyols).[31] Emulsifiers, such as carrageenan, are also suspect. That these substances are either food for or inhibitors of various strains of bacteria brings us back to discussion of the microbiome balance. This trend in conventional medicine seems to bridge the gap to the functional medicine approach.

A Functional View

Functional medicine views these conditions not so much as diseases but rather as symptoms of something more basic. I lump these conditions together because they have much in common. Besides being centered in the GI tract, they are typically called of "unknown cause" and all benefit from re-establishing microbial balance. Of course, genetic predisposition may be a factor in any or all, but as with any other health issue, diet, lifestyle, and our flora affect whether genes act up or stay dormant.

Research on these intestinal issues reflects the complexity of the situation because it is all over the map. For example, greater severity of IBS symptoms is linked to lower levels of vitamin B6.[32] (That may reflect a deficiency of probiotics which make B vitamins.) All varieties of these diseases have more in common than they do differences, so let's focus on probiotics for Crohn's Disease (CD) just as an example.

- Crohn's Disease (as well as IBD and UC) are more prevalent in less sunny climates. Vitamin D is an important balancer of immune function, and lack of the sunshine vitamin is now suspected as one causative factor of these diseases.[33]

- Another researcher adds these to the list of apparent causes: cigarette smoking, appendectomy, diet, stress, depression, and hormone imbalances.[34]

- Banana and broccoli fiber were shown to reduce the invasion of pathogenic *E-coli* bacteria into cells, but the common food additive Polysorbate 80 did the opposite.[35] (Polysorbate 80 is an emulsifier found, for example, in ice cream.)

How Probiotics Relate

The greatest weight of evidence recognized by mainstream medicine for successful intervention with probiotic supplements is for inflammatory intestinal conditions and pouchitis (an inflammatory problem following a type of colon surgery). As noted earlier, Japanese scientists believe that the meteoric rise in inflammatory bowel diseases in their country is due to reduced nutrition in the diet, overuse of antibiotics, and perhaps mostly to young folks no longer eating as many of the traditional fermented foods which are a source of probiotics and Postbiotics.[36]

An expert opinion reviewing the studies to date stated: "By far, the most convincing evidence was for the use of probiotics in IBS which reported that overall probiotics reduced the risk of symptom persistence by 21 percent."[37] A study of 108 IBS patients with bloating found a multi-strain probiotic effective and safe. A recent review of studies concluded: "Probiotics are effective treatments for IBS, although which individual species and strains are the most beneficial remains unclear."[38] That has to be a huge understatement. If fruits, vegetables, and whole grains make other people well but make IBS sufferers worse, we apparently need to know a lot more about what the microbiome balance issues are. We do know that IBS sufferers harbor more members of the phyla *Proteobacteria* and *Firmicutes*. Also, since lactate accumulates in bowel diseases, are they perhaps missing strains that use that as fuel and turn it into healing butyrate?

The fact that fecal microbiota transplant is a promising treatment for Inflammatory Bowel Disease provides clues to an answer.[39] A mixture of strains is typically helpful, and an animal study on the multi-strain cultured food probiotic complex discussed in the previous chapter showed impressive results with colitis and the accompanying tissue damage.[40] We hardly are accustomed to think of parasites as probiotics, but research is exploring the use of worms as a treatment for colitis.

Happily, there is a movement afoot to rely less on medications for these bowel diseases, and this concluding statement from an abstract seems to sum up the mood: "A broad spectrum of therapeutic tools, spanning from fecal transplantation, probiotics, prebiotics, microbial products, to microbe-tailored diets, may replace current IBD treatments."[41] Normal vitamin D processing is helpful to controlling colitis. Preliminary research indicates that probiotics may assist in that regard.[42] I certainly hope that we will soon know how to solve IBS without removing from the diet foods containing FODMAPs because those would otherwise be quite healthful.

Suggested Steps

There is little evidence for long term remission from use of the typical pharmaceutical medications, and the list of side effects from each one is alarming (let alone the drugs in combination). Given that also, in most cases these conditions are not immediately life threatening, a trial of a natural holistic approach seems very attractive. I've seen no indication that implementation of a gut restoration program as outlined here in *The Probiotic Cure* with carefully selected diet improvements, broad spectrum multi-strain probiotic supplements, and Aloe Vera, wouldn't be a very good place to start. There was a positive animal study result regarding colitis and good anecdotal reports with the use of the cultured food probiotic complex.[43] My guess would be the benefit was less from the probiotics and more from the postbiotics it contains.

Other Considerations

Enteric-coated peppermint oil capsules are a remedy worth a look.[44] Peppermint Plus by Enzymatic Therapy has a good reputation. IBgard is another readily available choice. An antioxidant extract of green tea was also shown to help IBS. The plant substance *resveratrol* is anti-inflammatory for the colon and inhibits colitis-associated colon cancer. In an animal study, rats were fed a diet with elevated amounts of high fructose corn syrup (HFCS). In animals supplemented with resveratrol (and quercetin) the HFCS caused less disruption of gut microbiota. They also experienced reduced serum insulin levels and weight gain.[45] But note, in too high a dose resveratrol negates benefits and can be an irritant.

MOOD AND STRESS

In Chapter 2 we discussed the research into mental health issues like depression, schizophrenia, and Alzheimer's disease, but this section is about more garden variety mood swings, stress, and problems with focus.

Conventional Treatment

Because there is little in the mainstream medical black bag specifically for these mild mood complaints, anti-depressants and anti-anxiety medicines may be prescribed even though they may be overkill for the indication, and a review of many studies shows that talk therapy works better and lasts longer.

A Functional View

Working to find and fix the cause is the more useful aim. Problems with mood and brain function can be a side effect of many medications. They may also result from a variety of conditions:

- blood sugar fluctuations: anxiousness before meals

- constipation: that dull "I can't think feeling"

- hormone imbalances: monthly blues

- liver disease: hepatic encephalopathy

- nutrient insufficiencies: confusion or PMS anxiety due to B6 deficiency or memory loss due to anemia or low B12

- sleep disturbance: crankiness and loss of zest for life

- toxicity: for example, "chemo brain"

- yeast overgrowth: boggy brain

How Probiotics Relate

On page 28 in regard to autism, we discussed the important role of the flora in helping maintain the integrity of the blood brain barrier. If that barrier is leaky, mood altering substances could pass from circulation into the brain. We've also covered probiotics' role in repairing all of the imbalances listed in the bullet points above. For example, inflammation is a factor in depression and mood problems. A healthy microbiome reduces inflammation. It also generates a healthful balance of neurotransmitters.

Neurotransmitters are signaling compounds that in the central nervous system affect mood and stress. As noted earlier, our microorganisms create many of these important chemicals. Not all of them cross the protective blood brain barrier and instead may affect the nervous system from a point somewhere else in the body. Links have actually been identified between specific neurotransmitters and microorganism strains shown to produce them. Some of those connections are shown in the following list along with a sample of what are typically complex and wide-ranging effects of that substance. The evidence does not yet support supplementing these strains to change mood, but I offer the list anyway as an example of how profoundly important the health and diversity of the microbiota is to our mood and behavior.

- **Acetylcholine**, attention (Lactobacillus)

- **Dopamine**, reward-motivated behavior (Bacillus, Serratia)

- **GABA** (gamma-Aminobutyric acid), calming (Lactobacillus, Bifidobacterium)

- **Norepinephrine**, flight or fight response (Escherichia, Bacilus, and Saccharomyces)

- **Serotonin**, cheeriness (Streptococcus, Escherichia, and Enterococcus)

Research on the gut brain access is in its infancy, but the preview we are witnessing is very exciting. This list gives hints to major breakthroughs that are in the wings.

- One study noted that "Alterations in gut microbial composition is associated with marked changes in behaviors relevant to mood, pain, and cognition."[60] Going a step further, transplanting the microbiome among mice was found to control whether they were bold and exploratory or timid and anxious.[61]

- The same article stated that the effect of our intestinal bacteria on the nervous system is so profound that it is now being called the "microbiome-brain-gut axis."

- A review of studies (which seemed quite enthusiastic about the prospect of using probiotics for depression) noted that probiotics communicate with the brain using various pathways—the nervous system, endocrine glands, and the immune system.[62]

- In a placebo-controlled study of healthy humans, those given multi-strain probiotics for a month experienced significantly less fixation on negative ideas and had fewer aggressive thoughts.[63]

- In a mouse experiment, continuing administration of the probiotic, *L. rhamnosus* (JB-1), reduced behaviors that indicate stress and anxiety. One of the researchers was quoted saying it was as though the mice were on Prozac. There were also measurable improvements in the way the nervous system signaling substances operated.[64]

- A whole new discipline is called "psychobiotics" to reflect the *two way street* between the gut microbes and the brain.

- Animal studies have linked probiotics to reduced stress. One human study showed that taking probiotics for two weeks before surgery lessened the stress of the surgery.[65] Another human study showed that simply supplementing prebiotics could reduce the effects of stress and improve outlook.[66]

- A type of dementia caused by liver cirrhosis was found to be improved by probiotics.[67]

Suggested Steps

To relieve stress, anxiety, mood problems, increase focus, in addition to working on intestinal probiotic balance, these help: assure adequate water intake, exercise consistently, and minimize the intake of refined starches and sugars that destabilize the supply of blood sugar to the brain.

Other Considerations

Improving blood levels of omega-3 fats appears to reduce brain shrinkage—surely a desirable outcome.[68] I always recommend products by Nordic Naturals as being quite clean and fresh. That is also an environmentally responsible company. Because virtually all vitamins and minerals have a role in the function of the nervous system, a multiple vitamin is good insurance. The Resource section, *see* page 207, recommends a book on brain function and a supplement that I use.

OSTEOPOROSIS

Osteoporosis is the most well-known bone-weakening condition. Our bodies continually remodel our skeleton, breaking down bone and hopefully rebuilding it stronger and better. Osteoporosis occurs when the rebuilding rate (making deposits) does not keep up with the breakdown rate (making withdrawals). Osteoporosis can cause us to become shorter, but the bigger fear is broken bones—especially broken hips which can become a life-threatening trauma. According to the National Osteoporosis Foundation (nof.org), the disease is responsible for two million broken bones a year.

Conventional Treatment

Television commercials feature movie stars touting bisphosphonate medications like Actonel, Boniva, Fosamax, and Reclast. The typical osteoporosis treatment is one of those drugs along with a calcium supplement, such as Caltrate. Fortunately, most mainstream doctors now also prescribe vitamin D3.

A Functional View

As discussed in the previous chapter, Celiac disease should always be ruled out with osteoporosis, but I don't know if that is done routinely in conventional practice. Bone thinning can also be caused by medications, such as corticosteroids (for example, Prednisone) taken for more than a short time. Those drugs can speed up the breakdown of bone, and slow its rebuilding—obviously a dangerous combination. The bisphosphonate drugs do make bone denser, but at the same time they become less flexible and therefore more brittle than bone built naturally. (You can visualize this problem if you think of a stick of chalk—it cannot bend even a little bit.) Thigh bone fractures are more common among those taking these medicines. There is also concern about the osteoporosis drugs' relatively rare but extremely serious side effects, such as death of the bone in the jaw.

As for supplementing calcium, it is at least curious that the U.S. has both the highest intake of calcium and the highest rates of osteoporosis on the planet. (There is more information on calcium in the Other Considerations section below.)

Lack of estrogen may be the most important factor in common bone weakening. Previously hormone replacement therapy (HRT) was given at least in part for this reason. That practice virtually stopped when it was shown that the HRT drugs increased cardiovascular risk. I agree with functional medicine doctors that the biggest problem was the *type* of medication that had been in use during the studies, and perhaps the way it was used. The estrogen in the studies was derived from pregnant horse urine, and it contained a variety of estrogen profiles, including some that were not exactly like the human forms. Another hormone, *progesterone,* was to be added to prevent uterine cancer. However, a synthetic *progestin* was prescribed that didn't offer all the protective benefits of the natural hormone. HRT may still be a very useful protocol if it uses hormones identical to the ones the body makes and in amounts sufficient to raise blood (or saliva) levels just to an age-appropriate normal level.

How Probiotics Relate

Many probiotic actions help bones. That includes, for example, improved nutrient absorption; creation of vitamin K2; detoxification support; inflammation reduction; antioxidant protection; assistance with hormone balancing; and boosting the energy to enable exercise. There are some other researched connections.

- An animal and laboratory study showed that one probiotic strain (*L. reuteri*) helped reduce bone loss in mice that were low in estrogen after ovary removal.[69]

- Interestingly, another study on the same strain showed benefit for male mice, but not for the females who still had their ovaries.[70]

- Other studies of probiotics and prebiotics in animals have shown bone benefits.[71] But a Japanese study of 157 human men and women (ages 20 to 70) seems more relevant. Improvements in bone mineral density were shown for both genders supplemented with the cultured food probiotic complex product.[72]

Suggested Steps

The sunshine nutrient, Vitamin D3, is critical to the absorption of calcium as well as hundreds of other reactions in the body. Americans are at great risk of vitamin D deficiency because food is not a good source, we live and work indoors, and we cover up with sunscreen when outdoors. The situation is even scarier for those with dark skin because they have built-in sunscreen. Standard lab reports of blood levels have been showing as *normal* a range of vitamin D that is far lower than *optimum*. Although the real danger is in having too *little* vitamin D, many doctors are still reluctant to suggest supplements of 4,000 to 7,000 IU which is the amount most people apparently need on a daily basis to achieve optimum blood levels. Visit the non-profit VitaminDCouncil.org site for more information.

Other Considerations

It takes a lot more than calcium and vitamin D to build bone. For example, magnesium is so important that, in my opinion, calcium should never be supplemented without it. Vitamin K2 is also critical because it helps direct calcium into bones rather than arteries. I often recommend Bone-Up by Jarrow Formulas because it contains those nutrients plus lesser known bone factors like zinc, manganese, and boron. Its special form of calcium (Microcrystalline Hydroxyapatite) is better suited to building bone than the type (basically ground rocks) contained in oft-prescribed products. Minerals in bone are held in a framework made of collagen. There are 3 different types of collagen—some are better for bone, hair, skin, nails, or joints. I suggest NeoCell, a brand that specializes in high quality collagen supplements customized for the various uses. Jarrow and NeoCell products are sold in most natural food stores.

Weight-bearing exercise is very important to building bone. The toxins in cigarette smoke should be avoided because among their other threats they sabotage the bone rebuilding process.

PSORIASIS

See **SKIN TROUBLES.**

REFLUX

See **ACID REFLUX.**

SINUSITIS

See **INFECTIONS.**

SKIN TROUBLES

Because people often judge us by what they see first, we are understandably very sensitive about the appearance of our skin. We should also care because the condition of the skin can mirror what is going on inside. This section focuses on eczema and psoriasis, but there is growing evidence that probiotics are helpful for acne and most of the information here would apply

Eczema is an inflammatory condition of the skin that is typically related to allergies and is more prevalent in children. It can involve some combination of redness, itching, swelling, flaking, cracking, and even oozing and bleeding. Psoriasis is similar in many ways, but skin cells can accumulate at the affected spots and appear a silvery-white. It is immune-related and can affect other parts of the body as is the case with psoriatic arthritis. Both conditions are subject to genetic predisposition.

Conventional Treatment

Neither condition is considered "curable," but children sometimes outgrow eczema. There may be a hundred or more medications for eczema, the most common of which are corticosteroids to reduce inflammation and anti-histamines to reduce itching. Moisturizers are also used. Treatment for psoriasis may include drugs called "biologics" that target certain immune cells or substances that they create. More severe cases may use systemic immune-suppressing drugs or meds that slow cell growth, including a chemotherapy drug, methotrexate. Light therapy may also be prescribed.

A Functional View

Psoriasis (even when moderate) is considered to be a risk factor for cardiovascular disease. Those with psoriasis or eczema are also more likely to suffer bone loss. What is going on here? Both skin conditions reflect general inflammation and are hard on health in that they cause stress. But, might another cause of the increased risk of heart disease and bone loss be not the skin issues, but rather the medications used for them? Both psoriasis and eczema are typically treated with corticosteroids. In the osteoporosis section (*see* page 172), we discussed the bone-weakening effects of those drugs, but they have other negative effects, including high blood pressure and weight gain. Many people know that topical corticosteroids can cause *external* problems, including thinning of the skin. They may not realize however that much of what is applied to the skin is *absorbed* into general circulation. The common effects of the biologic class of drugs may be respiratory infections and symptoms like the flu. More rarely, users can experience multiple sclerosis, seizures, and certain types of cancer.

With immune-suppressing drugs, patients run the obvious risk of having their immune system off duty when it is needed to fight infection or malignancy. With medications like methotrexate, cell replication is slowed, but so is tissue repair. Common side effects of that drug include blood in the urine or stools, bloody vomit, diarrhea, joint pain, stomach pain, and swelling of the feet. Less commonly, users may experience back pain, blurred vision, confusion, seizures, dizziness, shortness of breath, unusual bleeding, or weakness.

Functional medicine is interested in any effective natural approach to these conditions which reduces the need for these worrisome medications. They often find that repairing the gut solves skin problems.

How Probiotics Relate

Bacterial species on the skin are as diverse as in the gut, but not yet as well studied. It does appear that internally and topically probiotics can be useful against a number of skin diseases, including cancer. The authors of an article regarding friendly bacteria and skin cancer said "The human microbiome has recently gained prominence as a major factor in health and disease."[73] It is enlightening that probiotics taken internally shorten wound healing for burn patients.[74] As research shows, fresh glowing complexion comes from good health, and as we've seen, probiotics play a big part in achieving that as well as relief from chronic skin inflammation. There are even hints that we may see products promoting bacteria for beauty.

- Both psoriasis and eczema involve inflammation, and we know that probiotics help reduce inflammation in several ways. One study found that six to eight weeks of a probiotic (*B. infantis*) reduced the inflammatory marker CRP and one (TNF-?) targeted by some of the biologic drugs we just discussed.[75]

- Probiotics also help reduce immune overreactions, such as allergies. There seems to be a consensus that infants who develop eczema and other allergic manifestations have a less diverse microbiome. An analysis of 25 studies determined that probiotics were helpful for eczema, and that a mixture of strains was more effective than a single strain.[76]

- Since skin is our largest organ of elimination, it stands to reason that anything toxic in the body might irritate the skin on its way out. As we discovered, leaky gut allows allergens and toxic materials into the blood stream. Connecting the dots, it would seem logical to look for an association between probiotics and leaky gut with both diseases. A small study in 1991 showed a significant connection with intestinal permeability and psoriasis.[77] Unfortunately, I did not find that follow up studies have been conducted.

- Studies are beginning to show that one common thread between these and other diseases is a reduction in microbiome diversity. One study implies that maybe it isn't so much the *presence of pathogens* as the *loss of the benefits* provided by the good, such as certain fatty acids they make.[78]

- Some experts speculate that psoriasis, like Crohn's disease is a disordered immune reaction to certain bacteria.[79]

- One study showed benefit of a probiotic (*Lactobacillus rhamnosus GG*) against a common skin infection caused by *Staphylococcus aureus*.[80]

- There is also a good deal of interest in the microbiome *on* our skin. Topical probiotics can keep our "skin moist and make sure that if we get a wound that [dangerous] bacteria doesn't enter our bloodstream," as researcher Julia Segre of the National Institutes of Health pointed out.[81]

- Scientists are interested in using probiotics therapeutically, directly on the skin, as well as internally for conditions, such as eczema.[82]

- Analysis of dysbiosis of the skin may soon be used as a diagnostic tool.[83]

Suggested Steps

Psoriasis patients are helped by UV light therapy. Probably not coincidentally, they are also routinely found to be low in vitamin D. A good deal of evidence is accumulating that vitamin D is helpful in both eczema and psoriasis.

Other Considerations

Aloe Vera has been used to heal the skin since ancient times. A review of studies showed that while there are not many studying its use for psoriasis, in those that did, Aloe provided benefit and no adverse reactions. Many (if not most) commercial topical Aloe products contain very little Aloe gel. I have not found a better (or more reasonably priced) product than 99 percent Aloe Vera Gelly by Lily of the Desert. Coconut oil makes a cost-effective and beneficial moisturizer and has antimicrobial properties. Extra virgin organic coconut oil is now available as a private label in big club stores. Also, I have had excellent reports for improving general skin health and reducing irritations, such as those from razor burn with the use of a probiotic soap made in Japan from fermented plant extracts. (*See* Resources on page 207.)

STRESS

See **MOOD** and **STRESS**.

TOOTH DECAY

See **GUM DISEASE** and **TOOTH DECAY**.

ULCERATIVE COLITIS

See **IRRITABLE BOWEL ISSUES**.

ULCERS

Dr. Georges M. Halpern, MD, PhD (in his book *Ulcer Free!*) defines an ulcer clearly as "a deep lesion or crater sore on the mucosa or lining of the stomach or duodenal wall that is surrounded by acute inflammation." When we hear the term "ulcer" most people think of stomach ulcers which are also referred to as "gastric" ulcers. Actually, ulcerations are more common in the wall of the duodenum which is the part of the small intestine closest to the stomach. Besides blood loss from the ulcer, if the process isn't stopped, ulcerations can become potentially deadly perforations.

Conventional Treatment

The majority (up to 70 percent) of ulcers in either location are caused by infection with a bacterium, *Helicobacter Pylori (H. Pylori)*, and so the typical treatment has been a combination of strong antibiotics, bismuth, and acid-blocking medications. Unfortunately, the increasing incidence of antibiotic-resistant strains of *H. Pylori* has created problems for that approach. The next most common cause of ulcers is the use of non-steroidal anti-inflammatory drugs (NSAID's). In those cases the doctor can hopefully find a less damaging substitute for the NSAID's.

A Functional View

Of course, it is urgent to stop the bleeding of an ulcer. But, it also makes sense to find and address the initiating cause so that the ulcer does not *return*. The stomach is supposed to be protected against acid. So, if stomach ulcers are diagnosed, there must be some kind of imbalance affecting the integrity of the lining. For example, as we discussed with *H. Pylori* as a Double Agent, it is possible that the patient previously had insufficient stomach acid and/or insufficient probiotic strains that allowed *H. Pylori* to flourish. Or, nutritional deficiencies might have hampered the body's ability to keep up repair of the intestinal lining. Other subtle factors like food sensitivities and vitamin D insufficiency could be involved.

How Probiotics Relate

A review of all the jobs probiotics perform suggests many ways that they could help prevent and treat ulcers. Recent studies show, for one thing, they help absorb nutrients needed for repair of tissue. They also help reduce inflammation.

- Several studies show that various probiotics help to improve treatment of *H. Pylori*.[84]

- One study showed that a multi-strain probiotic (8 strains) used alone resolved the *H. Pylori* infection for roughly *one-third* of subjects. The researchers noted: "Probiotics survive in gastric environment competing with *H. Pylori*." And they added that "An adequate supplementation with probiotics might eradicate *H. Pylori*."[85]

- A lab study demonstrated that a cultured food probiotic complex was effective against *H. Pylori*.

- Probiotics help heal ulcers by reducing fungus that would otherwise slow healing.[86]

- Low levels of the hormone melatonin are linked to ulcers.[87] The majority of melatonin is made in the gut under the influence of probiotics.[88]

Suggested Steps

At the very least, probiotics should be used along with antibiotics if those are given. As devastating as those multiple strong antibiotics can be to the gut, I would consider an equally powerful combination of probiotics—*a full court press*. There is nothing wrong with combining the *S. Boulardii* friendly yeast supplement along with a high count freeze-dried multi-strain combination and the cultured food probiotic complex not only for its own benefits, but also to boost the effectiveness of the others.

Other Considerations

Deglycyrrhizinated licorice (DGL), Zinc-carnosine (as discussed in regard to leaky gut), and Mastic gum are all well researched ulcer remedies. Many functional medicine doctors are able to heal ulcers by using those supplements and probiotics without resorting to acid-blockers or antibiotics.

URINARY TRACT AND VAGINAL YEAST INFECTIONS

Urinary tract infections (UTI's) are also known as "acute cystitis" or "bladder infections." UTI's are considered the most common infection, generating more than seven million visits to the doctor's offices and one million to hospital emergency departments. Both men and women can be affected, but females are more likely to experience UTI's—almost one-half of us will suffer one. The annual cost is approximately $1.6 billion and that does not include UTI's contracted in the hospital. Infants, pregnant women, the elderly, diabetics, and those with multiple sclerosis are among those at increased risk.[89] Pathogenic bacteria or more rarely fungus or viruses can infect the mucous tissues anywhere along the urinary tract from the kidney on. Symptoms can include itching and/or pain and burning upon urination. In some cases there is severe pain in the lower abdomen or low back.

As many as three in four women will experience a *vaginal yeast* infection (usually caused by some variety of *Candida* yeast) and not surprisingly, the infections often occur after a round of antibiotics. Symptoms may be similar to UTI's, but usually with less pain and a vaginal discharge may be observed. This local overgrowth may be evidence of a systemic problem.

Conventional Treatment

Urinary tract infections are treated with antibiotics. Therefore a UTI might be followed by a vaginal yeast infection. Yeast infections are treated with antifungal drugs.

A Functional View

Very often in doctor's offices UTI's are diagnosed from the white cell count in the urine specimen without benefit of a lab culture to identify the offending organism. Therefore, it is likely that sometimes unnecessary antibiotics are prescribed or at least ones that are broader in spectrum than they need be.

How Probiotics Relate

Several probiotic strains have demonstrated a benefit against *both* vaginal yeast and bacterial UTI's. The urinary tract used to be considered sterile, but that view is changing. In the vagina, the normal friendly inhabitants are lactobacillus. Probiotics' varied roles in fighting pathogens and in boosting immune function come into play in this area as is shown by research findings.

- Scientists increasingly respect the role of lactic acid bacteria in maintaining urogenital health.[90]

- Oral capsules of two patented strains (*Lactobacillus rhamnosus*, GR-1 and *Lactobacillus reuteri*, RC-14) have been studied for twenty-five years. They have been shown to colonize and promote both vaginal and urinary tract health in part by keeping the pathogens from forming biofilms. They are available in the product Fem-Dophilus by Jarrow Formulas. It is sold in the cooler of most natural food stores.

- I know clinicians who get good results with soft gel multi-strain cultured food probiotic complex capsules used as a vaginal suppository at night. Success in a study using a multi-strain probiotic vaginally along with normal therapy adds credibility to this approach.[91] The suppository method can be used along with oral probiotics.

Suggested Steps

Some pathogens that infect the vagina and urinary tract come from the colon. To avoid contamination of that area, females should wipe with a motion that moves the toilet tissue strictly from front toward the back.

Other Considerations

Extract of cranberry has been shown to help prevent UTI's. That is apparently because it interferes with the pathogenic bacteria's ability to attach to the lining of the urinary tract. In at least some studies, low levels of vitamin D were associated with recurring UTI's.

VAGINAL YEAST INFECTIONS

See **URINARY TRACT** and **VAGINAL YEAST INFECTIONS.**

WEIGHT LOSS

There may be the most interest in this section because it was beginning to look like every single person in the U.S. would soon end up fat. It wouldn't add much value for me to list the discouraging statistics about the percentage of Americans (including children) that have become overweight and obese or to list the dire health consequences. We all know it is a major problem, so let's get right into what to do about it.

Conventional Treatment

Doctors and experts tell us to eat less and exercise more. Unfortunately, that seemingly logical advice seldom actually works. Approximately 95 out of 100 dieters ultimately fail and they regain the lost weight *plus more*. Diet pills may be prescribed in some cases. Stomach surgery of one kind or another has become the treatment of choice for upwards of 200,000 Americans per year. It has been known that a gene (FTO) is related to obesity. Recent research shows that it probably works by signaling food energy to be stored as fat. Not all overweight persons have this gene. We must look elsewhere for help while we wait for scientists to find a drug that turns off that switch but doesn't also disturb positive processes in the body. The much bigger pool of genetic information is in the microbiome which may control 25 percent of our metabolic machinery.

A Functional View

Functional medicine and clinical nutrition usually aim to improve health and thereby solve the *root cause* of excess weight. The concept is great but represents a tall order because overweight may actually be as many as 100 different diseases. For example, some of those root causes might include low thyroid function, imbalances of other hormones, nutrient deficiencies, poor blood sugar management, medication side effects, and emotional issues, such as stress. Sleep deprivation alone may be responsible for more obesity than overeating and lack of exercise. There are many more factors to consider.

- The average adult only requires about 1,300 calories a day to run their normal bodily functions. However, that average person eats 2,000 to 2,500 calories a day, meaning that they must somehow dispose of 40 to 50 percent of what they eat. That would theoretically require two hours a day of aerobics which is just not practical. There must be other factors at work.

- Soluble fiber (such as that in the skin of an apple or in beans) slows sugar absorption. Insoluble fiber (such as that from vegetables, grains, and the inside of an apple) provides satisfying bulk and food for bacteria. By helping us feel fuller, it has been shown that fiber may cause us to eat 15 percent less. It seems that most people have been on diets their whole life, so I never quite understood the concept of having an "appetizer." It might make more sense to eat an apple before lunch to kill your appetite.

- Diet pills are a temporary aid at best and unfortunately, on average, only generate between 4 percent to 8 percent weight loss beyond what a placebo (fake pill) would provide. Some of these meds have been recalled because they were too dangerous. Even natural appetite suppressants and metabolic stimulants are of limited and short term benefit.

- Surgery has risks, is expensive, and the reduced stomach size creates permanent nutrition challenges. However, there are some shockingly positive effects of Gastric Bypass surgery that will be discussed in the probiotic section.

- Counseling that encourages hefty folks to just accept and love their bodies may do some psychological good, but it ignores the long-term health risks that are linked to being overweight.

- Mindful eating helps us appreciate the food and more thorough chewing helps both satiety and digestion.

- For some reason there are flavor and aroma receptors not just in the mouth but also in other parts of the digestive tract. These receptors are apparently collecting information that may have something to do with feeling satisfied, and it appears the American diet is not making them happy.

- Our bodies obviously regulate the amount of blood in the circulatory system, the size of the liver, and so on very closely. What is less well-known is that the same is true of fat stores. One cause of obesity is a failure *of the system that regulates fat mass.* Fat mass is controlled by something akin to a thermostat that turns off the air-conditioner and turns on the heater to maintain a steady temperature. Similarly, the body guards its fat mass to keep it at a certain set point. It uses substances, such as ghrelin, to *increase* fat. Cholecystokinin (CCK), Peptide YY (PYY), insulin and amylin are used to *reduce* fat by affecting various functions, such as appetite, digestion, and metabolism. The body manipulates these signaling molecules based on input, such as reduced nutrient content in food, the fat cells themselves, and changes in insulin sensitivity. We now know that our microbes are perhaps a major factor in the ebb and flow of these chemicals.

- Improving gut microorganism balance is a relatively recent official addition to the functional medicine practitioner's little black bag.

How Probiotics Relate

When we focus first on improving health, normal body weight often follows. As it turns out, one reason for that outcome is that our efforts have helped overall health and the balance of gut bacteria. However, isolating specific bacteria designed for weight loss to supplement with is an entirely different matter. We'll get to the subject of strains on page 190, but first I'd like to explain some interesting research findings about gastric bypass surgery.

Lessons From Bariatric Surgery

After Roux-en-Y Gastric Bypass (RYGB) bariatric surgery, patients are less hungry, eat less sugar, and have fewer fat cravings. It is theorized that this type of surgery may actually trigger a change in the body's fat set points. Patients also often experience rapid loss of weight and fat that curiously cannot all be attributed to the reduction in calorie intake or altered nutrient absorption. They also gain healthier management of blood sugar. The mystery in these improvements may well be due to a changing of the bacterial guard.

I was intrigued by a lecture given by Lee Michael Kaplan, M.D., PH.D., Director of Obesity, Metabolism, and Nutrition Institute at Massachusetts General Hospital. (He is also an Associate Professor of Medicine at Harvard Medical School.) He was part of groundbreaking research designed to better explain the phenomenon. The study was done with germ-free mice. As you may recall, they are animals that do not have an intestinal microbiota and have been raised in a sterile environment. When these mice were implanted with a normal flora, they didn't eat more, but they did gain weight. Apparently, their new bacterial residents helped them extract more energy from the same amount of food.

When the mice were given RYGB surgery, they lost weight and the proportion of various strains of bacteria underwent a change. *Gammaproteobacteria* (*Escherichia*—a member of the phylum *Proteobacteria*) and *Verrucomicrobia* (*Akkermansia*) increased and maintained at the new higher levels. (Other research showed that after RYGB surgery the phylum *Bacteroidetes* also increases.) When that new post-surgery mouse microbiota was transplanted into mice that were still germ free, they lost weight and fat.[92] These changes are similar to those observed in the fecal microbiota of human RYGB subjects, and so the working theory is that this mouse study may explain what is happening to people too. RYGB surgery somehow causes changes in the gut bacteria that in turn play a significant role in weight loss. The hope is that a microbial method will soon be found to mimic the effect of RYGB without the surgery risk.

Mechanisms

It may seem improbable that these tiny bacteria and yeasts could have such a powerful effect on our body weight. We are just beginning to understand some of the specific functions that deliver the positive effects.

- Gut microorganisms are considered to be the equivalent of an endocrine organ like the thyroid gland which is critical to weight management. For example, probiotics and prebiotics are involved in regulating both the production of and cellular sensitivity to the ghrelin and leptin compounds that control our hunger and satiety. A lot of non-essential eating is related to mood, and low-calorie vegetables are not usually thought of as comfort food. As noted above in the section on mood and stress, our microorganisms create a variety of mood-normalizing substances.

- When *Bifidobacteria* digest fiber, butyrate is one result. That substance seems to suppress appetite. Acetate and propionate are other examples of bacteria-made short chain fatty acids that improve metabolism.

- It is a survival trait for microorganisms to drive us to feed them by generating cravings for the food they like, by altering how foods taste to us, and by altering our mood—for example, making us feel good or bad depending on whether or not we have satisfied their needs.[93]

- Yeast overgrowth, with its negative effects on metabolism, stimulation of cravings, and sapping of energy, is notorious for making its victims gain weight. Probiotics help control yeasts.

- Probiotics can manufacture CLA (Conjugated Linoleic Acid) which is often supplemented as a weight loss aid.[94]

- In Chapter 4 we discussed that probiotics can have a positive effect on insulin resistance, inflammation, nutrient absorption, hormone balance, energy (to exercise), detoxification, and other functions that have a positive effect on maintenance of a healthy body weight.

- As we saw earlier in Part Two, probiotics improve mood. This alone could be quite important since a great deal (if not the majority) of ill-advised eating is emotional in nature.

- Leaky gut may lead to weight gain and as demonstrated in Chapter 9, probiotics are crucial to controlling that condition.

- A great many medications list weight gain as a side effect. To the extent that probiotics solve health problems and obviate the need for medicine, they save us from those side effects.

Observational Studies

Not until The Human Microbiome Project did we have the tools to know that populations of bacteria might differ between the slim and the obese. This sampling of representative current science shows exciting promise. Don't worry if this seems a bit confusing. In fact, if it isn't confusing, I won't have reflected the situation accurately. Probiotic strains are listed were possible just to support a point I make in the Probiotic Strain Takeaway section (*see* page 190). In studies of the observational type, scientists simply look at factors as they currently are.

- It often said that general studies show that lean folks/animals have less (up to 50 percent) of the phyla *Firmicutes* than fat subjects and more (up to 50 percent) of the phyla *Bacteroidetes*; the obese theoretically the reverse. But, the situation seems more complex and there are some exceptions. In the following bullets, the names in brackets are the big groupings called phyla. I included them to make a point that may help us sort out oversimplifications sometimes thrown about.

- **Leanness** is associated with: *Christensenella (Firmicutes), Lactobacilli (Firmicutes), Bifidobacteria (Actinobacteria),* and *Verrucomicrobia (Akkermansia)*
- **Obesity** is associated with: *Erysipelotrichaceae (Firmicutes), Bacillus (Firmicutes), Eubacterium cylindroides, (Firmicutes), and enterobacter (Proteobacteria)*

    As will be discussed in the next section supplementing with *Lactobacilli* (a strain in *Firmicutes* the so-called "fat" phyla) increases beneficial strains in the lean category, such as *Bacteroidetes* and *bifidobacteria*

- As you can see, there are strains for both slimness and obesity in the phyla *Firmicutes*. Adults with higher levels of *Verrucomicrobia (Akkermansia)* were shown to have less fat and better blood sugar stability.[95] Specific stains are certainly of interest, but the overriding factor may be diversity. A study of Danish subjects, published in *Nature*, Aug 29, 2013, showed that there was a marked reduction in probiotic diversity among obese human subjects.

- We learned earlier in this book that infants *without* a diverse microbiome (because of antibiotic use or delivery by C-section) were more likely to become overweight later in childhood. Professor Tim Spector, a genetics expert at King's College in London, has followed 11,000 sets of *human* twins for over twenty years. He found that twins on restrictive weight loss diets were fatter and had microbiomes that were less diverse. Could the connection be that the limited variety of foods eaten on most weight loss regimes caused the reduction in diversity?

- Studies of twin mice pairs showed that the obese mice had a different assortment of gut bacteria and a loss of bacterial diversity compared to their lean twins.[96] Antibiotics cause farm animals and lab mice to gain weight. The drugs deplete the diversity of bacteria that would otherwise have kept the animal's weight normal. As noted in Chapter 2, when antibiotics are used to eradicate a stomach bug, body weight goes up.[97] Some scientists theorize that even the accumulation of the small amounts of second-hand antibiotics and anti-microbials in our food and water may be making us fat.[98]

Intervention Studies

In this type of study, researchers actually change a factor and measure the effect. Mice are often used because humans are so much harder to control and those studies are so much more costly. Twins are sometimes used to eliminate genetics as a factor.

- Professor Tim Spector, who was mentioned in the previous section, discovered that when twins are fed *identical diets* with the same number of added calories, one may gain up to *3 times as much weight,* and he attributed that to the differences in the flora.

- Germ-free mice were implanted with a complete assortment of microbes from human twins (one was lean and the other obese). The mice's weight soon reflected that of the donors. Mice usually pick up bacteria from those with whom they are housed. However, it was found that obese mice fed the rodent equivalent of the standard American diet were not able to acquire the lean producing bacteria from their skinny roommates.[99]

- It was shown that skinny mice can be made fat by sharing gut bacteria from fat mice. The fat mice showed an increase in members of the phylum *Firmicutes* and fewer from the phylum *Bacteroidetes.* That change seemed to allow them to pull more calories from food.[100] (We learned that ability can be a survival factor in the event of a famine, but Americans are usually *overfed* with calories at least.)

- Obese mice fed milk fermented with *Lactobacillus casei CRL 431 (Firmicutes)* lost more weight, had less fat in their livers, better immune function, and improved markers of metabolic function than the controls which were fed plain milk. Curiously, the supplemented mice also showed increased numbers of *Bacteroides (Bacteroidetes)* and *bifidobacteria (Actinobacteria)* which are members of different phyla.[101]

- Young rats were injected with a chemical to make them obese and develop metabolic syndrome. Administration of three probiotic strains: *Lactobacillus casei IMVB-7280 (Firmicutes)*, *Bifidobacterium animalis VKL (Actinobacteria)*, and *Bifidobacterium animalis VKB (Actinobacteria)* prevented those effects.[102]

- In a mouse study, supplementation with *Lactobacillus plantarum Strain K21 (Firmicutes)* reduced fat gain, decreased cholesterol and triglyceride levels, protected subjects from liver damage, and improved leaky gut.[103]

- A study found that humans fed a high fat, high calorie diet were protected from insulin-resistance by milk fermented with the probiotic *Lactobacillus casei Shirota (Firmicutes).*[104]

- A double blind human intervention study showed that supplementation of *Bifidobacterium breve B-3 (Actinobacteria)* for twelve weeks significantly lowered fat mass.[105]

- Supplementing *Lactobacillus paracasei subspecies paracasei L. casei W8 (Firmicutes)* reduced calorie intake, but it did not seem to change participants' feelings about their appetite.[106]

- In a recent study of obese menopausal women, supplementation with the probiotic *L. paracasei F19 (Firmicutes)* did not improve metabolic markers. However, supplementation with flaxseed mucilage over six weeks improved insulin sensitivity. That might be expected to lead to weight loss or at least better health. The mucilage also generated changes in 33 bacterial strains, but researchers did not think that explained the improvement in insulin sensitivity.[107]

- One study found that obese people were able to reduce the fat around their middle by 4.6 percent in twelve weeks by drinking a milk rich in *Lactobacillus gasseri SBT2055 (Firmicutes)*.[108]

- In another study, compared to diet-matched controls, participants experienced greater loss of body weight and body fat percentage when eating a multi-strain yogurt containing the probiotics *Lactobacillus acidophilus La5 (Firmicutes), Bifidobacterium BB12 (Actinobacteria), and Lactobacillus casei DN001 108 (Firmicutes)*.[109]

- Prebiotics are also important. A study was conducted of 58 obese postmenopausal women. They were divided groups consuming (1) a placebo; (2) high dose *L. paracasei F19;* or (3)10 grams of flaxseed mucilage daily. Over six weeks flaxseed mucilage enhanced the numbers of 33 types of intestinal bacteria and decreased 3 others. However, that change alone could not explain the improvements shown in insulin sensitivity.[110]

- A study compared microbiome changes in lab animals fed various diets. Not too surprisingly, the research showed that the animals on a high fat diet (37.5 percent of total calories as fat) consumed more calories and gained more weight in comparison to those on a low fat diet (10 percent of calories as fat). It is interesting that the bacteria of the mice whose diet was higher in *lard* ended up more closely resembling the *low fat* diet when compared to mice whose fat came from *milk* or *safflower* oil. Those eating lard also had less inflammation. We have known that oils high in omega-6 fatty acids, such as safflower oil, corn, and soy, are inflammatory. However, I for one was not aware that one reason for that inflammatory impact was the fats' effect on gut bacteria.[111]

- In that same study *Firmicutes* increased more with milk and vegetable oil feed than on lard. *Bacteroidetes* was dramatically higher in the animals on the low fat diet / high carbohydrate diet.

- Children supplemented for one month on a combination of probiotics and prebiotics improved body weight and blood fats compared to controls.[112]

Reviews of Studies

Scientists often look for common threads among a collection of studies done by others. From such a review they hope to make more definitive conclusions. One review study selected 61 out of 613 original pieces of research to review. The authors concluded that among the various studies of probiotics and pre-biotics, "the main effect observed was the increase in *bifidobacteria*, usually accompanied by weight loss and enhancement of parameters related to obesity."[113] Another review of studies found only 4 that met their criteria and did not find proof of a demonstrable effect of probiotics on weight loss.[114] What I find most puzzling is that the authors of the reviews somehow managed to come to conclusions when the studies used were all so different. They used different probiotics, prebiotics, and foods with different types of subjects over different time frames.

Probiotic Strain Takeaway

I wish I could say "swallow XYZ probiotic pill and the pounds will melt off." Unfortunately, the science just isn't there yet. As we've seen, many individual strains and sub-species of probiotics show weight loss benefit—even many that belong to the supposedly "fat phylum" *Firmicutes*. So, perhaps the main point to be taken from all of these studies is that the obese suffer from a poor diversity of bacterial strains in their intestines.[115] In virtually all studies, those with greater bacterial diversity had lower fasting blood sugar, lower insulin levels, and less body fat. That would imply that multistrain probiotic supplements would likely be of the most benefit as they were in the research. And it obviously makes a big difference what we feed our microbes. For example, we saw that flax is good and surprisingly lard may be preferable over vegetable oil. A study found that obese subjects who consumed at least 30 grams of fiber daily lost almost as much weight as those on a very restricted diet. We can guess that one reason for that effect was that the fiber encouraged beneficial bacteria.

The lack of scientific consensus will not prevent companies from marketing probiotic products claimed to benefit weight loss. For instance, after being annoyed by several spam emails for a diet product, I searched the internet for it. (I won't give the name for fear a casual reader might get the idea that I recommend it.) The product contains just a single bacterial strain, and I could find no studies supporting its use in dieting. All we know is that the strain is a spore former, and most reviews of the product were quite negative. Apparently any weight loss benefit would likely come from its stimulating herbal ingredient.

Suggested Steps

I suspect that some diet plans are self-defeating not only because they ignore the many divergent causes of excess listed early in this discussion of weight loss but also our responsibility to properly feed our probiotic team. In Chapter 7 we discussed the health importance of selecting foods for the kind bacteria that we want to flourish, and to avoid feeding harmful bacteria the foods that they like. It also appears crucial to eat foods that will consistently support the bacteria that encourage a lean body. Diet alone can change the balance of fat/lean producing strains. Even if a person could find supplements of the ideal leanness strains, they may well not stick around in the gut if the person lives on a junky diet. For example, one of the strains associated with leanness, *Verrucomicrobia (Akkermansia),* thrives on mucilage and fiber. (That strain may benefit us in part by creating substances that feed other friendly microorganisms.) On a steady diet of processed foods it would likely become depleted for lack of fuel.

Happily, we aren't talking about some bizarre diet, but rather the same nutritious foods that we should be eating anyway to prevent chronic disease. As it turns out, when we cut sweets and soft drinks to reduce the risk of diabetes, eat vegetables for their cancer protective properties, and exercise for our heart there is a multiplier effect from those activities because they also help our microbiome. For example, as I mentioned in the sections on yeast, those pathogens thrive on sugary, sweet, and starchy foods. Those are the same foods that also cause unstable blood sugar and set us up for diabetes, heart disease, cancer, and Alzheimer's disease—and of course, obesity. The more refined and processed those starchy/sweet foods are, the worse they are for us and our gut (both the inside and the one that hangs over our belts). Those highly processed foods by definition have the fewest nutrients. They also contain the most additives, which as you will recall includes emulsifiers with their negative effects on our probiotics and artificial sweeteners that reduce diversity. (By the way, most studies do not support the idea that artificial sweeteners help with weight loss.) A good diet can certainly have treats. For instance, chocolate (the darker the better) is considered food for good bacteria.

We can reduce our consumption of foods that we know are not good for us by keeping our brains from playing tricks on us. Brian Wansink, Ph.D., and his team at Cornell University have done remarkable, creative, and sometimes hilarious work showing how subtle clues change what we eat and how much. I listed his book in Resources on page 207, but a lot of valuable information is available free on the website foodpsychology.cornell.edu.

Eating quality non-processed proteins, vegetables, nuts, seeds, good fats, and whole fruits (less sweet is preferred) nourishes a better class of bacteria. Dairy and whole grains may be beneficial for those persons who tolerate them. (It might pay to be cautious of overdoing gluten in wheat, rye, and barley because of the concern that it seems to be a factor that worsens leaky gut. And some studies suggest that our microbiome does better on less meat and fat, but there are some confounding factors in those studies.) The foods just listed are part of the Mediterranean diet, which seems to lead to good health. I should point out that the Mediterranean diet is actually a *high fat* diet and is rich in fermented foods.

Other Considerations

Many medications can cause weight gain. For example, a study of 28,000 people over ten years found that those who took statin cholesterol-lowering drugs ate more and gained significantly more weight than those not taking the drug. Whether the drug affected the chemistry or the gut microbes or just caused a change in attitude, the fat was real.

CONCLUSION

In Part Two we have looked at how probiotics are related to improving an astonishing range of health problems. However, when we recall that we are each host to trillions of microorganisms in thousands of sub-strains with an enormous assortment of biochemical tasks, we are probably just seeing the tip of the iceberg. If the reader's pet peeve was not one of the complaints covered, there is nothing to lose and potentially much to gain by supporting gut health using the methods we've discussed. And, since many bacteria, some fungi, some parasites, and even some viruses can be *helpful*, we need to be very cautious about the use of strong drugs aimed at wiping out a whole category.

Conclusion

You may have noticed that the word "amazing" has just about been worn out. That's why I made a conscious effort not to use it to describe discoveries about the microbiome. But, that was a challenge because the word is truly appropriate in this case. Discovery of the impossibly huge and intricate contributions of our microscopic residents to health makes this an extremely exciting time. We certainly don't have all the answers yet, but at least we have begun to ask the right questions. Our little probiotic friends have gone from deep in the shadows to the cutting edge of an entirely new medical paradigm. Hopefully this book has given readers an improved view of that seismic shift.

Surely we all want to live full vibrant lives and die from simply having had too many birthdays. Unfortunately, the quality and quantity of our lives are too often shortened by chronic disease. It is great news that we can prevent and reverse most diseases by addressing their root causes and even alter the way our genes behave. Early nutritional healers observed that death and health both begin in the digestive tract. They were way ahead of their time even if they didn't know exactly what was going on in there. Science has begun filling in those information gaps as it broadens its focus from simply killing dangerous bacteria to also nurturing the ones that we so desperately need.

I had seen probiotics improve the health of my clients and family for decades. However, before digging into the science to document exactly how friendly bacteria prevent and reverse so many problems, I didn't properly appreciate how fundamental these microscopic allies are to our very life. Perhaps highlighting some of the benefits again will help assure that we don't become complacent about caring for them. Our friendly flora:

- boost the effectiveness of our own immune function

- create brain chemicals to improve mood and reduce appetite

- create selective antibiotics and antimicrobials that only attack the bad bacteria

- help digest our food and facilitate better absorption of nutrients

- improve detoxification

- increase energy

- manufacture important vitamins, such as vitamin K2

- protect us from leaky gut and fungus overgrowth, and in turn the many problems those can create

- reduce cholesterol and protect it from oxidation

- reduce inflammation

- suppress microorganisms that would make us fat

It is hard to exaggerate the importance of our good bacteria. We now know that they are actually a part of the body's instruction manual because their massive collective DNA supplies information that is not covered by our own genes. It seems that humans just didn't need to develop certain abilities because the bacteria were always handling those chores for us. With probiotics and good nutrition we can turn on our own beneficial genes and quiet the scary ones.

Sadly, there is a big chemical risk to our individual and societal microbiomes—pharmaceutical drugs. It is said that history is written by the winners. Until now, that would make the pharmaceutical companies the authors, given that *two-thirds* of Americans over age 65 take three or more drugs. Certainly we are grateful to have some modern drugs for emergencies and to give symptom relief to those unwilling or unable to solve their problems with changes in diet and lifestyle. But, TV commercials make it seem that there is something *wrong with us* if we do *not* have heartburn, erectile dysfunction, arthritis, depression, obesity, diabetes, obstructive lung disease, and so on. (Such degenerative problems may be *typical*, but they are far from *normal*.) While the actors in the commercials distract us by demonstrating how happily they get by now in spite of their disease, the audio cautions about frightening and even life-threatening side effects. (The ads don't even mention that most are hard on our good bacteria.) The side effects can lead to more drugs, putting the patient on a slippery slope to *polypharmacy* (taking many drugs), and *crisis medicine*.

Polypharmacy is obviously good business for drug companies. However, it is now apparent that a diverse natural blend of intestinal bacteria can resolve many health conditions that would otherwise require medication. I hope we do not see pushback from the powerful pharmaceutical industry. With history as a guide, that reaction could look something like what happened to herbs. Herbs used to be our medicines. While drugs can be blunt instruments that make the body do something that it isn't necessarily inclined to do, a whole complex herb (much like a nutrient or probiotic) might accomplish the same mission but do so more gently by supporting the body to do better what it would normally be inclined to do. Used properly, herbs seldom cause side effects. Very often a pharmaceutical company saw how therapeutic a particular herb was; isolated *one* of its molecular constituents; approximated it with a new-to-the-planet chemical; patented it and created a monopoly.

Of course, we wouldn't expect them to be *supportive* of the herbal competition—that would be like expecting the local car dealer to promote the idea of riding a bike to work. But, they used their powerful influence to have the herb condemned by medical schools and officials as being too crude. Herbs are now forbidden to make any claims for preventing or curing disease. It was easy enough to put pressure on herbs because FDA regulators are most comfortable when they can look at one molecule for a single effect over a short duration as they do with drug testing. Herbs are complex and that type of testing is not appropriate for them. It may also not be suitable to probiotics. Harvard's Lee Kaplan, MD, PHD made a very telling point when he said, "even drugs don't fit the drug model" because they have wide-ranging effects, but typically only one is studied.

If probiotics followed the pattern of herbs and becoming prescription drugs, higher prices will result. Worse yet, we might see attempts to limit the use of our handy non-prescription probiotics. When the government does get around to crafting probiotic regulations, we must be alert to any efforts to force probiotics into that drug model. Their action against Phillips' probiotics (discussed in the Introduction) hints that they might be naturally inclined to go that route.

However, we do want the government to be on alert for unfair profiteering—something such as a snack manufacturer lacing its product with a bacterial strain to increase our cravings for snacks. (That is not far-fetched because whistle blowers have exposed similar tactics with chemical additives.) Since patentable uniqueness is so motivating to industry, it concerns me that we will see genetic modification of probiotic bacteria (GMB's or designer bugs) with unknown, unintended long-term consequences. Hopefully the FDA will keep a lid on that.

The massive industry that has been created to treat our illnesses has itself already become one of our biggest threats to wellness and is a reason that the U.S. remains the unhealthiest nation in the developed world. That is in spite of spending twice as much on "health care" (more accurately "disease care"). A group of concerned doctors surveyed the medical literature and showed that the combination of medication side effects, hospital-acquired infections, medical mistakes, and so forth add up to an annual death total greater than that from heart disease.[116] Learn more about efforts to protect us at patientsafetyamerica.com

If it wasn't such serious business, given the weight of science on the risks of antibiotics and the *benefits of probiotics,* it would be hilarious that mainstream medicine still seems more comfortable giving *antibiotics* than *probiotics.* But, alas, the natural approach versus pharmaceuticals is not really a fair fight. As an example of a problem that is all too common, in 2015 Nexium makers payed a $7.9 million fine to settle charges that it offered kickbacks to insure that its product was prescribed. Even more fundamentally, pharmaceutical companies pay to train doctors to use their products, but physicians have to pay out of their own pockets for training in nutrition and natural methods.

In spite of the lopsided odds, many mainstream doctors are now finding that simply handing out ever greater numbers of prescriptions for an ever increasing list of symptoms isn't the healing mission that they signed up for. Most physicians appreciate the health benefits of diet and exercise, but the current system does not reimburse them to take the time to counsel patients about them. It ends up just easier to follow the official cookbook known as the "standard of care," and that usually means more drugs.

Functional medicine is a good deal for patient, practitioner, and society. It is a gentler and more patient-centered way of practicing, and it is significantly more rewarding for doctors. They see real cures and patients who *thrive* instead of just *survive.* This discipline teaches about balance; about what goes on at the cellular level; and the concept that we lose health slowly over time due to the gradual accumulation of small insults from inadequate nutrition, toxins, and imbalanced intestinal flora. It is the medical equivalent of an airline pilot who leaves New York headed for Los Angeles. She/he makes a number of small course corrections to account for changing conditions, and thereby avoids ending up in Alaska by mistake. Doctors who are inspired to practice functional medicine often are much more satisfied and become less reliant on insurance reimbursements. Unfortunately, patients who rely solely on health insurance may not currently have access to a functional medicine doctor or even a Certified Clinical Nutritionist.

But, anyone can apply the principles discussed in this book as an excellent start to better health and vitality. We don't have to wait the decades it may take for mainstream medicine to reach some arbitrary end point of scientific agreement. There is potentially fantastic benefit and no harm in doing a sensible probiotic reboot right now. Author/nurse, Tana Amen, a fan of probiotics, tells her children to treat their friendly bacteria as though they were *beloved pets*. What a great idea! We should make looking out for their welfare a permanent part of our lifestyle.

However, probiotics can only go so far to protect us if we smoke or drink to excess. They are not a substitute for exercising or for drinking sufficient water or for changing jobs if the one that we have is too stressful. Probiotics can't keep us from texting while we drive.

Glossary

acidophilus. A long studied and popular strain of lactic acid probiotic bacteria. Its proper name is *Lactobacillus acidophilus*.

adhesion. The colonization of microorganisms in the intestinal tract, in contrast to strains of bacteria that are transient (just passing through).

aerobic bacteria. They need oxygen to grow.

anaerobic bacteria. These will die if exposed to oxygen. ("Facultative anaerobes" can grow with, or without oxygen.)

antibiotic. The word means "against life" and is a substance that kills microorganisms. In generic medical terminology that can include fungi and parasites. However, "antibiotic" is typically used to mean to anti-*bacterial* drugs. They are not effective against viruses, but they are often being prescribed for colds and flu anyway. Most antibiotics prescribed are mycotoxins produced by fungi. Although some have a narrow range of action, many are "broad spectrum" meaning that they kill friendly bacteria along with the pathogenic ones.

antibiotic-resistance. Bacteria develop the ability to survive antibiotic treatment. This is a dangerous world-wide threat caused by the overuse of antibiotics.

antioxidant. An antidote to oxidants. Oxidants are also known as free radicals that can be generated by radiation, smoking, toxins, and even normal processes in the body. These unstable entities can damage our cells, probiotics, DNA, and nutrients. Antioxidants can be vitamins, minerals, enzymes, or nutrients from plants. Glutathione is known as the master antioxidant.

atopic dermatitis. The medical name for chronic or relapsing non-contagious, inflammatory, itchy skin disorders. Eczema is often used as a synonym.

bacteria. The name of a domain of single cell microorganisms. They come in a variety of shapes and sizes and are found almost everywhere on earth. There may be millions of types with wide-ranging activities.

bacteriocins. *Selective* antimicrobials created by bacteria to fight their enemies that often happen to also be our disease-causing enemies.

bacterium. The singular of bacteria.

bifidobacterium. Anaerobic bacteria that grow in the intestines of mammals. Several strains are used as probiotics. They are members of the phylum *Actinobacteria*.

biofilms. Mixed colonies of microorganisms protected under slimy coverings. Various species contribute specialized functions to the commune. Those near the surface protect the organisms in the middle from threats, such as antibiotics and basically feed them. In return, those in the middle might secrete a growth factor that benefits the border guards. But, since both residents compete for resources, either one can withdraw its support when their survival is threatened. This is a relatively new and exciting field of study.[1]

biogenics. Sometimes this term is applied to the bacteriocins, enzymes, organic acids, vitamins, and other substances created by probiotics. However, because "biogenics" is also used for other substances produced by plants and animals, I prefer my term "Postbiotics."

candida. A type of yeast that can get out of control in the intestinal tract, the respiratory tract, or other parts of the body and cause serious symptoms. Yeasts commonly grow to a problematic scale because antibiotics have killed our probiotics. Yeast overgrowth is difficult to diagnose in the typical medical office because the symptoms are often subtle, varied, and seemingly unrelated to the gut. To determine whether or not you have an overgrowth of yeast, you may find the questionnaire in the back of this book helpful, *see* page 211.

c-diff. *Clostridium difficile* is a bacterial disease that can cause intractable and potentially lethal diarrhea when the bacteria have become resistant to common antibiotics. Fecal Microbiota Transplantation (FMT) is presently the most effective treatment for critical cases.

CFU. *See* colony forming units.

colony forming units. This usually means the number of probiotic cells that were bottled. With freeze-dried bacteria that figure would usually be much greater than the number that would be expected to have survived processing with sufficient vigor, to be capable of reproducing in the digestive tract.

commensal. One organism benefits from another without affecting it. Although the term is often applied to our friendly bacteria, it seems outdated now that we know the benefits are a two-way street.

cultured food probiotic complex. The type of supplement that most closely resembles fermented foods. The capsules contain the Postbiotics created over years of fermentation as well as live organisms and their food supply consisting of mixed fruits, vegetables, seaweeds, and herbs. This type will contain fewer CFU's, but be better able to support the person's own unique flora.

diversity. In the gut, flora refers to the importance of a wide variety of bacterial types because each has its own benefits, and the variety avoids allowing any single strain to get out of hand.

eczema. A chronic inflammatory skin condition also known as atopic dermatitis. Functional medicine practitioners link this condition to the gut.

enteric. Having to do with the human gastrointestinal tract. "Enteric coating" usually means a coating applied to bacteria or a capsule to protect it from stomach and bile acids.

enterotypes. A way of referring to the broad community in a particular microbiome.

FDA. *See* Food and Drug Administration.

fecal transplant/fecal microbiota transplantation. The insertion into an ill person's GI tract the bacterial content from the digestive tract of a healthy person. Although most commonly used for *C-Diff*, it has also been suggested for conditions ranging from obesity and autism to mental illness. That suggests the new respect that probiotics are attaining.

fermented foods/beverages. Foods or liquids that have been changed by bacteria or yeasts over time. Fermented foods can become more digestible and nutrient-dense as well as less allergenic. Pickling and brewing are examples of the process.

flora. The entire collection of organisms in the intestinal tract. Most commonly used to refer to the friendly bacteria. *See* microbiome.

FMT. *See* fecal transplant/fecal microbiota transplantation.

Food and Drug Administration. The U.S. government agency charged with protecting us from dangerous and unproven drugs and contaminated food. They have a huge job and insufficient funding. However, many studies show that they are too friendly with drug companies, and they have evidenced a historic bias against natural remedies.

FOS. *See* fructooligosaccharides.

fructooligosaccharides. Indigestible fibers added to supplements as a prebiotic. In amounts greater than 10 grams a day causes gas and bloating in some people.

functional medicine. A philosophy of health practice that according to functionalmedicine.org, "addresses the underlying causes of disease using a systems-oriented approach and engaging both patient and practitioner in a therapeutic partnership."

fungi. The plural of fungus. These planimals (sort of like plants and sort of like animals) include yeasts. They can be either friendly or pathogenic. *Candida* is the most well-known health issue related to them.

glutathione. The "master antioxidant" that recycles other antioxidants, such as vitamins C and E as well as coenzyme Q10. It is required to make and repair DNA. Glutathione reduces inflammation and detoxifies pesticides and heavy metals. It is thought of as an anti-aging substance that diminishes the effects of stress as well as improves energy and brain function. It is made in the body but often in insufficient quantities, due for example to age, alcohol, and disease. Food and oral supplements are not good sources. The bacterial strain *Lactobacillus fermentum ME-3* has been shown to raise blood levels.

gluten. A somewhat sticky protein found in wheat, barley, and rye. For persons with Celiac disease it causes serious disease, but may also be problematic for a much larger percentage of the public, not just from undiagnosed sensitivity, but also because it may lead to relaxing of the tight junctions between cells in the intestinal lining.

h. pylori. *See* helicobacter pylori.

healthy user bias. A factor that skews conclusions from scientific studies. Data can be misleading if researchers study one factor, but do not adequately control for the other things a person might be eating or doing. For example, a person who eats more fruits, vegetables, and fiber may also eat fewer food additives and practice yoga.

helicobacter pylori. A strain of bacteria that is the cause of the most prevalent infection worldwide. Oddly, although it is blamed for 70 percent of ulcers, it causes no symptoms for most people, and the absence of it is associated with other problems.

hygiene hypothesis. A theory advanced by David Strachan in 1989 to describe the idea that we have become so sanitation-minded that we are killing off entire species of bacteria that we need for health.

inulin. A type of indigestible fiber (a fructan or long chains of simple sugars called polysaccharides) added to supplements as a prebiotic. It is typically derived from chicory or artichoke and seems to boost the *numbers* of probiotics but *not their diversity.*

lactic acid bacteria. So named because they can turn lactose (milk sugar) and other sugars into lactic acid. Some strains are used in the making of yogurt, cheese, sauerkraut, and other foods and beverages.

lactobacillus. Rod shaped bacteria that comprise most of the probiotic group called lactic acid bacteria. Some strains can live with or without oxygen, and they are found in the mouth, GI tract, vagina, and nasal cavity.

lactobacillus fermentum ME-3. A strain of probiotic isolated from the GI tract of a healthy one year old Estonian child. Is noted mainly for its ability to increase blood levels of the master antioxidant glutathione, but it also increases another antioxidant, superoxide dismutase (SOD). *ME-3* has been shown to withstand stomach and bile acids and to implant in the digestive tract.

leaky gut syndrome. A double whammy condition where the lining of the intestine (1) no longer acts as an effective barrier against the seepage of pathogens, toxins, and food components from the gut into blood circulation and (2) reduces the absorption into circulation of necessary nutrients. In this state of hyper permeability, villi are flattened and the tight junctions between cells are loosened. Yeast is a common cause of the problem, and the result can be a worsening of almost any health condition imaginable.

meta-analysis. A type of study that reviews a number of similar studies to find trends that support broad-based conclusions.

metabolite. A product of some type of metabolism (a chemical reaction in the body). Bacteria make a great many metabolites (such as short chain fatty acids, bacteriocins, enzymes, vitamins, signaling molecules, and so on). I include those, bacterial cell walls and DNA in the term "Postbiotics."

methicillin-resistant staphylococcus aureus. A strain of pathogenic bacteria that no longer responds to antibiotics. Originally, known mainly as a hospital-acquired infection, it is now also contracted in nursing homes, prisons, and even gyms.

microbiome. The collection of all microorganisms living in and on the body. It and "microbiota" are fancier terms for flora. The microbiome weighs several pounds; contains 100 times as many cells as our own; consists of several thousand subspecies; and provides up to 1,000 as much DNA as the human genome. The dominant species in the microbiome are from the phyla *Bacteroidetes* and *Firmicutes*.

microbiota. For all practical purposes, the same as "microbiome" or "flora."

microorganisms. Microscopic life forms.

microvilli. Small protrusions on villi that add additional surface area for the absorption of nutrients in the intestines. In the colon they may absorb mostly water. *See also* villi.

mitochondria. Known as the tiny energy factories inside cells, these organelles contain a substantial amount of DNA (different from that in our own cells) that is apparently inherited from our mother's mitochondria. Scientists believe mitochondria may have originally been bacteria that became permanent residents providing benefit to humans in turn for a place to live.

MRSA. *See methicillin-resistant staphylococcus aureus.*

mutualistic. Co-operation between organisms.

mycotoxins. Toxic substances produced by fungi. These can form on crops or be made by yeasts inside our bodies.

neurotransmitter. A chemical that the body makes to send a message to a nerve or the brain or that is sent from nerve tissues to cells to activate them in some way.

nosocomial. An infection acquired in a hospital or clinic.

pasteurization. The heating of food to kill bacteria.

placebo. A fake inactive substance or procedure used in a study to provide a comparison with the active subject of the study. As it turns out, because of the powerful mind/body connection, the "placebo effect" can be quite powerful. In some studies the placebo beats a medicine. Interestingly, for FDA drug approval, new medicines only need to be compared to other drugs, not to placebo.

prebiotics. Food for bacteria. The types of bacteria that flourish depend greatly on the food we provide. In the best cases this is the fiber and nutrients supplied in fruits, vegetables, spices, herbs, and seaweeds. In supplement pills prebiotics are more often inulin or FOS.

probiotics. Microorganisms that provide benefits to the host, either naturally occurring in the body or taken as supplements. These can be bacteria or more rarely, yeast cells.

postbiotics. A wide variety of substances made by probiotics as well as some remnants of the probiotics. These may include selective antimicrobials, enzymes, vitamins, organic acids, signaling compounds, amino acids, neurotransmitters, short chain fatty acids, as well as the cell walls and DNA from bacteria that are no longer active.

quorum sensing. The process whereby microorganisms take inventory of the numbers of their own kind and communicate that information using unique chemical "words" and specialized receptors. When they *sense* they have sufficient number (a *quorum*) they may change their behavior. That may be what is going on when yeasts change form during an overgrowth in the GI tract.

species. Near the bottom of the hierarchy in taxonomy. A fairly specific description. Sub-species are more specific yet. *See* also taxonomy.

strains. Term used interchangeably with species and often sub-species.

sub-clinical. Imbalances in the body that are not sufficiently advanced to show up on typical clinical tests. Although they might be detected by specialized testing these imbalances often stay under the radar and lead to disease later. Examples would be nutrition insufficiencies, toxic accumulations, and some thyroid issues. Sometimes there are visible signs, such as in the case of a vitamin C deficiency that can cause bleeding gums, but the situation is not serious enough to be diagnosed as scurvy.

sub-species. Names given to microorganisms when there are noticeable changes to a species, but the alterations are not sufficient to warrant declaring it an entirely new species.

symbiotic. This is a very broad term covering various types of interactions among groups. It is a bit confusing to use in regard to our friendly flora because it is broad and sometimes used to cover even parasitic relationships.

synbiotics. Combinations of prebiotics and probiotics.

taxonomy. In biology a system of relative identification that uses a hierarchy of ever more specific levels. In this listing of the levels, brackets demonstrate a specific example: life (versus rocks), domain (bacteria), phylum (*Firmicutes*), class (*Bacilli*), family (*Lactobacillaceae*), genus (*Lactobacillus*), species (*Lactobacillus acidophilus*), and sub-species (*Lactobacillus acidophilus La5*).

toll receptors. Like a guard checking ID's at the entrance to a restricted building, the intestinal track checks out bacteria using something called toll receptors or pattern recognition receptors to determine if they are friend or foe. If these PRR's are damaged, mouse studies show that intestinal imbalance, inflammation, and even obesity may result.[2]

United States Department of Agriculture. An agency charged with the often conflicting responsibilities of promoting good nutrition while also supporting U.S. agribusiness.

USDA. *See* United States Department of Agriculture.

villi. Tiny protrusions on the membranes lining the intestines. They greatly increase the surface area available for the absorption of nutrients in the small intestine. Similar structures in the large intestine have been thought to mainly absorb water, but that idea may be revisited. On these villi are even finer protrusions called microvilli. Both can be flattened out by "leaky gut."

viruses. Bits of genetic material that infect cells of plants, animals, and bacteria and cause the host to do whatever is in the interests of the virus.

Resources

HEALTH MEDIA

Healthy by Nature Show with Martie Whittekin, CCN
Website: HBNShow.com
Source of a free health Library (articles on various aspects of health and resources for finding holistic practitioners), information on the show, e-news, and a book store that sells some of the books below

Know the Cause with Doug Kaufmann
Website: KnowTheCause.com
Syndicated health television show

The People's Pharmacy
Website: PeoplesPharmacy.com
Syndicated radio program, newspaper column, and web resources

Total Wellness Newsletter by Sherry Rogers, MD
Website: prestigepublishing.com
Phone: (Toll Free) 1-800-846-6687
(exceptionally well documented newsletter)

RECOMMENDED BOOKS

Appleton, Nancy, PhD. *Killer Colas: The Hard Truth About Soft Drinks*. Garden City Park, New York: Square One Publishers, 2011.

Bentley, Nancy Lee. *Truly Cultured: Rejuvenating Taste, Health and Community with Naturally Fermented Foods*. Nancy Lee Bentley, 2008 (Contains easy recipes and a lot of helpful information on fermented foods.)

Crook, William G., MD. *The Yeast Connection Handbook: How Yeasts Can Make You Feel Sick All Over and the Steps You Need to Take to Regain Your Health*. Garden City Park, New York: Square One Publishers, 2007.

Gittleman, Ann Louise, Ph.D. CNS. *Guess What Came to Dinner: Parasites and Your Health*. New York: Penguin Publishing Group, 2001.

Halpern, Georges M., MD, PhD. *Ulcer Free*. Garden City Park, New York: Square One Publishers, 2006.

Kaufmann, Doug. *The Fungus Link: An Introduction to Fungal Disease Including the Initial Phase Diet.* Rockwall, Texas: MediaTrition, 2000.

Murray, Michael T., N.D. and Pizzorno, Joseph, ND. *Encyclopedia of Natural Medicine,* 2nd Edition. New York: Three Rivers Press, 1997.

Rheaume-Bleue, Kate. *Vitamin K2 and the Calcium Paradox.* Hoboken, New Jersey: John Wiley & Sons, 2011. (This book also discusses the work of pioneering dentist Weston A. Price.)

Smith, Kyle, DC. *Brighter Mind.* Brighter Mind Media Group, Ltd. 2011

Wansink, Brian Ph.D. *Slim by Design: Mindless Eating Solutions for Everyday Life.* William Morrow, 2014.

Whittekin, Martie CCN. *Natural Alternative to Nexium, Maalox, Tagament, Prilosec & Other Acid Blockers: What to Use to Relieve Acid Reflux, Heartburn, and Gastric Ailments Medications.* Garden City, New York: Square One Publishers, 2012.

PRODUCTS AND SOURCES

Please remember that I do not work for any product manufacturer or retailer. The products I mention are ones that I know to be of uniquely superior quality and effectiveness as well as being the ones I have used myself and would provide to my family. Because the emphasis with these items is on *value* rather than *cheap price,* they will likely not be found in the mass/big box discount market but rather in natural food stores. For more updated information on products go HBNShow.com/TheProbioticCure.

Dr. Ohhira's Probiotics (Original and Professional).
This is the cultured food probiotic complex supplement discussed in the book. It is made with 12 strains fermented for years with dozens of nutritious plant materials. The culture medium, probiotics, and Postbiotics are all included in the capsule. Information on the probiotic soap (Kampuku Beauty Bar) and a store locator at EssentialFormulas.com

Fem-Dophilus by Jarrow Formulas
Contains two probiotic strains, *Lactobacillus rhamnosus, GR-1* and *Lactobacillus reuteri, RC-14.* It is an oral supplement that has been shown in over twenty-five years of research to promote health of the urinary tract and vagina.

Friendly Yeast. *Saccharomyces Boulardii*+MOS by Jarrow Formulas.
This product is *not harmed by antibiotics.* MOS (MannanOligoSaccharides) in the product is an oligosaccharide that can discourage pathogenic bacteria from adhering to the cells lining the GI tract. This or other brands of the yeast are available in most natural food stores.

Memory Works
A supplement created by the author of *Brighter Mind* and the originator of well-known Focus Factor. I find it not only makes me feel sharper but also reduces my sweet cravings. Available at xenesta.com/healthy.

Organic Fiber Prebiotic
Created by a doctor who tests for GI issues. The products are made with whole organic blueberries and muscadine grapes. Order direct at theorganic alternative.com.

Propolis Plus
This is Brazilian green propolis with antioxidants and probiotics formulated by Dr. Ohhira. Find a store locator at EssentialFormulas.com

Probimune
Liquid multi-strain probiotic in a dropper bottle. Order from YoungHealth .com or call 800-770-4470.

Stomach Formula by Lily of the Desert
This contains Aloe Vera that is very rich in high molecular weight poly-saccharides that is blended with digestion-soothing herbs and minerals. The company also makes organic Aloe Vera. Available in most natural food stores nationwide.

SUPPLIER OF PROBIOTIC STRAINS

UASLabs has thirty years of experience in probiotic formulation and has won several awards. They supply a large selection of well researched bacteria to a number of high quality brands both retail and health professional private labels. Most importantly, the company adheres strictly to the guidelines of Good Manufacturing Practices. Learn more at uaslabs.com.

Reg'Activ
This is the brand that contains *Lactobacillus fermentum ME-3*, the strain shown to over twenty years of research increase glutathione levels. Reg'Activ has been on the market for many years as a cardiovascular formula sold only in Europe. Recently, it has become available in the U.S. in three combinations with nutrients specifically for Cardio Wellness, Immune/Vitality, and Detox/ Liver Health. Find a store locator at Essential Formulas.com

USEFUL LINKS

DirtDoctor.com
Source of non-toxic organic approaches for home, garden, and landscape.

Enterolab.com
EnteroLab is a registered and fully accredited clinical laboratory specializing in the analysis of intestinal specimens for food sensitivities (such as gluten) that cause a variety of symptoms and diseases.

EWG.org
The Environmental Working Group is a great source of information about avoiding toxins in food and skin care products.

FunctionalMedicine.org
Information on a type of medicine frequently referred to in this book.

HBNShow.com/TheProbioticCure
This is a direct link to this book.

JustLabelIt.org
Information about Genetically Modified Foods.

NonGMOProject.org
Information about Genetically Modified Foods.

SaveAntibiotics.org
Campaign on Human Health and Industrial Farming by the Pew Charitable Trusts.

TheVitalityNetwork.com
This online, on-demand video library includes a number of video segments by the author on topics like heartburn, diet, and many individual food categories, such as sugar.

VitaminDCouncil.org
Non-profit source of vitamin D information.

Zip code locator of who represents you in Washington, DC
https://www.opencongress.org/people/zipcodelookup

Candida Questionnaire and Score Sheet

Complete this comprehensive questionnaire to determine if your health problems are likely related to an overgrowth of yeast. The score of the questionnaire will give you at least a general idea. A nutrition-oriented health professional can also perform lab tests to confirm the connection. However, many will simply use a trial of the yeast-controlling program because it is not risky, does not cost much, and may well improve your health in any case. See Chapter 9 for more information about the effect of yeast and remedies. If symptoms persist, consult your doctor.

SECTION A: History. These are factors that promote the growth of Candida Albicans and that frequently are found in people with yeast-related health problems. Circle the score for those that questions to which you answer "yes."

	Point Score
Have you taken tetracyclines or other antibiotics for acne for *one month or longer*?	35
Have you at any time in your life taken broad-spectrum antibiotics or other antibacterial medication for respiratory, urinary, or other infections for *two months or longer,* or in shorter courses four or more times in a one-year period?	35
Have you taken a broad-spectrum antibiotic drug—even in a single dose?	6
Have you, at any time in your life, been bothered by persistent prostatitis, vaginitis, or other problems affecting your reproductive organs?	25
Are you bothered by memory or concentration problems—do you sometimes feel boggy brained or spaced out?	20
Do you feel "sick all over" yet, in spite of visits to many different physicians, the causes haven't been found?	25

	Point Score
Have you been pregnant *two or more* times?	5
Have you been pregnant *one time* only?	3
Have you taken birth control pills for *more than two years*?	15
Have you taken birth control pills for *six months to two years*?	8
Have you taken steroids orally, injected, or inhaled for *more than two weeks*?	15
Have you taken steroids orally, injected, or inhaled for *two weeks or less*?	6
Do perfumes, insecticides, fabric shops, and other chemicals provoke *moderate to severe* symptoms?	20
Do perfumes, insecticides, fabric shops, and other chemicals provoke *mild* symptoms?	5
Does tobacco smoke really bother you?	10
Are your symptoms worse on damp, muggy days, or in moldy places like basements or barns?	20
Have you had *severe or persistent* athlete's foot, ring worm, "jock itch," or other chronic fungus infections of the skin or nails?	20
Have you had *mild to moderate* athlete's foot, ring worm, "jock itch," or other chronic fungus infections of the skin or nails?	10
Do you crave sugar and/or starch?	10

TOTAL OF ALL POINTS CIRCLED IN SECTION A:

SECTION B: Major Symptoms. These symptoms are often present in persons with yeast-related health problems. For each of the symptoms in this section, check the appropriate column indicating your experience. If you do not have the symptom at all, make no mark.

Symptoms	Occasional or Mild	Frequent or Moderately Severe	Severe or Disabling
Abdominal pain			
Attacks of anxiety or crying			
Bloating, belching, or intestinal gas			

Symptoms	Occasional or Mild	Frequent or Moderately Severe	Severe or Disabling
Constipation and/or diarrhea			
Cramps and/or other menstrual irregularities			
Cystitis (urinary tract infection) or interstitial cystitis			
Depression or manic depression			
Endometriosis or infertility			
Fatigue or lethargy			
Feeling of being "drained"			
Headache			
Heartburn, acid reflux			
Hypothyroidism (for example, thinning hair, dry skin, fatigue, weight gain, cold hands or feet, or low body temperature)			
Impotence			
Loss of sexual desire or feeling			
Muscle aches			
Muscle weakness or paralysis			
Numbness, burning, or tingling			
Pain and/or swelling in joints			
Premenstrual tension			
Shaking or irritable when hungry			
Troublesome vaginal burning, itching, or discharge			
Total number of marks in each column			
Multiply the number above by the points assigned to each column	× 3	× 6	× 9
Total points in each column			
TOTAL OF ALL COLUMNS IN SECTION B:			

SECTION C: Other Symptoms. These symptoms are sometimes seen in people with yeast-related problems. They also may be caused by other conditions. Again, for each of the symptoms in this section, put a mark in the appropriate column indicating your experience. If you do not have the symptom, make no mark.

Symptoms	Occasional or Mild	Frequent or Moderately Severe	Severe or Disabling
Bad breath			
Burning or tearing eyes			
Burning on urination			
Chronic hives (urticaria)			
Cough or recurrent bronchitis			
Dizziness/loss of balance			
Drowsiness, including inappropriate drowsiness			
Dry mouth or throat			
Ear pain or deafness			
Eczema, itching eyes			
Foot, hair, or body odor not relieved by washing			
Frequent mood swings			
Indigestion or heartburn			
Insomnia			
Irritability			
Laryngitis, loss of voice			
Mouth rashes, including "white" tongue			
Mucus in stools			
Nasal congestion or postnasal drip			
Nasal itching			
Pain or tightness in chest			

Symptoms	Occasional or Mild	Frequent or Moderately Severe	Severe or Disabling
Poor coordination			
Pressure above ears—feeling of head swelling			
Psoriasis			
Rectal itching			
Recurrent infections or fluid in ears			
Sensitivity to milk, wheat, corn, or other common foods			
Sinus problems—tenderness of cheekbones or forehead			
Sore throat			
Spots in front of eyes or erratic vision			
Tendency to bruise easily			
Urinary frequency or urgency			
Wheezing or shortness of breath			
Total number of marks in each column			
Multiply the number above by the points assigned to each column	× 1	× 2	× 3
Total points in each column			

TOTAL OF ALL COLUMNS IN SECTION C:

Section A _____

+ Section B _____

+ Section C _____

= GRAND TOTAL _____

See the results of your score on the following page.

TOTAL SCORES

Scores in women will run slightly higher, as seven items in the questionnaire apply exclusively to women, while only two apply exclusively to men.

For Women:

180 and up   Yeast-connected health problems are **almost certainly** present.

120 to 179   Yeast-connected health problems are **probably** present.

60 to 119   Yeast-connected health problems are **possibly** present.

59 or lower   Yeasts are **less likely** to be the cause of health problems.

For Men:

140 and up   Yeast-connected health problems are **almost certainly** present.

90 to 139   Yeast-connected health problems are **probably** present.

40 to 89   Yeast-connected health problems are **possibly** present.

39 or lower   Yeasts are **less likely** to be the cause of health problems.

This questionnaire has been adapted and updated from *The Yeast Connection Handbook,* by William G. Crook, MD, published by Square One Publishers, Garden City Park, New York, reprinted by permission of the publisher. I highly recommend this book if you have a high score on the questionnaire.

References

PREFACE

1. Dietert RR. "The Microbiome in Early Life: Self-Completion and Microbiota Protection as Health Priorities." *Birth Defects Res B Dev Reprod Toxicol.* 2014 Jul 10. doi: 10.1002/bdrb.21116.

2. Saei AA1, Barzegari A. "The microbiome: the forgotten organ of the astronaut's body—probiotics beyond terrestrial limits." *Future Microbiol.* 2012 Sep;7(9):1037-46. doi: 10.2217/fmb.12.82.

3. Xu J, Gordon JI. "Honor thy symbionts." *Proc Natl Acad Sci U S A.* 2003 Sep 2;100(18):10452-9.

4. Barzegari A, Saeedi N, Saei AA. "Shrinkage of the human core microbiome and a proposal for launching microbiome biobanks." *Future Microbiol.* 2014 May;9:639-56. doi: 10.2217/fmb.14.22.

5. Melling D. "General practitioners roles and experiences with functional foods containing probiotics and plant sterols." *Prim Health Care Res Dev.* 2014 Aug 7:1-9. [Epub ahead of print]

INTRODUCTION

1. Elmer GW. "Probiotics: 'living drugs'." *Am J Health Syst Pharm.* 2001 Jun 15;58(12):1101-9.

2. Wikoff WR, Anfora AT, Liu J, Schultz PG, Lesley SA, Peters EC, Siuzdak G. "Metabolomics analysis reveals large effects of gut microflora on mammalian blood metabolites." *Proc Natl Acad Sci U S A.* 2009 Mar 10;106(10):3698-703. doi: 10.1073/pnas.0812874106.

3. Braat H, Rottiers P, Hommes DW, Huyghebaert N, Remaut E, Remon JP, van Deventer SJ, Neirynck S, Peppelenbosch MP, Steidler L. "A phase I trial with transgenic bacteria expressing interleukin-10 in Crohn's disease." *Clin Gastroenterol Hepatol.* 2006 Jun;4(6):754-9. Epub 2006 May 22.

CHAPTER ONE

1. Turnbaugh P., Ley R., Hamady M., Fraser-Liggett C., Knight R., Gordon J. "The human microbiome project: exploring the microbial part of ourselves in a changing world." *Nature.* 2007 October 18; 449(7164): 804–810. doi:10.1038/nature06244

2. Walsh CJ, Guinane CM, O'Toole PW, Cotter PD. "Beneficial modulation of the gut microbiota." *FEBS Lett.* 2014 Mar 26. pii: S0014-5793(14)00254-3. doi: 10.1016/j.febslet.2014.03.035.

3. Grice E, Kong H, Conlan S, Deming C, Davis J, Young A, NISC Comparative Sequencing Program, Bouffard G, Blakesley R, Murray P, Green E, Turner M, Segre J. "Topographical and Temporal Diversity of the Human Skin Microbiome" *Science* 29 May 2009: Vol. 324 no. 5931 pp. 1190–1192.

4. Lauran Neergaard . "Scientists find bacterial zoo thrives in our skin." *Associated Press*, May 28, 2009

5. Xu J, Mahowald MA, Ley RE, Lozupone CA, Hamady M, Martens EC, Henrissat B, Coutinho PM, Minx P, Latreille P, Cordum H, Van Brunt A, Kim K, Fulton RS, Fulton LA, Clifton SW, Wilson RK, Knight RD, Gordon JI. "Evolution of symbiotic bacteria in the distal human intestine." *PLoS Biol.* 2007 Jul;5(7):e156.

6. Fierer N, Lauber CL, Zhou N, McDonald D, Costello EK, Knight R. "Forensic identification using skin bacterial communities." *Proc Natl Acad Sci U S A.* 2010 Apr 6;107(14):6477-81. doi: 10.1073/pnas.1000162107.

7. Barzegari A, Saei AA. "Designing probiotics with respect to the native microbiome." *Future Microbiol.* 2012 May;7(5):571-5. doi: 10.2217/fmb.12.37.

8. Lax S, Smith DP, Hampton-Marcell J, Owens SM, Handley KM, Scott NM, Gibbons SM, Larsen P, Shogan BD, Weiss S, Metcalf JL, Ursell LK, Vázquez-Baeza Y, Van Treuren W, Hasan NA, Gibson MK, Colwell R, Dantas G, Knight R, Gilbert JA. "Longitudinal analysis of microbial interaction between humans and the indoor environment." *Science.* 2014 Aug 29;345(6200): 1048–52. doi: 10.1126/science.1254529.

9. Ley RE, Hamady M, Lozupone C, Turnbaugh PJ, Ramey RR, Bircher JS, Schlegel ML, Tucker TA, Schrenzel MD, Knight R, Gordon JI. "Evolution of mammals and their gut microbes." *Science.* 2008 Jun 20;320(5883):1647-51. doi: 10.1126/science.1155725.

10. Karunasena E1 McMahon KW, Kurkure PC, Brashears MM. "A comparison of cell mediators and serum cytokines transcript expression between male and female mice infected with Mycobacterium avium subspecies paratuberculosis and/or consuming probiotics." *Pathog Dis.* 2014 Jul 9. doi: 10.1111/2049-632X.12193.

11. Duffy LC, Raiten DJ, Hubbard VS, Starke-Reed P. "Progress and Challenges in Developing Metabolic Footprints from Diet in Human Gut Microbial Cometabolism." *J Nutr.* 2015 Apr 1. pii: jn194936. [Epub ahead of print]

CHAPTER TWO

1. Sharma R, Kapila R, Dass G, Kapila S. "Improvement in Th1/Th2 immune homeostasis, antioxidative status and resistance to pathogenic E. coli on consumption of probiotic Lactobacillus rhamnosus fermented milk in aging mice." *Age (Dordr).* 2014 Aug;36(4):9686. doi: 10.1007/s11357-014-9686-4.

2. Matsumoto M, Kurihara S. "Probiotics-induced increase of large intestinal luminal polyamine concentration may promote longevity." *Med Hypotheses.* 2011 Oct;77(4):469-72. doi: 10.1016/j.mehy.2011.06.011.

3. Satoh T, Murata M, Iwabuchi N, Odamaki T, Wakabayashi H, Yamauchi K, Abe F, Xiao JZ. "Effect of Bifidobacterium breve B-3 on skin photoaging induced by chronic UV irradiation in mice." *Benef Microbes.* 2015 Mar 25:1-8. [Epub ahead of print]

4. Zhao L, Qiao X, Zhu J, Zhang X, Jiang J, Hao Y, Ren F. "Correlations of fecal bacterial communities with age and living region for the elderly living in Bama, Guangxi, China." *J Microbiol.* 2011 Apr;49(2):186-92. doi: 10.1007/s12275-011-0405-x.

5. von Mutius E, Vercelli D. "Farm living: effects on childhood asthma and allergy." *Nat Rev Immunol.* 2010 Dec;10(12):861-8. doi: 10.1038/nri2871.

6. Hansbro PM, Starkey MR, Kim RY, Stevens RL, Foster PS, Horvat JC. "Programming of the lung by early-life infection." *J Dev Orig Health Dis.* 2012 Jun;3(3):153-158.

7. Peng J, Narasimhan S, Marchesi JR, Benson A, Wong FS, Wen L. "Long term effect of gut microbiota transfer on diabetes development." *J Autoimmun.* 2014 Apr 22. pii: S0896–8411(14)00069-9. doi: 10.1016/j.jaut.2014.03.005.

8. Magrone T, Jirillo E. "The Interleukin-17/Interleukin-22 Innate Axis in the Gut as a New Drug Target in Allergic-Inflammatory and Autoimmune Diseases. A Working Hypothesis." *Endocr Metab Immune Disord Drug Targets.* 2014 Mar 24.

9. Alipour B, Homayouni-Rad A, Vaghef-Mehrabany E, Sharif SK, Vaghef-Mehrabany L, Asghari-Jafarabadi M, Nakhjavani MR, Mohtadi-Nia J. "Effects of Lactobacillus casei supplementation on disease activity and inflammatory cytokines in rheumatoid arthritis patients: a randomized double-blind clinical trial." *Int J Rheum Dis.* 2014 Jun;17(5):519-27. doi: 10.1111/1756-185X.12333.

10. Bedaiwi MK, Inman RD. "Microbiome and probiotics: link to arthritis." *Curr Opin Rheumatol.* 2014 Jul;26(4):410-5. doi: 10.1097/BOR.0000000000000075.

11. Rashid T, Wilson C, Ebringer A. "The link between ankylosing spondylitis, Crohn's disease, Klebsiella, and starch consumption." *Clin Dev Immunol.* 2013;2013:872632. doi: 10.1155/2013/872632. Epub 2013 May 27.

12. Baxter NT, Zackular JP, Chen GY, Schloss PD. "Structure of the gut microbiome following colonization with human feces determines colonic tumor burden." *Microbiome.* 2014 Jun 17;2:20. doi: 10.1186/2049-2618-2-20.

13. Zackular JP, Rogers MA, Ruffin MT 4th, Schloss PD. "The Human Gut Microbiome as a Screening Tool for Colorectal Cancer." *Cancer Prev Res (Phila).* 2014 Aug 7. [Epub ahead of print]

14. Zhong L, Zhang X, Covasa M. "Emerging roles of lactic acid bacteria in protection against colorectal cancer." *World J Gastroenterol.* 2014 Jun 28;20(24):7878-7886.

15. Linsalata M, Orlando A, Russo F. "Pharmacological and dietary agents for colorectal cancer chemoprevention: Effects on polyamine metabolism (Review)." *Int J Oncol.* 2014 Aug 14. doi: 10.3892/ijo.2014.2597.

16. Touchefeu Y, Montassier E, Nieman K, Gastinne T, Potel G, Bruley des Varannes S, Le Vacon F, de La Cochetière MF. "Systematic review: the role of the gut microbiota in chemotherapy- or radiation-induced gastrointestinal mucositis - current evidence and potential clinical applications." *Aliment Pharmacol Ther.* 2014 Jul 11. doi: 10.1111/apt.12878.

17. Hu J, Wang C, Ye L, Yang W, Huang H, Meng F, Shi S, Ding Z. "Anti-tumour immune effect of oral administration of Lactobacillus plantarum to CT26 tumour-bearing mice." *J Biosci.* 2015 Jun;40(2):269-79.

18. Ahn J, Sinha R, Pei Z, Dominianni C, Wu J, Shi J, Goedert JJ, Hayes RB, Yang L. "Human gut microbiome and risk for colorectal cancer." *J Natl Cancer Inst.* 2013 Dec 18;105(24):1907-11. doi: 10.1093/jnci/djt300.

19. Aragón F, Carino S, Perdigón G, de Moreno de LeBlanc A. "Inhibition of Growth and Metastasis of Breast Cancer in Mice by Milk Fermented With Lactobacillus casei CRL 431." *J Immunother.* 2015 Jun;38(5):185-96. doi: 10.1097/CJI.0000000000000079.

20. Wang SM, Zhang LW, Fan RB, Han X, Yi HX, Zhang LL, Xue CH, Li HB, Zhang YH, Shigwedha N. "Induction of HT-29 cells apoptosis by lactobacilli isolated from fermented products." *Res Microbiol.* 2014 Apr;165(3):202-14. doi: 10.1016/j.resmic.2014.02.004.

21. Feyisetan O, Tracey C, Hellawell GO. "Probiotics, dendritic cells and bladder cancer." *BJU Int.* 2012 Jun;109(11):1594-7. doi: 10.1111/j.1464-410X.2011.10749.x.

22. Azam R, Ghafouri-Fard S, Tabrizi M, Modarressi MH, Ebrahimzadeh-Vesal R, Daneshvar M, Mobasheri MB, Motevaseli E. "Lactobacillus acidophilus and Lactobacillus crispatus culture supernatants downregulate expression of cancer-testis genes in the MDA-MB-231 cell line." *Asian Pac J Cancer Prev.* 2014;15(10):4255-9.

23. Aragón F, Perdigón G, de Moreno de LeBlanc A. "Modification in the diet can induce beneficial effects against breast cancer." *World J Clin Oncol.* 2014 Aug 10;5(3):455-64. doi: 10.5306/wjco.v5.i3.455.

24. Oliveira Silva E, Cruz de Carvalho T, Parshikov IA, Alves dos Santos R, Silva Emery F, Jacometti Cardoso Furtado NA. "Cytotoxicity of lapachol metabolites produced by probiotics." *Lett Appl Microbiol.* 2014 Jul;59(1):108-14. doi: 10.1111/lam.12251.

25. Nami Y, Abdullah N, Haghshenas B, Radiah D, Rosli R, Khosroushahi AY. "Assessment of probiotic potential and anticancer activity of newly isolated vaginal bacterium Lactobacillus plantarum 5BL." *Microbiol Immunol.* 2014 Sep;58(9):492-502. doi: 10.1111/1348-0421.12175.

26. Mandair D, Rossi RE2 Pericleous M, Whyand T, Caplin ME. "Prostate cancer and the influence of dietary factors and supplements: a systematic review." *Nutr Metab (Lond).* 2014 Jun 16;11:30. doi: 10.1186/1743-7075-11-30.

27. Nowak A, Kuberski S, Libudzisz Z. "Probiotic lactic acid bacteria detoxify N-nitrosodimethylamine." *Food Addit Contam Part A Chem Anal Control Expo Risk Assess.* 2014 Jul 10.

28. Stubbe CE, Valero M. "Complementary strategies for the management of radiation therapy side effects." *J Adv Pract Oncol.* 2013 Jul;4(4):219-31.

29. Sanaie S, Ebrahimi-Mameghani M, Mahmoodpoor A, Shadvar K, Golzari SE. "Effect of a Probiotic Preparation (VSL#3) on Cardiovascular Risk Parameters in Critically-Ill Patients." *J Cardiovasc Thorac Res.* 2013;5(2):67-70. doi: 10.5681/jcvtr.2013.014.

30. Khalesi S, Sun J, Buys N, Jayasinghe R. "Effect of Probiotics on Blood Pressure : A Systematic Review and Meta-Analysis of Randomized, Controlled Trials." *Hypertension.* 2014 Jul 21. pii: HYPERTENSIONAHA.114.03469. [Epub ahead of print]

31. Taranto MP, Medici M, Perdigon G, Ruiz Holgado AP, Valdez GF. "Evidence for hypocholesterolemic effect of Lactobacillus reuteri in hypercholesterolemic mice." *J Dairy Sci.* 1998 Sep;81(9):2336-40.

32. Agerholm-Larsen L, Raben A, Haulrik N, Hansen AS, Manders M, Astrup A. "Effect of 8 week intake of probiotic milk products on risk factors for cardiovascular diseases." *Eur J Clin Nutr.* 2000 Apr;54(4):288-97.

33. Kumar M, Rakesh S, Nagpal R, Hemalatha R, Ramakrishna A, Sudarshan V, Ramagoni R, Shujauddin M, Verma V, Kumar A, Tiwari A, Singh B, Kumar R. "Probiotic Lactobacillus rhamnosus GG and Aloe vera gel improve lipid profiles in hypercholesterolemic rats." *Nutrition.* 2013 Mar;29(3):574-9. doi: 10.1016/j.nut.2012.09.006.

34. Ahn HY, Kim M, Chae JS, Ahn YT, Sim JH, Choi ID, Lee SH, Lee JH. "Supplementation with two probiotic strains, Lactobacillus curvatus HY7601 and Lactobacillus plantarum KY1032, reduces fasting triglycerides and enhances apolipoprotein A-V levels in non-diabetic subjects with hypertriglyceridemia." *Atherosclerosis.* 2015 Jun 18;241(2):649-656. doi: 10.1016/j.atherosclerosis.2015.06.030. [Epub ahead of print]

35. Rerksuppaphol S, Rerksuppaphol L. "A Randomized Double-blind Controlled Trial of Lactobacillus acidophilus Plus Bifidobacterium bifidum versus Placebo in Patients with Hypercholesterolemia." *J Clin Diagn Res.* 2015 Mar;9(3):KC01-4. doi: 10.7860/JCDR/2015/11867.5728.

36. Shimizu M, Hashiguchi M, Shiga T, Tamura HO, Mochizuki M. "Meta-Analysis: Effects of Probiotic Supplementation on Lipid Profiles in Normal to Mildly Hypercholesterolemic Individuals." *PLoS One.* 2015 Oct 16;10(10):e0139795. doi: 10.1371/journal.pone.0139795.

37. Guardamagna O, Amaretti A, Puddu PE, Raimondi S, Abello F4 Cagliero P, Rossi M. "Bifidobacteria supplementation: Effects on plasma lipid profiles in dyslipidemic children." *Nutrition.* 2014 Jul-Aug;30(7-8):831-6. doi: 10.1016/j.nut.2014.01.014.

38. Barreto FM, Colado Simão AN, Morimoto HK, Batisti Lozovoy MA, Dichi I, da Silva H, Miglioranza L. "Beneficial effects of Lactobacillus plantarum on glycemia and homocysteine levels in postmenopausal women with metabolic syndrome." *Nutrition.* 2014 Jul-Aug;30(7-8):939-42. doi: 10.1016/j.nut.2013.12.004.

39. Schlienger JL, Paillard F, Lecerf JM, Romon M, Bonhomme C, Schmitt B, Donazzolo Y, Defoort C, Mallmann C, Le Ruyet P, Bresson JL. "Effect on blood lipids of two daily servings of Camembert cheese. An intervention trial in mildly hypercholesterolemic subjects." *Int J Food Sci Nutr.* 2014 Aug 6:1-6. [Epub ahead of print]

40. Kiessling G, Schneider J, Jahreis G. "Long-term consumption of fermented dairy products over 6 months increases HDL cholesterol." *Eur J Clin Nutr.* 2002 Sep;56(9):843-9.

41. Rai AK, Debetto P, Sala FD. "Molecular regulation of cholesterol metabolism: HDL-based intervention through drugs and diet." *Indian J Exp Biol.* 2013 Nov;51(11):885-94.

42. Lam V, Su J, Koprowski S, Hsu A, Tweddell JS, Rafiee P, Gross GJ, Salzman NH, Baker JE. "Intestinal microbiota determine severity of myocardial infarction in rats." *FASEB J.* 2012 Apr;26(4):1727-35. doi: 10.1096/fj.11-197921.

43. Gan XT, Ettinger G, Huang CX, Burton JP, Haist JV, Rajapurohitam V, Sidaway JE, Martin G, Gloor GB, Swann JR, Reid G, Karmazyn M. "Probiotic administration attenuates myocardial hypertrophy and heart failure after myocardial infarction in the rat." *Circ Heart Fail.* 2014 May;7(3):491-9. doi:10.1161/CIRCHEARTFAILURE.113.000978.

44. Larsen N, Vogensen FK, van den Berg FW, Nielsen DS, Andreasen AS, Pedersen BK, Al-Soud WA, Sørensen SJ, Hansen LH, Jakobsen M. "Gut microbiota in human adults with type 2 diabetes differs from non-diabetic adults." *PLoS One.* 2010 Feb 5;5(2):e9085. doi: 10.1371/journal.pone.0009085.

45. Savcheniuk O, Kobyliak N, Kondro M, Virchenko O, Falalyeyeva T, Beregova T. "Short-term periodic consumption of multiprobiotic from childhood improves insulin sensitivity, prevents development of non-alcoholic fatty liver disease and adiposity in adult rats with glutamate-induced obesity." *BMC Complement Altern Med.* 2014 Jul 16;14(1):247. [Epub ahead of print]

46. Vrieze A, Van Nood E, Holleman F, Salojärvi J, Kootte RS, Bartelsman JF, Dallinga-Thie GM, Ackermans MT, Serlie MJ, Oozeer R, Derrien M, Druesne A, Van Hylckama Vlieg JE, Bloks VW, Groen AK, Heilig HG, Zoetendal EG, Stroes ES, de Vos WM, Hoekstra JB, Nieuwdorp M. "Transfer of intestinal microbiota from lean donors increases insulin sensitivity in individuals with metabolic syndrome." *Gastroenterology.* 2012 Oct;143(4):913-6.e7. doi: 10.1053/j.gastro.2012.06.031.

47. Razmpoosh E, Javadi M, Ejtahed HS, Mirmiran P. "Probiotics as beneficial agents in the management of diabetes mellitus: a systematic review." *Diabetes Metab Res Rev.* 2015 May 11. doi: 10.1002/dmrr.2665. [Epub ahead of print]

48. Davis-Richardson AG, Triplett EW. "A model for the role of gut bacteria in the development of autoimmunity for type 1 diabetes." *Diabetologia*. 2015 Jul;58(7):1386-93. doi: 10.1007/s00125-015-3614-8.

49. Gomes AC, Bueno AA, de Souza RG, Mota JF1. "Gut microbiota, probiotics and diabetes." *Nutr J*. 2014 Jun 17;13:60. doi: 10.1186/1475-2891-13-60.

50. He C, Shan Y, Song W. "Targeting gut microbiota as a possible therapy for diabetes." *Nutr Res*. 2015 Mar 14. pii: S0271-5317(15)00060-3. doi: 10.1016/j.nutres.2015.03.002. [Epub ahead of print]

51. Taghizadeh M, Asemi Z. "Effects of synbiotic food consumption on glycemic status and serum hs-CRP in pregnant women: a randomized controlled clinical trial." *Hormones (Athens)*. 2014 Jul;13(3):398-406. doi: 10.14310/horm.2002.1489.

52. Mohamadshahi M, Veissi M, Haidari F, Shahbazian H, Kaydani GA, Mohammadi F. "Effects of probiotic yogurt consumption on inflammatory biomarkers in patients with type 2 diabetes." *Bioimpacts*. 2014;4(2):83-8. doi: 10.5681/bi.2014.007. Epub 2014 Jun 11.

53. Su Y, Zhang B, Su L. "CD4 detected from Lactobacillus helps understand the interaction between Lactobacillus and HIV." *Microbiol Res*. 2013 Jun 12;168(5):273-7. doi: 10.1016/j.micres.2012.12.004.

54. Yang OO, Kelesidis T, Cordova R, Khanlou H. "Immunomodulation of Antiretroviral Drug-Suppressed Chronic HIV-1 Infection in an Oral Probiotic Double-Blind Placebo-Controlled Trial." *AIDS Res Hum Retroviruses*. 2014 Aug 15. [Epub ahead of print]

55. Gautam N, Dayal R, Agarwal D, Kumar R, Singh TP, Hussain T, Singh SP. "Role of Multivitamins, Micronutrients and Probiotics Supplementation in Management of HIV Infected Children." *Indian J Pediatr*. 2014 Apr 24. [Epub ahead of print]

56. Hu H, Merenstein DJ, Wang C, Hamilton PR, Blackmon ML, Chen H, Calderone RA, Li D. "Impact of eating probiotic yogurt on colonization by Candida species of the oral and vaginal mucosa in HIV-infected and HIV-uninfected women." *Mycopathologia*. 2013 Oct;176(3-4):175-81. doi: 10.1007/s11046-013-9678-4.

57. Hummelen R, Changalucha J, Butamanya NL, Koyama TE, Cook A, Habbema JD, Reid G. "Effect of 25 weeks probiotic supplementation on immune function of HIV patients." *Gut Microbes*. 2011 Mar-Apr;2(2):80-5. Epub 2011 Mar 1.

58. Gupta R. "Lack of demonstrated safety and efficacy of probiotics in HIV patients." *HIV Med*. 2013 Sep;14(8):516. doi: 10.1111/hiv.12037.

59. http://www.cdc.gov/hai/surveillance/

60. http://www.cdc.gov/hai/pdfs/hai/infections_deaths.pdf

61. Jarvis WR, Schlosser J, Jarvis AA, Chinn RY. "National point prevalence of Clostridium difficile in US health care facility inpatients, 2008." *Am J Infect Control*. 2009 May;37(4):263-70. doi: 10.1016/j.ajic.2009.01.001.

62. Kondepudi KK, Ambalam P, Karagin PH, Nilsson I, Wadström T, Ljungh A. "A novel multistrain probiotic and synbiotic supplement for prevention of Clostridium difficile infection in a murine model." *Microbiol Immunol*. 2014 Jul 25. doi: 10.1111/1348-0421.12184.

63. Ray S, Dasgupta AK. "Probiotics as cheater cells: Parameter space clustering for individualized prescription." *J Theor Biol*. 2014 Jul 24. pii: S0022-5193(14)00416-0. doi: 10.1016/j.jtbi.2014.07.019. [Epub ahead of print]

64. Boonma P, Spinler JK, Venable SF, Versalovic J, Tumwasorn S. "Lactobacillus rhamnosus L34 and Lactobacillus casei L39 suppress Clostridium difficile-induced IL-8 production by colonic epithelial cells." *BMC Microbiol*. 2014 Jul 2;14(1):177. doi: 10.1186/1471-2180-14-177.

65. Maziade PJ, Pereira P, Goldstein EJ. "A Decade of Experience in Primary Prevention of Clostridium difficile Infection at a Community Hospital Using the Probiotic Combination Lactobacillus acidophilus CL1285, Lactobacillus casei LBC80R, and Lactobacillus rhamnosus CLR2 (Bio-K+)." *Clin Infect Dis*. 2015 May 15;60 Suppl 2:S144-7. doi: 10.1093/cid/civ178.

66. Sikorska H, Smoragiewicz W. "Role of probiotics in the prevention and treatment of meticillin-resistant Staphylococcus aureus infections." *Int J Antimicrob Agents*. 2013 Dec;42(6):475-81. doi: 10.1016/j.ijantimicag.2013.08.003. Epub 2013 Sep 7.

67. http://www.cdc.gov/hai/surveillance/

68. Barraud D, Bollaert PE, Gibot S. "Impact of the administration of probiotics on mortality in critically ill adult patients: a meta-analysis of randomized controlled trials." *Chest*. 2013 Mar;143(3):646-55. doi: 10.1378/chest.12-1745.

69. Rossi M, Johnson DW, Morrison M, Pascoe E, Coombes JS, Forbes JM, McWhinney BC, Ungerer JP, Dimeski G, Campbell KL. "SYNbiotics Easing Renal failure by improving Gut microbiologY (SYNERGY): a protocol of placebo-controlled randomised cross-over trial." *BMC Nephrol*. 2014 Jul 4;15:106. doi: 10.1186/1471-2369-15-106.

70. Pavan M. "Influence of prebiotic and probiotic supplementation on the progression of chronic kidney disease." *Minerva Urol Nefrol*. 2014 Jul 3. [Epub ahead of print]

71. Lau WL, Kalantar-Zadeh K, Vaziri ND. "The Gut as a Source of Inflammation in Chronic Kidney Disease." *Nephron*. 2015;130:92-8. doi: 10.1159/000381990. Epub 2015 May 9.

72. Kaufman DW, Kelly JP, Curhan GC, Anderson TE, Dretler SP, Preminger GM, Cave DR. "Oxalobacter formigenes may reduce the risk of calcium oxalate kidney stones." *J Am Soc Nephrol*. 2008 Jun;19(6):1197-203. doi: 10.1681/ASN.2007101058.

73. Siener R, Bangen U, Sidhu H, Hönow R, von Unruh G, Hesse A. "The role of Oxalobacter formigenes colonization in calcium oxalate stone disease." *Kidney Int*. 2013 Jun;83(6):1144-9. doi: 10.1038/ki.2013.104.

74. Kumar P, Ranawade AV, Kumar NG. "Potential Probiotic Escherichia coli 16 Harboring the Vitreoscilla Hemoglobin Gene Improves Gastrointestinal Tract Colonization and Ameliorates Carbon Tetrachloride Induced Hepatotoxicity in Rats." *Biomed Res Int*. 2014;2014:213574. doi: 10.1155/2014/213574. Epub 2014 Jun 19.

75. Singh AK, Pandey SK, Naresh Kumar G. "Pyrroloquinoline Quinone-Secreting Probiotic Escherichia coli Nissle 1917 Ameliorates Ethanol-Induced Oxidative Damage and Hyperlipidemia in Rats." *Alcohol Clin Exp Res*. 2014 Jul;38(7):2127-37. doi: 10.1111/acer.12456. Epub 2014 Jun 13.

76. Xu J, Ma R, Chen LF, Zhao LJ, Chen K, Zhang RB. "Effects of probiotic therapy on hepatic encephalopathy in patients with liver cirrhosis: an updated meta-analysis of six randomized controlled trials." *Hepatobiliary Pancreat Dis Int*. 2014 Aug;13(4):354-60.

77. Fukui H. "Gut-liver axis in liver cirrhosis: How to manage leaky gut and endotoxemia." *World J Hepatol*. 2015 Mar 27;7(3):425-42. doi: 10.4254/wjh.v7.i3.425.

78. Stadlbauer V, Mookerjee RP, Hodges S, Wright GA, Davies NA, Jalan R. "Effect of probiotic treatment on deranged neutrophil function and cytokine responses in patients with compen-

sated alcoholic cirrhosis." *J Hepatol*. 2008 Jun;48(6):945-51. doi: 10.1016/j.jhep.2008.02.015. Epub 2008 Mar 25.

79. Lee do K, Kang JY, Shin HS, Park IH, Ha NJ. "Antiviral activity of Bifidobacterium adolescentis SPM0212 against Hepatitis B virus." *Arch Pharm Res*. 2013 Dec;36(12):1525-32. doi: 10.1007/s12272-013-0141-3. Epub 2013 May 9.

80. Sharma K, Malik B, Goyal AK, Rath G. "Development of probiotic-based immunoparticles for pulmonary immunization against Hepatitis B." *J Pharm Pharmacol*. 2014 Jul 16. doi: 10.1111/jphp.12247. [Epub ahead of print]

81. Plaza-Diaz J, Gomez-Llorente C, Abadia-Molina F, Saez-Lara MJ, Campaña-Martin L, Muñoz-Quezada S, Romero F, Gil A, Fontana L. "Effects of Lactobacillus paracasei CNCM I-4034, Bifidobacterium breve CNCM I-4035 and Lactobacillus rhamnosus CNCM I-4036 on hepatic steatosis in Zucker rats." *PLoS One*. 2014 May 22;9(5):e98401. doi: 10.1371/journal.pone.0098401.

82. Miura K, Ohnishi H. "Role of gut microbiota and Toll-like receptors in nonalcoholic fatty liver disease." *World J Gastroenterol*. 2014 Jun 21;20(23):7381-7391.

83. Mayer EA, Tillisch K, Gupta A. "Gut/brain axis and the microbiota." *J Clin Invest*. 2015 Mar 2;125(3):926-38. doi: 10.1172/JCI76304.

84. Jeong JJ, Kim KA, Ahn YT, Sim JH, Woo JY, Huh CS, Kim DH. "Probiotic mixture KF attenuates age-dependent memory deficit and lipidemia in Fischer 344 rats." *J Microbiol Biotechnol*. 2015 May 14. [Epub ahead of print]

85. Fond G, Boukouaci W, Chevalier G, Regnault A, Eberl G, Hamdani N, Dickerson F, Macgregor A, Boyer L, Dargel A, Oliveira J, Tamouza R, Leboyer M. "The 'psychomicrobiotic': Targeting microbiota in major psychiatric disorders: A systematic review." *Pathol Biol (Paris)*. 2014 Nov 2. pii: S0369-8114(14)00163-1. doi: 10.1016/j.patbio.2014.10.003. [Epub ahead of print]

86. Tillisch K. "The effects of gut microbiota on CNS function in humans." *Gut Microbes*. 2014 May 1;5(3):404-410.

87. Braniste V, Al-Asmakh M, Kowal C, Anuar F, Abbaspour A, Tóth M, Korecka A, Bakocevic N, Ng LG, Kundu P, Gulyás B, Halldin C, Hultenby K, Nilsson H, Hebert H, Volpe BT, Diamond B, Pettersson S. "The gut microbiota influences blood-brain barrier permeability in mice." *Sci Transl Med*. 2014 Nov 19;6(263):263ra158. doi: 10.1126/scitranslmed.3009759.

88. Rosenfeld CS. "Microbiome Disturbances and Autism Spectrum Disorders." *Drug Metab Dispos*. 2015 Apr 7. pii: dmd.115.063826. [Epub ahead of print]

89. Pärtty A, Kalliomäki M, Wacklin P, Salminen S, Isolauri E. "A possible link between early probiotic intervention and the risk of neuropsychiatric disorders later in childhood: a randomized trial." *Pediatr Res*. 2015 Mar 11. doi: 10.1038/pr.2015.51. [Epub ahead of print]

90. Hsiao EY, McBride SW, Hsien S, Sharon G, Hyde ER, McCue T, Codelli JA, Chow J, Reisman SE, Petrosino JF, Patterson PH, Mazmanian SK. "Microbiota modulate behavioral and physiological abnormalities associated with neurodevelopmental disorders." *Cell*. 2013 Dec 19;155(7):1451-63. doi: 10.1016/j.cell.2013.11.024.

91. Ringel-Kulka T, Kotch JB, Jensen ET, Savage E, Weber DJ. "Randomized, Double-Blind, Placebo-Controlled Study of Synbiotic Yogurt Effect on the Health of Children." *J Pediatr*. 2015 Apr 1. pii: S0022-3476(15)00158-4. doi: 10.1016/j.jpeds.2015.02.038. [Epub ahead of print]

92. Holmqvist S, Chutna O, Bousset L, Aldrin-Kirk P, Li W, Björklund T, Wang ZY, Roybon L,

Melki R, Li JY. "Direct evidence of Parkinson pathology spread from the gastrointestinal tract to the brain in rats." *Acta Neuropathol.* 2014 Oct 9. [Epub ahead of print]

93. Forsyth CB, Shannon KM, Kordower JH, Voigt RM, Shaikh M, Jaglin JA, Estes JD, Dodiya HB, Keshavarzian A. "Increased intestinal permeability correlates with sigmoid mucosa alpha-synuclein staining and endotoxin exposure markers in early Parkinson's disease." *PLoS One.* 2011;6(12):e28032. doi: 10.1371/journal.pone.0028032.

94. Cassani E, Privitera G, Pezzoli G, Pusani C, Madio C, Iorio L, Barichella M. "Use of probiotics for the treatment of constipation in Parkinson's disease patients." *Minerva Gastroenterol Dietol.* 2011 Jun;57(2):117-21.

95. Severance EG, Yolken RH, Eaton WW. "Autoimmune diseases, gastrointestinal disorders and the microbiome in schizophrenia: more than a gut feeling." *Schizophr Res.* 2014 Jul 14. pii: S0920-9964(14)00319-3. doi: 10.1016/j.schres.2014.06.027.

96. Dickerson FB, Stallings C, Origoni A, Katsafanas E, Savage CL, Schweinfurth LA, Goga J, Khushalani S, Yolken RH. "Effect of probiotic supplementation on schizophrenia symptoms and association with gastrointestinal functioning: a randomized, placebo-controlled trial." *Prim Care Companion CNS Disord.* 2014;16(1). pii: PCC.13m01579. doi: 10.4088/PCC.13m01579. Epub 2014 Feb 13.

97. Yang Y, Guo Y, Kan Q, Zhou XG, Zhou XY, Li Y. "A meta-analysis of probiotics for preventing necrotizing enterocolitis in preterm neonates." *Braz J Med Biol Res.* 2014 Sep;47(9):804-10.

98. Hua XT, Tang J, Mu DZ. ["Effect of oral administration of probiotics on intestinal colonization with drug-resistant bacteria in preterm infants"]. *Zhongguo Dang Dai Er Ke Za Zhi.* 2014 Jun;16(6):606-9.

99. AlFaleh K, Anabrees J. "Probiotics for prevention of necrotizing enterocolitis in preterm infants." *Cochrane Database Syst Rev.* 2014 Apr 10;4:CD005496. doi: 10.1002/14651858.CD005496 .pub4.

100. Said MB, Hays S, Maucort-Boulch D, Oulmaati A, Hantova S, Loys CM, Jumas-Bilak E, Picaud JC. "Gut microbiota in preterm infants with gross blood in stools: A prospective, controlled study." *Early Hum Dev.* 2014 Aug 12;90(10):579-585. doi: 10.1016/j.earlhumdev.2014 .07.004.

101. Zhonghua Wei Zhong Bing Ji Jiu Yi Xue. "The effects of early enteral nutrition with addition of probiotics on the prognosis of patients suffering from severe acute pancreatitis." 2013 Apr;25(4):224-8. doi: 10.3760/cma.j.issn.2095-4352.2013.04.011.

102. Ivey KL, Hodgson JM, Kerr DA, Thompson PL, Stojceski B, Prince RL. "The effect of yoghurt and its probiotics on blood pressure and serum lipid profile; a randomised controlled trial." *Nutr Metab Cardiovasc Dis.* 2014 Aug 1. pii: S0939-4753(14)00255-5. doi: 10.1016/ j.numecd.2014.07.012. [Epub ahead of print]

103. Taibi A, Comelli EM. "Practical approaches to probiotics use." *Appl Physiol Nutr Metab.* 2014 Aug;39(8):980-6. doi: 10.1139/apnm-2013-0490

CHAPTER THREE

1. Lukjancenko O, Wassenaar TM, Ussery DW. "Comparison of 61 sequenced Escherichia coli genomes." *Microb Ecol.* 2010 Nov;60(4):708-20. doi: 10.1007/s00248-010-9717-3.

2. Deriu E, Liu JZ, Pezeshki M, Edwards RA, Ochoa RJ, Contreras H, Libby SJ, Fang FC,

Raffatellu M. "Probiotic bacteria reduce salmonella typhimurium intestinal colonization by competing for iron." *Cell Host Microbe.* 2013 Jul 17;14(1):26-37. doi: 10.1016/j.chom.2013.06.007.

3. Jerry Adler and Jeneen Interlandi, *Newsweek Magazine* October 29, 2007

4. Kwak MK, Liu R, Kwon JO, Kim MK, Kim AH, Kang SO. "Cyclic dipeptides from lactic acid bacteria inhibit proliferation of the influenza A virus." *J Microbiol.* 2013 Dec;51(6):836-43. doi: 10.1007/s12275-013-3521-y.

5. Aboubakr HA, El-Banna AA, Youssef MM, Al-Sohaimy SA, Goyal SM. "Antiviral Effects of Lactococcus lactis on Feline Calicivirus, A Human Norovirus Surrogate." *Food Environ Virol.* 2014 Aug 17. [Epub ahead of print]

6. Barr JJ, Auro R, Furlan M, Whiteson KL, Erb ML, Pogliano J, Stotland A, Wolkowicz R, Cutting AS, Doran KS, Salamon P, Youle M, Rohwer F. "Bacteriophage adhering to mucus provide a non-host-derived immunity." *Proc Natl Acad Sci U S A.* 2013 Jun 25;110(26):10771-6. doi: 10.1073/pnas.1305923110.

7. Woo J, Ahn J. "Assessment of synergistic combination potential of probiotic and bacteriophage against antibiotic-resistant Staphylococcus aureus exposed to simulated intestinal conditions." *Arch Microbiol.* 2014 Jul 12. [Epub ahead of print]

8. Kaufmann D, Jennings L, Curtis L. "Fungi and their mycotoxins: an underappreciated role in cancers." *Oncology News,* Nov-Dec 2014:164-166

9. Nyanzi R, Awouafack MD, Steenkamp P, Jooste PJ, Eloff JN. "Anticandidal activity of cell extracts from 13 probiotic Lactobacillus strains and characterisation of lactic acid and a novel fatty acid derivative from one strain." *Food Chem.* 2014 Dec 1;164:470-5. doi: 10.1016/j.food chem.2014.05.067.

10. Ben Salah-Abbès J, Abbès S, Jebali R, Haous Z, Oueslati R. "Potential preventive role of lactic acid bacteria against Aflatoxin M1 immunotoxicity and genotoxicity in mice." *J Immunotoxicol.* 2014 Apr 17:1-8. [Epub ahead of print]

11. Rawal S, Bauer MM, Mendoza KM, El-Nezami H, Hall JR, Kim JE, Stevens JR, Reed KM, Coulombe RA Jr. "Aflatoxicosis chemoprevention by probiotic Lactobacillius and lack of effect on the major histocompatibility complex." *Res Vet Sci.* 2014 Jun 13. pii: S0034-5288(14)00170-2. doi: 10.1016/j.rvsc.2014.06.008.

12. Dinleyici EC, Kara A, Ozen M, Vandenplas Y. "Saccharomyces boulardii CNCM I-745 in different clinical conditions." *Expert Opin Biol Ther.* 2014 Jul 4:1-17. [Epub ahead of print]

13. Gouriet F, Million M, Henri M, Fournier PE, Raoult D. "Lactobacillus rhamnosus bacteremia: an emerging clinical entity." *Eur J Clin Microbiol Infect Dis.* 2012 Sep;31(9):2469-80. doi: 10.1007/s10096-012-1599-5.

14. Simkins J, Kaltsas A, Currie BP. "Investigation of inpatient probiotic use at an academic medical center." *Int J Infect Dis.* 2013 May;17(5):e321-4. doi: 10.1016/j.ijid.2012.11.010.

15. Moore WE, Cato EP, Holdeman LV. "Some current concepts in intestinal bacteriology." *Am J Clin Nutr.* 1978 Oct;31(10 Suppl):S33-42.

16. Xu J, Gordon JI. "Honor thy symbionts." *Proc Natl Acad Sci U S A.* 2003 Sep 2;100(18):10452-9.

17. Wexler HM. "Bacteroides: the good, the bad, and the nitty-gritty." *Clin Microbiol Rev.* 2007 Oct;20(4):593-621.

18. Hojsak I, Kolacek S. "Is Helicobacter pylori always a 'bad guy'?" *Curr Pharm Des.* 2014;20(28):4517-20.

19. Chacko Y, Holtmann GJ. "Helicobacter pylori eradication and weight gain: has it opened a Pandora's box?" *Aliment Pharmacol Ther.* 2011 Jul;34(2):256. doi: 10.1111/j.1365-2036.2011.04704.x.

20. Galan MV, Kishan AA, Silverman AL. "Oral broccoli sprouts for the treatment of Helicobacter pylori infection: a preliminary report." *Dig Dis Sci.* 2004 Aug;49(7-8):1088-90.

21. Amer EI, Mossallam SF, Mahrous H. "Therapeutic enhancement of newly derived bacteriocins against Giardia lamblia." *Exp Parasitol.* 2014 Nov;146:52-63. doi: 10.1016/j.exppara.2014.09.005.

22. Oliveira-Sequeira TC, David ÉB, Ribeiro C, Guimarães , Masseno AP, Katagiri S, Sequeira JL. "Effect of Bifidobacterium animalis on mice infected with Strongyloides venezuelensis." *Rev Inst Med Trop Sao Paulo.* 2014 Mar-Apr;56(2):105-9. doi: 10.1590/S0036-46652014000200003.

CHAPTER FOUR

1. Randal Bollinger R, Barbas AS, Bush EL, Lin SS, Parker W. "Biofilms in the large bowel suggest an apparent function of the human vermiform appendix." *J Theor Biol.* 2007 Dec 21;249(4):826-31.

2. Jackson HT, Mongodin EF, Davenport KP, Fraser CM, Sandler AD, Zeichner SL. "Culture-independent evaluation of the appendix and rectum microbiomes in children with and without appendicitis." *PLoS One.* 2014 Apr 23;9(4):e95414. doi: 10.1371/journal.pone.0095414.

3. Moore WE, Holdeman LV. "Human fecal flora: the normal flora of 20 Japanese-Hawaiians." *Appl Microbiol.* 1974 May;27(5):961-79.

4. Turnbaugh P., Ley R., Hamady M., Fraser-Liggett C., Knight R., Gordon J. "The human microbiome project: exploring the microbial part of ourselves in a changing world." *Nature.* 2007 October 18; 449(7164): 804–810. doi:10.1038/nature06244

5. Fijan S. "Microorganisms with claimed probiotic properties: an overview of recent literature." *Int J Environ Res Public Health.* 2014 May 5;11(5):4745-67. doi: 10.3390/ijerph110504745.

6. Schnorr SL, Candela M, Rampelli S, Centanni M, Consolandi C, Basaglia G, Turroni S, Biagi E, Peano C, Severgnini M, Fiori J, Gotti R, De Bellis G, Luiselli D, Brigidi P, Mabulla A, Marlowe F, Henry AG, Crittenden AN. "Gut microbiome of the Hadza hunter-gatherers." *Nat Commun.* 2014 Apr 15;5:3654. doi: 10.1038/ncomms4654.

7. Xu J, Mahowald MA, Ley RE, Lozupone CA, Hamady M, Martens EC, Henrissat B, Coutinho PM, Minx P, Latreille P, Cordum H, Van Brunt A, Kim K, Fulton RS, Fulton LA, Clifton SW, Wilson RK, Knight RD, Gordon JI. "Evolution of symbiotic bacteria in the distal human intestine." *PLoS Biol.* 2007 Jul;5(7):e156.

8. Barbour A, Philip K. "Variable characteristics of bacteriocin-producing Streptococcus salivarius strains isolated from Malaysian subjects." *PLoS One.* 2014 Jun 18;9(6):e100541. doi: 10.1371/journal.pone.0100541.

9. Corthésy B, Gaskins HR, Mercenier A. "Cross-talk between probiotic bacteria and the host immune system." *J Nutr.* 2007 Mar;137(3 Suppl 2):781S-90S.

10. Ray S, Dasgupta AK. "Probiotics as cheater cells: Parameter space clustering for individualized prescription." *J Theor Biol.* 2014 Jul 24. pii: S0022-5193(14)00416-0. doi: 10.1016/j.jtbi.2014.07.019. [Epub ahead of print]

11. Soltan Dallal MM, Mojarrad M, Baghbani F, Raoofian R, Mardaneh J, Salehipour Z. "Effects of Probiotic Lactobacillus acidophilus and Lactobacillus casei on Colorectal Tumor Cells Activity"(CaCo-2). *Arch Iran Med.* 2015 Mar;18(3):167-72. doi: 0151803/AIM.006.

12. Hooper L, Stappenbeck T, Hong C, Gordon J. "Angiogenins: a new class of microbicidal proteins involved in innate immunity." *Nat Immunol*. 2003 Mar;4(3):269-73.

13. Kol A, Foutouhi S, Walker NJ, Kong NT, Weimer BC, Borjesson DL. "Gastrointestinal Microbes Interact with Canine Adipose-Derived Mesenchymal Stem Cells In Vitro and Enhance Immunomodulatory Functions." *Stem Cells Dev*. 2014 Jun 26. [Epub ahead of print]

14. AlFaleh K, Anabrees J. "Probiotics for prevention of necrotizing enterocolitis in preterm infants." *Cochrane Database Syst Rev*. 2014 Apr 10;4:CD005496. doi: 10.1002/14651858 .CD005496.pub4.

15. Pontier-Bres R, Munro P, Boyer L, Anty R, Imbert V, Terciolo C, André F, Rampal P, Lemichez E, Peyron JF, Czerucka D. "Saccharomyces boulardii Modifies Salmonella Typhimurium Traffic and Host Immune Responses along the Intestinal Tract." *PLoS One*. 2014 Aug 13;9(8):e103069. doi: 10.1371/journal.pone.0103069.

16. Chen X, Yang G, Song JH, Xu H, Li D, Goldsmith J, Zeng H, Parsons-Wingerter PA, Reinecker HC, Kelly CP. "Probiotic yeast inhibits VEGFR signaling and angiogenesis in intestinal inflammation." *PLoS One*. 2013 May 13;8(5):e64227. doi: 10.1371/journal.pone.0064227.

17. Aragón F, Carino S, Perdigón G, de Moreno de LeBlanc A. "The administration of milk fermented by the probiotic Lactobacillus casei CRL 431 exerts an immunomodulatory effect against a breast tumour in a mouse model." *Immunobiology*. 2014 Jun;219(6):457-64. doi: 10.1016/ j.imbio.2014.02.005.

18. Ahmed A, Dachang W, Lei Z, Jianjun L, Juanjuan Q, Yi X. "Effect of Lactobacillus species on Streptococcus mutans Biofilm formation." *Pak J Pharm Sci*. 2014 Sep;27(5 Spec No):1523-8.

19.Nowak A, Kuberski S, Libudzisz Z. "Probiotic lactic acid bacteria detoxify N-nitrosodimethylamine." *Food Addit Contam Part A Chem Anal Control Expo Risk Assess*. 2014 Jul 10.

20. Apás AL, González SN, Arena ME. "Potential of goat probiotic to bind mutagens." *Anaerobe*. 2014 Aug;28:8-12. doi: 10.1016/j.anaerobe.2014.04.004.

21. Trinder M, Bisanz JE, Burton JP, Reid G. "Probiotic lactobacilli: a potential prophylactic treatment for reducing pesticide absorption in humans and wildlife." *Benef Microbes*. 2015 Jun 30:1-8. [Epub ahead of print]

22. Rodes L, Saha S, Tomaro-Duchesneau C, Prakash S. "Microencapsulated Bifidobacterium longum subsp. infantis ATCC 15697 Favorably Modulates Gut Microbiota and Reduces Circulating Endotoxins in F344 Rats." *Biomed Res Int*. 2014;2014:602832. doi: 10.1155/2014/602832.

23. Ramezani A, Raj DS. "The gut microbiome, kidney disease, and targeted interventions." *J Am Soc Nephrol*. 2014 Apr;25(4):657-70. doi: 10.1681/ASN.2013080905.

24. Duncan S, Richardson A, Kaul P, Holmes R, Allison M, Stewart C. "Oxalobacter formigenes and its potential role in human health." *Appl Environ Microbiol*. 2002 Aug;68(8):3841-7.

25. Lin R, Jiang Y, Zhao X, Guan Y, Qian W, Fu XC, Ren HY, Hou XH. "Four types of Bifidobacteria trigger autophagy response in intestinal epithelial cells." *J Dig Dis*. 2014 Aug 13. doi: 10.1111/1751-2980.12179. [Epub ahead of print]

26. Hill MJ. "Intestinal flora and endogenous vitamin synthesis." *Eur J Cancer Prev*. 1997 Mar;6 Suppl 1:S43-5.

27. Ranji P, Akbarzadeh A, Rahmati-Yamchi M. "Associations of Probiotics with Vitamin D and Leptin Receptors and their Effects on Colon Cancer." *Asian Pac J Cancer Prev*. 2015;16(9):3621-7.

28. Jones ML, Martoni CJ, Prakash S. "Oral supplementation with probiotic L. reuteri NCIMB

30242 increases mean circulating 25-hydroxyvitamin D: a post hoc analysis of a randomized controlled trial." *J Clin Endocrinol Metab.* 2013 Jul;98(7):2944-51. doi: 10.1210/jc.2012-4262.

29. Pereira-Caro G, Oliver CM, Weerakkody R, Singh T, Conlon M, Borges G, Sanguansri L, Lockett T, Roberts SA, Crozier A, Augustin MA. "Chronic administration of a microencapsulated probiotic enhances the bioavailability of Orange juice flavanones in humans." *Free Radic Biol Med.* 2015 Mar 20. pii: S0891-5849(15)00122-7. doi: 10.1016/j.freeradbiomed.2015.03.010. [Epub ahead of print]

30. García-Mantrana I, Monedero V, Haros M. "Reduction of Phytate in Soy Drink by Fermentation with Lactobacillus casei Expressing Phytases From Bifidobacteria." *Plant Foods Hum Nutr.* 2015 May 24. [Epub ahead of print]

31. García-Mantrana I, Monedero V, Haros M. "Reduction of Phytate in Soy Drink by Fermentation with Lactobacillus casei Expressing Phytases From Bifidobacteria." *Plant Foods Hum Nutr.* 2015 May 24. [Epub ahead of print]

32. Persichetti E, De Michele A, Codini M, Traina G. "Antioxidative capacity of Lactobacillus fermentum LF31 evaluated in vitro by oxygen radical absorbance capacity assay." *Nutrition.* 2014 Jul-Aug;30(7-8):936-8. doi: 10.1016/j.nut.2013.12.009.

33. Verma A, Shukla G. "Synbiotic (Lactobacillus rhamnosus+Lactobacillus acidophilus+inulin) attenuates oxidative stress and colonic damage in 1,2 dimethylhydrazine dihydrochloride-induced colon carcinogenesis in Sprague-Dawley rats: a long-term study." *Eur J Cancer* Prev. 2014 Jul 14. [Epub ahead of print]

34. Kullisaar T, Songisepp E, Aunapuu M, Kilk K, Arend A, Mikelsaar M, Rehema A, Zilmer M. "Complete glutathione system in probiotic Lactobacillus fermentum ME-3." *Prikl Biokhim Mikrobiol.* 2010 Sep-Oct;46(5):527-31.

35. Centanni M, Turroni S, Rampelli S, Biagi E, Quercia S, Consolandi C, Severgnini M, Brigidi P, Candela M. "Bifidobacterium animalis ssp. lactis BI07 modulates the tumor necrosis factor alpha-dependent imbalances of the enterocyte-associated intestinal microbiota fraction." *FEMS Microbiol Lett.* 2014 Jun 25. doi: 10.1111/1574-6968.12515. [Epub ahead of print]

36. Jialal I, Rajamani U. "Endotoxemia of Metabolic Syndrome: A Pivotal Mediator of Meta-Inflammation." *Metab Syndr Relat Disord.* 2014 Aug 27. [Epub ahead of print]

37. Jardim-Perassi BV, Arbab AS, Ferreira LC, Borin TF, Varma NR, Iskander AS, Shankar A, Ali MM, de Campos Zuccari DA. "Effect of melatonin on tumor growth and angiogenesis in xenograft model of breast cancer." *PLoS One.* 2014 Jan 9;9(1):e85311. doi: 10.1371/journal.pone.0085311.

38. Chen CQ, Fichna J, Bashashati M, Li YY, Storr M. "Distribution, function and physiological role of melatonin in the lower gut." *World J Gastroenterol.* 2011 Sep 14;17(34):3888-98. doi: 10.3748/wjg.v17.i34.3888.

39. Wong RK, Yang C, Song GH, Wong J, Ho KY. "Melatonin Regulation as a Possible Mechanism for Probiotic (VSL#3) in Irritable Bowel Syndrome: A Randomized Double-Blinded Placebo Study." *Dig Dis Sci.* 2014 Aug 5. [Epub ahead of print]

40. Wall R, Cryan JF, Ross RP, Fitzgerald GF, Dinan TG, Stanton C. "Bacterial neuroactive compounds produced by psychobiotics." *Adv Exp Med Biol.* 2014;817:221-39. doi: 10.1007/978-1-4939-0897-4_10.

41. Shing CM, Peake JM, Lim CL, Briskey D, Walsh NP, Fortes MB, Ahuja KD, Vitetta L. "Effects

of probiotics supplementation on gastrointestinal permeability, inflammation and exercise performance in the heat." *Eur J Appl Physiol.* 2014 Jan;114(1):93-103. doi: 10.1007/s00421-013-2748-y.

42. Ohhira I, Kawasaki M, Araki N, Inokihara K, Matsubara T, Iwasaki H. "The Influences on the VO; max of Athletes Taking (Ohhira) Lactic Acid Bacteria." Kurashiki University of Science and the Arts, Kurashiki, Japan, Research Institution of Okayama Life Science, Okayama, Japan and Sanyo Gakuen University, Okayama, Japan (1997).

43. Art T, Votion D, McEntee K, Amory H, Linden A, Close R, Lekeux P. "Cardio-respiratory, haematological and biochemical parameter adjustments to exercise: effect of a probiotic in horses during training." *Vet Res.* 1994;25(4):361-70.

44. Vitetta L, Hall S, Linnane AW. "Live probiotic cultures and the gastrointestinal tract: symbiotic preservation of tolerance whilst attenuating pathogenicity." *Front Cell Infect Microbiol.* 2014 Oct 15;4:143. doi: 10.3389/fcimb.2014.00143.

45. Ishimwe N, Daliri EB, Lee BH, Fang F, Du G. "The perspective on cholesterol lowering mechanisms of probiotics." *Mol Nutr Food Res.* 2014 Nov 18. doi: 10.1002/mnfr.201400548. [Epub ahead of print]

46. Tuohy KM, Fava F, Viola R. "'The way to a man's heart is through his gut microbiota'— dietary pro- and prebiotics for the management of cardiovascular risk." *Proc Nutr Soc.* 2014 May;73(2):172-85. doi: 10.1017/S0029665113003911.

47. Shokryazdan P, Sieo CC, Kalavathy R, Liang JB, Alitheen NB, Faseleh Jahromi M, Ho YW. "Probiotic Potential of Lactobacillus Strains with Antimicrobial Activity against Some Human Pathogenic Strains." *Biomed Res Int.* 2014;2014:927268. Epub 2014 Jul 3.

CHAPTER FIVE

1. Foti JJ, Devadoss B, Winkler JA, Collins JJ, Walker GC. "Oxidation of the guanine nucleotide pool underlies cell death by bactericidal antibiotics." *Science.* 2012 Apr 20;336(6079):315-9. doi: 10.1126/science.1219192.

2. Tamim HM, Hanley JA, Hajeer AH, Boivin JF, Collet JP. "Risk of breast cancer in relation to antibiotic use." *Pharmacoepidemiol Drug Saf.* 2008 Feb;17(2):144-50.

3. Wirtz HS, Buist DS, Gralow JR, Barlow WE, Gray S, Chubak J, Yu O, Bowles EJ, Fujii M, Boudreau DM. "Frequent antibiotic use and second breast cancer events." *Cancer Epidemiol Biomarkers Prev.* 2013 Sep;22(9):1588-99. doi: 10.1158/1055-9965.EPI-13-0454.

4. Boursi B, Mamtani R, Haynes K, Yang YX. "The effect of past antibiotic exposure on diabetes risk." *Eur J Endocrinol.* 2015 Mar 24. pii: EJE-14-1163. [Epub ahead of print]

5. Cohen JS. "Peripheral neuropathy associated with fluoroquinolones." *Ann Pharmacother.* 2001 Dec;35(12):1540-7.

6. Mortensen EM, Halm EA, Pugh MJ, Copeland LA, Metersky M, Fine MJ, Johnson CS, Alvarez CA, Frei CR, Good C, Restrepo MI, Downs JR, Anzueto A. "Association of azithromycin with mortality and cardiovascular events among older patients hospitalized with pneumonia." *JAMA.* 2014 Jun 4;311(21):2199-208. doi: 10.1001/jama.2014.4304.

7. Fayock K, Voltz M, Sandella B, Close J, Lunser M, Okon J. "Antibiotic precautions in athletes." *Sports Health.* 2014 Jul;6(4):321-5. doi: 10.1177/1941738113506553.

8. Bhat RV, Deshmukh CT. "A study of Vitamin K status in children on prolonged antibiotic therapy." *Indian Pediatr.* 2003 Jan;40(1):36-40.

9. Conly J, Stein K. "Reduction of vitamin K2 concentrations in human liver associated with the use of broad spectrum antimicrobials." *Clin Invest Med.* 1994 Dec;17(6):531-9.

10. Johnson CC, Ownby DR, Alford SH, Havstad SL, Williams LK, Zoratti EM, Peterson EL, Joseph CL. "Antibiotic exposure in early infancy and risk for childhood atopy." *J Allergy Clin Immunol.* 2005 Jun;115(6):1218-24.

11. Bailey LC, Forrest CB, Zhang P, Richards TM, Livshits A, DeRusso PA. "Association of antibiotics in infancy with early childhood obesity." *JAMA Pediatr.* 2014 Nov 1;168(11):1063-9. doi: 10.1001/jamapediatrics.2014.1539.

12. http://www.pewtrusts.org/en/research-and-analysis/fact-sheets/2014/05/05/antibiotics-and-industrial-farming-101

13. Wall Street Journal online, May 22, 2013

14. Kenealy T, Arroll B. "Antibiotics for the common cold and acute purulent rhinitis." *Cochrane Database Syst Rev.* 2013 Jun 4;6:CD000247.

15. Garbutt JM, Banister C, Spitznagel E, Piccirillo JF. "Amoxicillin for acute rhinosinusitis: a randomized controlled trial." *JAMA.* 2012 Feb 15;307(7):685-92.

16. Wald ER, Applegate KE, Bordley C, Darrow DH, Glode MP, Marcy SM, Nelson CE, Rosenfeld RM, Shaikh N, Smith MJ, Williams PV, Weinberg ST. "Clinical Practice Guideline for the Diagnosis and Management of Acute Bacterial Sinusitis in Children Aged 1 to 18 Years." *Pediatrics.* 2013 Jun 24. [Epub ahead of print]

17. Albert, RH. "Diagnosis and treatment of acute bronchitis." *Am Fam Physician.* 2010 Dec 1;82(11):1345-50.

18. Pichichero ME1, Green JL, Francis AB, Marsocci SM, Murphy ML. "Outcomes after judicious antibiotic use for respiratory tract infections seen in a private pediatric practice." *Pediatrics.* 2000 Apr;105(4 Pt 1):753-9.

19. Coco AS1, Horst MA, Gambler AS. "Trends in broad-spectrum antibiotic prescribing for children with acute otitis media in the United States, 1998-2004." *BMC Pediatr.* 2009 Jun 24;9:41. doi: 10.1186/1471-2431-9-41.

20. Coco A1, Vernacchio L, Horst M, Anderson A. "Management of acute otitis media after publication of the 2004 AAP and AAFP clinical practice guideline." *Pediatrics.* 2010 Feb;125(2):214-20. doi: 10.1542/peds.2009-1115.

21. Linder JA, Doctor JN, Friedberg MW, Reyes Nieva H, Birks C, Meeker D, Fox CR. "Time of Day and the Decision to Prescribe Antibiotics." *JAMA Intern Med.* 2014 Oct 6. doi: 10.1001/jamainternmed.2014.5225. [Epub ahead of print] As reported in The New York Times October 27, 2014

22. http://www.cdc.gov/getsmart/healthcare/

23. U.S. Food and Drug Administration, *FDA Annual Report on Antimicrobials Sold or Distributed for Food-Producing Animals in 2011,* Feb. 5, 2013, http://www.fda.gov/AnimalVeterinary/NewsEvents/CVMUpdates/ucm338178.htm .

24. Karen Meister, supervisory congressional affairs specialist, U.S. Food and Drug Administration, letter to Representative Louise Slaughter (D-NY), April 19, 2011.

25. Preservation of Antibiotics for Medical Treatment Act of 2009, hearing on H.R. 1549 before the U.S. House of Representatives Committee on Rules, statement of Frank M. Aarestrup and Henrik Wegener, National Food Institute, Technical University of Denmark, Soborg, July 13,

2009, http://www.livablefutureblog.com/wp-content/uploads/2009/08/testimony-of-dr-frank-moller-aarestrup-1.pdf.

26. Nordstrom L, Liu CM, Price LB. "Foodborne urinary tract infections: a new paradigm for antimicrobial-resistant foodborne illness." *Front Microbiol.* 2013 Mar 6;4:29. doi: 10.3389/fmicb.2013.00029.

27. Dallas Morning News April 21, 2012

28. http://toxics.usgs.gov/pubs/FS-027-02/

29. Lenoir-Wijnkoop I, Gerlier L, Bresson JL, Le Pen C, Berdeaux G. "Public Health and Budget Impact of Probiotics on Common Respiratory Tract Infections: A Modelling Study." *PLoS One.* 2015 Apr 10;10(4):e0122765. doi: 10.1371/journal.pone.0122765.

CHAPTER SIX

1. Obad J, ?u?kovi? J, Kos B. "Antimicrobial activity of ibuprofen: New perspectives on an "Old" non-antibiotic drug." *Eur J Pharm Sci.* 2015 Apr 25;71:93-8. doi: 10.1016/j.ejps.2015.02.011.

2. Clarke SF, Murphy EF, O'Sullivan O, Lucey AJ, Humphreys M, Hogan A, Hayes P, O'Reilly M, Jeffery IB, Wood-Martin R, Kerins DM, Quigley E, Ross RP, O'Toole PW, Molloy MG, Falvey E, Shanahan F, Cotter PD. "Exercise and associated dietary extremes impact on gut microbial diversity." *Gut.* 2014 Jun 9. pii: gutjnl-2013-306541. doi: 10.1136/gutjnl-2013-306541.

3. Booyens J, Thantsha MS. "Fourier transform infra-red spectroscopy and flow cytometric assessment of the antibacterial mechanism of action of aqueous extract of garlic (Allium sativum) against selected probiotic Bifidobacterium strains." *BMC Complement Altern Med.* 2014 Aug 6;14(1):289.

4. Zhang W Jiang S1, Qian D, Shang EX, Duan JA. "Analysis of interaction property of caly-cosin-7-O-?-D-glucoside with human gut microbiota." *J Chromatogr B Analyt Technol Biomed Life Sci.* 2014 Jul 15;963:16-23. doi: 10.1016/j.jchromb.2014.05.015.

5. Sharma K, Malik B, Goyal AK, Rath G. "Development of probiotic-based immunoparticles for pulmonary immunization against Hepatitis B." *J Pharm Pharmacol.* 2014 Jul 16. doi: 10.1111/jphp.12247.

6. http://www.homeopathycenter.org/news/homeoprophylaxis-human-records-studies-and-trials

7. Foxman EF, Storer JA, Fitzgerald ME, Wasik BR, Hou L, Zhao H, Turner PE, Pyle AM, Iwasaki A. "Temperature-dependent innate defense against the common cold virus limits viral replication at warm temperature in mouse airway cells." *Proc Natl Acad Sci U S A.* 2015 Jan 20;112(3):827-32. doi: 10.1073/pnas.1411030112.

8. http://www.nbcnews.com/id/41838546/ns/health-childrens_health/t/e-coli-found-percent-shopping-carts/#.U-exp2OCUTA

9. Associated Press September 19, 2014.

10. Nordstrom L, Liu CM, Price LB. "Foodborne urinary tract infections: a new paradigm for antimicrobial-resistant foodborne illness." *Front Microbiol.* 2013 Mar 6;4:29. doi: 10.3389/fmicb.2013.00029.

11. *Consumer Reports On Health*, November 2014.

12. Kanno T, Matsuki T, Oka M, Utsunomiya H, Inada K, Magari H, Inoue I, Maekita T, Ueda K, Enomoto S, Iguchi M, Yanaoka K, Tamai H, Akimoto S, Nomoto K, Tanaka R, Ichinose M.

"Gastric acid reduction leads to an alteration in lower intestinal microflora." *Biochem Biophys Res Commun.* 2009 Apr 17;381(4):666-70.

13. Ibid.

14. "Hands Across America" by David Owen, *The New Yorker Magazine*, March 4, 2013.

15. de Vendômois JS, Roullier F, Cellier D, Séralini GE. "A comparison of the effects of three GM corn varieties on mammalian health." *Int J Biol Sci.* 2009 Dec 10;5(7):706-26.

16. Gress S, Lemoine S, Séralini GE, Puddu PE. "Glyphosate-Based Herbicides Potently Affect Cardiovascular System in Mammals: Review of the Literature." *Cardiovasc Toxicol.* 2014 Sep 23. [Epub ahead of print]

17. http://www.iuss.org/19th percent20WCSS/Symposium/pdf/1807.pdf

18. Samsel A, Seneff S. "Glyphosate, pathways to modern diseases II: Celiac sprue and gluten intolerance." *Interdiscip Toxicol.* 2013 Dec;6(4):159-84. doi: 10.2478/intox-2013-0026.

19. Mesnage R, Defarge N, Spiroux de Vendômois J, Séralini GE. "Major pesticides are more toxic to human cells than their declared active principles." *Biomed Res Int.* 2014;2014:179691. doi: 10.1155/2014/179691.

20. Chassaing B, Koren O, Goodrich JK, Poole AC, Srinivasan S, Ley RE, Gewirtz AT. "Dietary emulsifiers impact the mouse gut microbiota promoting colitis and metabolic syndrome." *Nature.* 2015 Mar 5;519(7541):92-6. doi: 10.1038/nature14232.

21. Dufault R, LeBlanc B, Schnoll R, Cornett C, Schweitzer L, Wallinga D, Hightower J, Patrick L, Lukiw WJ. "Mercury from chlor-alkali plants: measured concentrations in food product sugar." *Environ Health.* 2009 Jan 26;8:2. doi: 10.1186/1476-069X-8-2.

22. [REFERENCE MISSING]

23. Suez J, Korem T, Zeevi D, Zilberman-Schapira G, Thaiss CA, Maza O, Israeli D, Zmora N, Gilad S, Weinberger A, Kuperman Y, Harmelin A, Kolodkin-Gal I, Shapiro H, Halpern Z, Segal E, Elinav E. "Artificial sweeteners induce glucose intolerance by altering the gut microbiota." *Nature.* 2014 Oct 9;514(7521):181-6. doi: 10.1038/nature13793.

24. Abou-Donia MB, El-Masry EM, Abdel-Rahman AA, McLendon RE, Schiffman SS. "Splenda alters gut microflora and increases intestinal p-glycoprotein and cytochrome p-450 in male rats." *J Toxicol Environ Health A.* 2008;71(21):1415-29.

25. Esmerino EA, Cruz AG, Pereira EP, Rodrigues JB, Faria JA, Bolini HM. "The influence of sweeteners in probiotic Petit Suisse cheese in concentrations equivalent to that of sucrose." *J Dairy Sci.* 2013 Sep;96(9):5512-21. doi: 10.3168/jds.2013-6616.

26. Deni?a I, Semjonovs P, Fomina A, Treimane R, Linde R. "The influence of stevia glycosides on the growth of Lactobacillus reuteri strains." *Lett Appl Microbiol.* 2014 Mar;58(3):278-84. doi: 10.1111/lam.12187.

27. Gandhi A, Cui Y, Zhou M, Shah NP. "Effect of KCl substitution on bacterial viability of Escherichia coli (ATCC 25922) and selected probiotics." *J Dairy Sci.* 2014 Jul 23. pii: S0022-0302(14)00501-3. doi: 10.3168/jds.2013-7681.

CHAPTER SEVEN

1. Aagaard K, Ma J, Antony KM, Ganu R, Petrosino J, Versalovic J. "The placenta harbors a unique microbiome." *Sci Transl Med.* 2014 May 21;6(237):237ra65. doi: 10.1126/scitranslmed.3008599.

2. Lif Holgerson P, Harnevik L, Hernell O, Tanner AC, Johansson I. "Mode of birth delivery affects oral microbiota in infants." *J Dent Res*. 2011 Oct;90(10):1183-8. doi: 10.1177/0022034511418973.

3. Huh SY, Rifas-Shiman SL, Zera CA, Edwards JW, Oken E, Weiss ST, Gillman MW. "Delivery by caesarean section and risk of obesity in preschool age children: a prospective cohort study." *Arch Dis Child*. 2012 Jul;97(7):610-6. doi: 10.1136/archdischild-2011-301141.

4. Smaill FM, Grivell RM. "Antibiotic prophylaxis versus no prophylaxis for preventing infection after cesarean section." *Cochrane Database Syst Rev*. 2014 Oct 28;10:CD007482. doi: 10.1002/14651858.CD007482.pub3.

5. Mathew JL. "Effect of maternal antibiotics on breast feeding infants." *Postgrad Med J*. 2004 Apr;80(942):196-200.

6. Ajslev TA, Andersen CS, Gamborg M, Sørensen TI, Jess T. "Childhood overweight after establishment of the gut microbiota: the role of delivery mode, pre-pregnancy weight and early administration of antibiotics." *Int J Obes (Lond)*. 2011 Apr;35(4):522-9. doi: 10.1038/ijo.2011.27.

7. Underwood MA, German JB, Lebrilla CB, Mills DA. "Bifidobacterium longum subspecies infantis: champion colonizer of the infant gut." *Pediatr Res*. 2014 Oct 10. doi: 10.1038/pr.2014.156. [Epub ahead of print]

8. Mastromarino P, Capobianco D, Miccheli A, Praticò G, Campagna G, Laforgia N, Capursi T, Baldassarre ME. "Administration of a multi-strain probiotic product (VSL#3) to women in the perinatal period differentially affects breast milk beneficial microbiota in relation to mode of delivery." *Pharmacol Res*. 2015 Mar 31;95-96C:63-70. doi: 10.1016/j.phrs.2015.03.013. [Epub ahead of print]

9. Endo A, P?rtty A, Kalliom?ki M, Isolauri E, Salminen S. "Long-term monitoring of the human intestinal microbiota from the 2nd week to 13 years of age." *Anaerobe*. 2014 Jun 13;28C:149-156. doi: 10.1016/j.anaerobe.2014.06.006.

10. Clemente JC, Pehrsson EC, Blaser MJ, Sandhu K, Gao Z, Wang B, Magris M, Hidalgo G, Contreras M, Noya-Alarcón Ó, Lander O, McDonald J, Cox M, Walter J, Oh PL, Ruiz JF, Rodriguez S, Shen N, Song SJ, Metcalf J, Knight R, Dantas G, Dominguez-Bello MG. "The microbiome of uncontacted Amerindians." *Sci Adv*. 2015 Apr 3;1(3). pii: e1500183.

11. Hesselmar B, Aberg N, Aberg B, Eriksson B, Björkstén B. "Does early exposure to cat or dog protect against later allergy development?" *Clin Exp Allergy*. 1999 May;29(5):611-7.

12. Sneed RS, Cohen S, Turner RB, Doyle WJ. "Parenthood and host resistance to the common cold." *Psychosom Med*. 2012 Jul-Aug;74(6):567-73. doi: 10.1097/PSY.0b013e31825941ff.

13. Bloomfield S, Stanwell-Smith R, Crevel R, Pickup J. "Too clean, or not too clean: the Hygiene Hypothesis and home hygiene" *Clin Exp Allergy*. Apr 2006; 36(4): 402–425.

14. Schnorr SL, Candela M, Rampelli S, Centanni M, Consolandi C, Basaglia G, Turroni S, Biagi E, Peano C, Severgnini M, Fiori J, Gotti R, De Bellis G, Luiselli D, Brigidi P, Mabulla A, Marlowe F, Henry AG, Crittenden AN. "Gut microbiome of the Hadza hunter-gatherers." *Nat Commun*. 2014 Apr 15;5:3654. doi: 10.1038/ncomms4654.

15. Wu GD, Compher C, Chen EZ, Smith SA, Shah RD, Bittinger K, Chehoud C, Albenberg LG, Nessel L, Gilroy E, Star J, Weljie AM, Flint HJ, Metz DC, Bennett MJ, Li H, Bushman FD, Lewis JD. "Comparative metabolomics in vegans and omnivores reveal constraints on diet-dependent gut microbiota metabolite production." *Gut*. 2014 Nov 26. pii: gutjnl-2014-308209. doi: 10.1136/gutjnl-2014-308209.

16. Claesson MJ, Jeffery IB, Conde S, Power SE, O'Connor EM, Cusack S, Harris HM, Coakley

M, Lakshminarayanan B, O'Sullivan O, Fitzgerald GF, Deane J, O'Connor M, Harnedy N, O'Connor K, O'Mahony D, van Sinderen D, Wallace M, Brennan L, Stanton C, Marchesi JR, Fitzgerald AP, Shanahan F, Hill C, Ross RP, O'Toole PW. "Gut microbiota composition correlates with diet and health in the elderly." *Nature.* 2012 Aug 9;488(7410):178-84. doi: 10.1038/nature11319.

17. Couch RD, Dailey A, Zaidi F, Navarro K, Forsyth CB, Mutlu E, Engen PA, Keshavarzian A. "Alcohol induced alterations to the human fecal VOC metabolome." *PLoS One.* 2015 Mar 9;10(3):e0119362. doi: 10.1371/journal.pone.0119362.

18. David LA, Maurice CF, Carmody RN, Gootenberg DB, Button JE, Wolfe BE, Ling AV, Devlin AS, Varma Y, Fischbach MA, Biddinger SB, Dutton RJ, Turnbaugh PJ. "Diet rapidly and reproducibly alters the human gut microbiome." *Nature.* 2014 Jan 23;505(7484):559-63. doi: 10.1038/nature12820.

19. Caesar R, Tremaroli V, Kovatcheva-Datchary P, Cani PD, Bäckhed F. "Crosstalk between Gut Microbiota and Dietary Lipids Aggravates WAT Inflammation through TLR Signaling." *Cell Metab.* 2015 Aug 26. pii: S1550-4131(15)00389-7. doi: 10.1016/j.cmet.2015.07.026. [Epub ahead of print]

20. Chassaing B, Miles-Brown JP, Pellizzon M, Ulman E, Ricci M, Zhang L, Patterson AD, Vijay-Kumar M, Gewirtz AT. "Lack of soluble fiber drives diet-induced adiposity in mice." *Am J Physiol Gastrointest Liver Physiol.* 2015 Jul 16:ajpgi.00172.2015. doi: 10.1152/ajpgi.00172.2015.

21. Sutherland J, Miles M, Hedderley D, Li J, Devoy S, Sutton K, Lauren D. "In vitro effects of food extracts on selected probiotic and pathogenic bacteria." *Int J Food Sci Nutr.* 2009 Dec;60(8):717-27. doi: 10.3109/09637480802165650.

22. Ono H, Nishio S, Tsurii J, Kawamoto T, Sonomoto K, Nakayama J. "Effects of Japanese pepper and red pepper on the microbial community during nukadoko fermentation." *Biosci Microbiota Food Health.* 2015;34(1):1-9. doi: 10.12938/bmfh.2014-011.

23. Vásquez A, Forsgren E, Fries I, Paxton RJ, Flaberg E, Szekely L, Olofsson TC. "Symbionts as major modulators of insect health: lactic acid bacteria and honeybees." *PLoS One.* 2012;7(3):e33188. doi: 10.1371/journal.pone.0033188.

24. Hilimire MR, DeVylder JE, Forestell CA. "Fermented foods, neuroticism, and social anxiety: An interaction model." *Psychiatry Res.* 2015 Aug 15;228(2):203-8. doi: 10.1016/j.psychres .2015.04.023. Epub 2015 Apr 28.

25. Kanai T, Matsuoka K, Naganuma M, Hayashi A, Hisamatsu T. "Diet, microbiota, and inflammatory bowel disease: lessons from Japanese foods." *Korean J Intern Med.* 2014 Jul;29(4):409-15. doi: 10.3904/kjim.2014.29.4.409.

26. Abdhul K, Ganesh M, Shanmughapriya S, Kanagavel M, Anbarasu K, Natarajaseenivasan K. "Antioxidant activity of exopolysaccharide from probiotic strain Enterococcus faecium (BDU7) from Ngari." *Int J Biol Macromol.* 2014 Jul 22. pii: S0141-8130(14)00501-7. doi: 10.1016/j.ijbiomac.2014.07.026.

27. Larsson SC, Andersson SO, Johansson JE, Wolk A. "Cultured milk, yogurt, and dairy intake in relation to bladder cancer risk in a prospective study of Swedish women and men." *Am J Clin Nutr.* 2008 Oct;88(4):1083-7.

28. Wu GD, Compher C, Chen EZ, Smith SA, Shah RD, Bittinger K, Chehoud C, Albenberg LG, Nessel L, Gilroy E, Star J, Weljie AM, Flint HJ, Metz DC, Bennett MJ, Li H, Bushman FD, Lewis JD. "Comparative metabolomics in vegans and omnivores reveal constraints on diet-dependent

gut microbiota metabolite production." *Gut*. 2014 Nov 26. pii: gutjnl-2014-308209. doi: 10.1136/gutjnl-2014-308209.

29. Berlec A. "Novel techniques and findings in the study of plant microbiota: search for plant probiotics." *Plant Sci*. 2012 Sep;193-194:96-102. doi: 10.1016/j.plantsci.2012.05.010.

30. Kwak MK, Liu R, Kwon JO, Kim MK, Kim AH, Kang SO. "Cyclic dipeptides from lactic acid bacteria inhibit proliferation of the influenza A virus." *J Microbiol*. 2013 Dec;51(6):836-43. doi: 10.1007/s12275-013-3521-y.

31. Park KY, Jeong JK, Lee YE, Daily JW 3rd. "Health benefits of kimchi (Korean fermented vegetables) as a probiotic food." *J Med Food*. 2014 Jan;17(1):6-20. doi: 10.1089/jmf.2013.3083.

32. V?na I, Semjonovs P, Linde R, Deni?a I. "Current evidence on physiological activity and expected health effects of kombucha fermented beverage." *J Med Food*. 2014 Feb;17(2):179-88. doi: 10.1089/jmf.2013.0031.

33. Tannock GW. "A special fondness for lactobacilli." *Appl Environ Microbiol*. 2004 Jun;70(6):3189-94.

CHAPTER EIGHT

1. Marcinkevicius EV, Shirasu-Hiza MM. "Message in a biota: gut microbes signal to the circadian clock." *Cell Host Microbe*. 2015 May 13;17(5):541-3. doi: 10.1016/j.chom.2015.04.013.

2. Adams CA. "The probiotic paradox: live and dead cells are biological response modifiers." *Nutr Res Rev*. 2010 Jun;23(1):37-46. doi: 10.1017/S0954422410000090.

3. Rachmilewitz D, Katakura K, Karmeli F, Hayashi T, Reinus C, Rudensky B, Akira S, Takeda K, Lee J, Takabayashi K, Raz E. "Toll-like receptor 9 signaling mediates the anti-inflammatory effects of probiotics in murine experimental colitis." *Gastroenterology*. 2004 Feb;126(2):520-8.

4. Vasama M, Kumar H, Salminen S, Haskard CA. "Removal of paralytic shellfish toxins by probiotic lactic Acid bacteria." *Toxins (Basel)*. 2014 Jul 18;6(7):2127-36. doi: 10.3390/toxins6072127.

5. Quigley EM, Shanahan F. "The future of probiotics for disorders of the brain-gut axis." *Adv Exp Med Biol*. 2014;817:417-32. doi: 10.1007/978-1-4939-0897-4_19.

6. Loh TC, Choe DW, Foo HL, Sazili AQ, Bejo MH. "Effects of feeding different postbiotic metabolite combinations produced by Lactobacillus plantarum strains on egg quality and production performance, faecal parameters and plasma cholesterol in laying hens." *BMC Vet Res*. 2014 Jul 5;10(1):149. doi: 10.1186/1746-6148-10-149.

7. Kulakova IuV, Aleshkin AV, Afanas'ev SS, Zhilenkova OG. "[Development of polycomponent metabolite probiotic].[Article in Russian]" *Zh Mikrobiol Epidemiol Immunobiol*. 2013 Sep-Oct;(5):80-6.

8. Burke KE, Lamont JT. "Fecal transplantation for recurrent Clostridium difficile infection in older adults: a review." *J Am Geriatr Soc*. 2013 Aug;61(8):1394-8. doi: 10.1111/jgs.12378.

9. Austin M, Mellow M, Tierney WM. "Fecal microbiota transplantation in the treatment of Clostridium difficile infections." *Am J Med*. 2014 Jun;127(6):479-83. doi: 10.1016/j.amjmed.2014.02.017.

10. van Nood E, Vrieze A, Nieuwdorp M, Fuentes S, Zoetendal EG, de Vos WM, Visser CE, Kuijper EJ, Bartelsman JF, Tijssen JG, Speelman P, Dijkgraaf MG, Keller JJ. "Duodenal infusion of donor feces for recurrent Clostridium difficile." *N Engl J Med*. 2013 Jan 31;368(5):407-15. doi: 10.1056/NEJMoa1205037.

11. Ianiro G, Bibbò S, Gasbarrini A, Cammarota G. "Therapeutic modulation of gut microbiota: current clinical applications and future perspectives." *Curr Drug Targets*. 2014;15(8):762-70.

12. No authors listed. "Critical Views in Gastroenterology and Hepatology: Fecal Microbiota Transplantation: Where Is It Leading?" *Gastroenterol Hepatol (N Y)*. 2014 May;10(5):307-9.

13. Kulp W, Rettger L. "Comparative Study of Lactobacillus acidophilus and Lactobacillus bulgaricus." *J Bacteriol*. Jul 1924; 9(4): 357–395.

14. Fairfax MR, Lephart PR, Salimnia H. "Weissella confusa: problems with identification of an opportunistic pathogen that has been found in fermented foods and proposed as a probiotic." *Front Microbiol*. 2014 Jun 12;5:254. doi: 10.3389/fmicb.2014.00254.

15. Hell M, Bernhofer C, Stalzer P, Kern JM, Claassen E. "Probiotics in Clostridium difficile infection: reviewing the need for a multi-strain probiotic." *Benef Microbes*. 2013 Mar 1;4(1):39-51. doi: 10.3920/BM2012.0049.

16. Berlec A. "Novel techniques and findings in the study of plant microbiota: search for plant probiotics." *Plant Sci*. 2012 Sep;193-194:96-102. doi: 10.1016/j.plantsci.2012.05.010.

17. Cananzi FC, Mudan S, Dunne M, Belonwu N, Dalgleish AG. "Long-term survival and outcome of patients originally given Mycobacterium vaccae for metastatic malignant melanoma." *Hum Vaccin Immunother*. 2013 Nov;9(11):2427-33.

18. Tannock GW, Munro K, Harmsen HJ, Welling GW, Smart J, Gopal PK. "Analysis of the fecal microflora of human subjects consuming a probiotic product containing Lactobacillus rhamnosus DR20." *Appl Environ Microbiol*. 2000 Jun;66(6):2578-88.

19. Senz M, van Lengerich B, Bader J, Stahl U. "Control of cell morphology of probiotic Lactobacillus acidophilus for enhanced cell stability during industrial processing." *Int J Food Microbiol*. 2014 Sep 22;192C:34-42. doi: 10.1016/j.ijfoodmicro.2014.09.015.

20. Santivarangkna C, Kulozik U, Foerst P. "Inactivation mechanisms of lactic acid starter cultures preserved by drying processes." *J Appl Microbiol*. 2008 Jul;105(1):1-13. doi: 10.1111/j.1365-2672.2008.03744.x.

21. Muller C, Mazel V2, Dausset C, Busignies V, Bornes S, Nivoliez A, Tchoreloff P. "Study of the lactobacillus rhamnosus lcr35 properties after compression and proposition of a model to predict tablet stability." *Eur J Pharm Biopharm*. 2014 Aug 13. pii: S0939-6411(14)00239-2. doi: 10.1016/j.ejpb.2014.07.014. [Epub ahead of print]

22. Song H, Yu W, Liu X, Ma X. "Improved probiotic viability in stress environments with post-culture of alginate-chitosan microencapsulated low density cells." *Carbohydr Polym*. 2014 Aug 8;108:10-6. doi: 10.1016/j.carbpol.2014.02.084.

23. Rad AH, Mehrabany EV, Alipoor B, Mehrabany LV. The comparison of food and supplement as probiotic delivery vehicles. *Crit Rev Food Sci Nutr*. 2014 Aug 13. [Epub ahead of print]

24. Robitaille G, Champagne CP. "Growth-promoting effects of pepsin- and trypsin-treated caseinomacropeptide from bovine milk on probiotics." *J Dairy Res*. 2014 Aug;81(3):319-24. doi: 10.1017/S0022029914000247.

25. He Y, Chen Z, Liu X, Wang C, Lu W. "Influence of Trace Elements Mixture on Bacterial Diversity and Fermentation Characteristics of Liquid Diet Fermented with Probiotics under Air-Tight Condition." *PLoS One*. 2014 Dec 8;9(12):e114218. doi: 10.1371/journal.pone.0114218.

26. van Zanten GC, Krych L, Röytiö H, Forssten S, Lahtinen SJ, Al-Soud WA, Sørensen S, Svensson B, Jespersen L, Jakobsen M. "Synbiotic Lactobacillus acidophilus NCFM and cellobiose does not affect human gut bacterial diversity but increases abundance of lactobacilli, bifidobacteria and branched-chain fatty acids: a randomized, double-blinded cross-over trial." *FEMS Microbiol Ecol.* 2014 Aug 7. doi: 10.1111/1574-6941.12397.

27. Tee W, Nazaruddin R, Tan Y, Ayob M "Effects of encapsulation on the viability of potential probiotic Lactobacillus plantarum exposed to high acidity condition and presence of bile salts." *Food Sci Technol Int.* 2014 Sep;20(6):399-404. doi: 10.1177/1082013213488775.

28. An H, Douillard FP, Wang G, Zhai Z, Yang J, Song S, Cui J, Ren F, Luo Y, Zhang B, Hao Y. "Integrated transcriptomic and proteomic analysis of the bile stress response in a centenarian-originated probiotic Bifidobacterium longum BBMN68." *Mol Cell Proteomics.* 2014 Jun 25. pii: mcp.M114.039156. [Epub ahead of print]

29. Würth R, Lagkouvardos I, Clavel T, Wilke J, Foerst P, Kulozik U, Haller D, Hörmannsperger G. "Physiological relevance of food grade microcapsules: Impact of milk protein based microcapsules on inflammation in mouse models for inflammatory bowel diseases." *Mol Nutr Food Res.* 2015 Apr 30. doi: 10.1002/mnfr.201400885. [Epub ahead of print]

30. Wong A, Ngu DY, Dan LA, Ooi A, Lim RL. "Detection of antibiotic resistance in probiotics of dietary supplements." *Nutr J.* 2015 Sep 14;14:95. doi: 10.1186/s12937-015-0084-2.

31. Itoh T, Miyake Y, Onda A, Kubo J, Ando M, Tsukamasa Y, Takahata M. "Immunomodulatory effects of heat-killed Enterococcus faecalis TH10 on murine macrophage cells." *Microbiologyopen.* 2012 Dec;1(4):373-80. doi: 10.1002/mbo3.41.

CHAPTER NINE

1. Warshaw AL, Walker WA, Cornell R, Isselbacher KJ. "Small intestinal permeability to macromolecules. Transmission of horseradish peroxidase into mesenteric lymph and portal blood." *Lab Invest.* 1971 Dec;25(6):675-84.

2. DeMeo MT, Mutlu EA, Keshavarzian A, Tobin MC. "Intestinal permeation and gastrointestinal disease." *J Clin Gastroenterol.* 2002 Apr;34(4):385-96.

3. Vaarala O. "Human intestinal microbiota and type 1 diabetes." Curr Diab Rep. 2013 Oct;13(5):601-7. doi: 10.1007/s11892-013-0409-5.

4. Nouri M, Bredberg A, Weström B, Lavasani S. "Intestinal barrier dysfunction develops at the onset of experimental autoimmune encephalomyelitis, and can be induced by adoptive transfer of auto-reactive T cells." *PLoS One.* 2014 Sep 3;9(9):e106335. doi: 10.1371/journal.pone.0106335.

5. Severance EG, Yolken RH, Eaton WW. "Autoimmune diseases, gastrointestinal disorders and the microbiome in schizophrenia: more than a gut feeling." *Schizophr Res.* 2014 Jul 14. pii: S0920-9964(14)00319-3. doi: 10.1016/j.schres.2014.06.027.

6. Smythies L, Smythies J. "Microbiota, the immune system, black moods and the brain—melancholia updated." *Front Hum Neurosci.* 2014 Sep 15;8:720. doi: 10.3389/fnhum.2014.00720.

7. Patrick Hanaway, MD. Textbook of Functional Medicine, adapted as a Continuing Medical Education Module, "Balance of Flora, Galt, and Mucosal Integrity." *Innovision Communications,* September 1, 2006.

8. Nébot-Vivinus M, Harkat C, Bzioueche H, Cartier C, Plichon-Dainese R, Moussa L, Eutamene H, Pishvaie D, Holowacz S, Seyrig C, Piche T, Theodorou V. "Multispecies probiotic protects gut barrier function in experimental models." *World J Gastroenterol.* 2014 Jun 14;20(22):6832-43. doi: 10.3748/wjg.v20.i22.6832.

9. Zeng J, Li YQ, Zuo XL, Zhen YB, Yang J, Liu CH. "Clinical trial: effect of active lactic acid bacteria on mucosal barrier function in patients with diarrhoea-predominant irritable bowel syndrome." *Aliment Pharmacol Ther.* 2008 Oct 15;28(8):994-1002. doi: 10.1111/j.1365-2036.2008 .03818.x.

10. Liu ZH, Huang MJ, Zhang XW, Wang L, Huang NQ, Peng H, Lan P, Peng JS, Yang Z, Xia Y, Liu WJ, Yang J, Qin HL, Wang JP. "The effects of perioperative probiotic treatment on serum zonulin concentration and subsequent postoperative infectious complications after colorectal cancer surgery: a double-center and double-blind randomized clinical trial." *Am J Clin Nutr.* 2013 Jan;97(1):117-26. doi: 10.3945/ajcn.112.040949.

11. Croft DN. *Proc. R. Soc. Med.* 63,1221–1224 (1970)

12. Croft DN, Cotton PB. *Digestion* 8,144–160. (1973)

13. Langmead L, Makins RJ, Rampton DS. "Anti-inflammatory effects of aloe vera gel in human colorectal mucosa in vitro." *Aliment Pharmacol Ther.* 2004 Mar 1;19(5):521-7.

14. Watari I, Oka S, Tanaka S, Aoyama T, Imagawa H, Shishido T, Yoshida S, Chayama K. "Effectiveness of polaprezinc for low-dose aspirin-induced small-bowel mucosal injuries as evaluated by capsule endoscopy: a pilot randomized controlled study." *BMC Gastroenterol.* 2013 Jul 4;13:108. doi: 10.1186/1471-230X-13-108.

15. Mahmood A, FitzGerald AJ, Marchbank T, Ntatsaki E, Murray D, Ghosh S, Playford RJ. "Zinc carnosine, a health food supplement that stabilises small bowel integrity and stimulates gut repair processes." *Gut.* 2007 Feb;56(2):168-75.

16. Bertrand J, Ghouzali I, Guérin C, Bôle-Feysot C, Gouteux M, Déchelotte P, Ducrotté P, Coëffier M. "Glutamine Restores Tight Junction Protein Claudin-1 Expression in Colonic Mucosa of Patients With Diarrhea-Predominant Irritable Bowel Syndrome." JPEN *J Parenter Enteral Nutr.* 2015 May 13. pii: 0148607115587330. [Epub ahead of print]

17. Karaku?a-Juchnowicz H, Szachta P, Opolska A, Morylowska-Topolska J, Ga??cka M, Juchnowicz D, Krukow P, Zofia L. "The role of IgG hypersensitivity in the pathogenesis and therapy of depressive disorders." *Nutr Neurosci.* 2014 Sep 30. [Epub ahead of print]

18. Fasano A. "Zonulin, regulation of tight junctions, and autoimmune diseases." *Ann N Y Acad Sci.* 2012 Jul;1258:25-33. doi: 10.1111/j.1749-6632.2012.06538.x.

19. Orlando A, Linsalata M, Notarnicola M, Tutino V, Russo F. "Lactobacillus GG restoration of the gliadin induced epithelial barrier disruption: the role of cellular polyamines." *BMC Microbiol.* 2014 Jan 31;14:19. doi: 10.1186/1471-2180-14-19.

20. Assa A, Vong L, Pinnell LJ, Avitzur N, Johnson-Henry KC, Sherman PM. "Vitamin D deficiency promotes epithelial barrier dysfunction and intestinal inflammation." *J Infect Dis.* 2014 Oct 15;210(8):1296-305. doi: 10.1093/infdis/jiu235.

21. Guimarães MD, Marchiori E, de Souza Portes Meirelles G, Hochhegger B, Santana PR, Gross JL, Bitencourt AG, Boonsirikamchai P, Godoy MC. "Fungal infection mimicking pulmonary malignancy: clinical and radiological characteristics." *Lung.* 2013 Dec;191(6):655-62. doi: 10.1007/s00408-013-9506-0.

22. Skrobik Y, Laverdiere M. "Why Candida sepsis should matter to ICU physicians." *Crit Care Clin.* 2013 Oct;29(4):853 64. doi: 10.1016/j.ccc.2013.06.007.

23. Rucklidge JJ. "Could yeast infections impair recovery from mental illness? A case study using micronutrients and olive leaf extract for the treatment of ADHD and depression." *Adv Mind Body Med.* 2013 Summer;27(3):14-8.

24. Kuwaki S, Ohhira I, Takahata M, Murata Y, Tada M. "Antifungal activity of the fermentation product of herbs by lactic acid bacteria against tinea." *J Biosci Bioeng.* 2002;94(5):401-5.

25. Demirel G, Celik IH, Erdeve O, Saygan S, Dilmen U, Canpolat FE. "Prophylactic Saccharomyces boulardii versus nystatin for the prevention of fungal colonization and invasive fungal infection in premature infants." *Eur J Pediatr.* 2013 Oct;172(10):1321-6. doi: 10.1007/s00431-013-2041-4.

26. Murzyn A, Krasowska A, Stefanowicz P, Dziadkowiec D, ?ukaszewicz M. "Capric acid secreted by S. boulardii inhibits C. albicans filamentous growth, adhesion and biofilm formation." *PLoS One.* 2010 Aug 10;5(8):e12050. doi: 10.1371/journal.pone.0012050.

27. Mattila HR, Rios D, Walker-Sperling VE, Roeselers G, Newton IL. "Characterization of the active microbiotas associated with honey bees reveals healthier and broader communities when colonies are genetically diverse." *PLoS One.* 2012;7(3):e32962. doi: 10.1371/journal.pone.0032962.

PART TWO

1. Antoniou T, Macdonald E, Hollands S, Gomes T, Mamdani M, Garg A, Paterson J, Juurlink D. "Proton pump inhibitors and the risk of acute kidney injury in older patients: a population-based cohort study" *CMAJ Open* 2015;Apr;3:E166-E171.

2. Fujimori S. "What are the effects of proton pump inhibitors on the small intestine?" *World J Gastroenterol.* 2015 Jun 14;21(22):6817-9. doi: 10.3748/wjg.v21.i22.6817.

3. Namin BM, Daryani NE, Mirshafiey A, Yazdi MK, Soltan Dallal MM. "The effect of probiotics on the expression of Barrett's oesophagus biomarkers." *J Med Microbiol.* 2015 Feb 9. pii: jmm.0.000039. doi: 10.1099/jmm.0.000039. [Epub ahead of print]

4. Igarashi M, Nagano J, Tsuda A, Suzuki T, Koike J, Uchida T, Matsushima M, Mine T, Koga Y. "Correlation between the Serum Pepsinogen I Level and the Symptom Degree in Proton Pump Inhibitor-Users Administered with a Probiotic." *Pharmaceuticals (Basel).* 2014 Jun 25;7(7):754-64. doi: 10.3390/ph7070754.

5. Kalliomäki M, Salminen S, Arvilommi H, Kero P, Koskinen P, Isolauri E. "Probiotics in primary prevention of atopic disease: a randomised placebo-controlled trial." *Lancet.* 2001 Apr 7;357(9262):1076-9.

6. Enomoto T, Sowa M, Nishimori K, Shimazu S, Yoshida A, Yamada K, Furukawa F, Nakagawa T, Yanagisawa N, Iwabuchi N, Odamaki T, Abe F, Nakayama J, Xiao JZ. "Effects of Bifidobacterial Supplementation to Pregnant Women and Infants in the Prevention of Allergy Development in Infants and on Fecal Microbiota." *Allergol Int.* 2014 Jul 25. [Epub ahead of print]

7. Tang ML, Ponsonby AL, Orsini F, Tey D, Robinson M, Su EL, Licciardi P, Burks W, Donath S. "Administration of a probiotic with peanut oral immunotherapy: A randomized trial." *J Allergy Clin Immunol.* 2015 Mar;135(3):737-744.e8. doi: 10.1016/j.jaci.2014.11.034.

8. Bakshi A, Stephen S, Borum ML, Doman DB. "Emerging therapeutic options for celiac disease: potential alternatives to a gluten-free diet." *Gastroenterol Hepatol* (N Y). 2012 Sep;8(9):582-8.

9. Visser J, Rozing J, Sapone A, Lammers K, Fasano A. "Tight junctions, intestinal permeability, and autoimmunity: celiac disease and type 1 diabetes paradigms." *Ann N Y Acad Sci.* 2009 May;1165:195-205. doi: 10.1111/j.1749-6632.2009.04037.x.

10. de Sousa Moraes LF, Grzeskowiak LM, de Sales Teixeira TF, Gouveia Peluzio Mdo C.

"Intestinal microbiota and probiotics in celiac disease." *Clin Microbiol Rev.* 2014 Jul;27(3):482-9. doi: 10.1128/CMR.00106-13.

11. Sarno M, Lania G, Cuomo M, Nigro F, Passannanti F, Budelli A, Fasano F, Troncone R, Auricchio S, Barone MV, Nigro R, Nanayakkara M. "Lactobacillus paracasei CBA L74 interferes with gliadin peptides entrance in Caco-2 cells." *Int J Food Sci Nutr.* 2014 Jul 17:1-7. [Epub ahead of print]

12. Golfetto L, Senna FD, Hermes J, Beserra BT, França Fda S, Martinello F. "Lower bifidobacteria counts in adult patients with celiac disease on a gluten-free diet." *Arq Gastroenterol.* 2014 Apr;51(2):139-43.

13. Klemenak M, Dolin?ek J, Langerholc T, Di Gioia D, Mi?eti?-Turk D. "Administration of Bifidobacterium breve Decreases the Production of TNF-? in Children with Celiac Disease." *Dig Dis Sci.* 2015 Jul 2. [Epub ahead of print]

14. http://www.nlm.nih.gov/medlineplus/druginfo/meds/a601104.html

15. Wan XY, Luo M, Li XD, He P, Wu MC. "Inhibitory effects of taurine and oat fiber on intestinal endotoxin release in rats." *Chem Biol Interact.* 2010 Mar 30;184(3):502-4. doi: 10.1016/j.cbi .2009.12.031.

16. Koenig R, Dickman JR, Kang C, Zhang T, Chu YF, Ji LL. "Avenanthramide supplementation attenuates exercise-induced inflammation in postmenopausal women." *Nutr J.* 2014 Mar 19;13:21. doi: 10.1186/1475-2891-13-21.

17. Guo W, Nie L, Wu D, Wise ML, Collins FW, Meydani SN, Meydani M. "Avenanthramides inhibit proliferation of human colon cancer cell lines in vitro." *Nutr Cancer.* 2010;62(8):1007-16. doi: 10.1080/01635581.2010.492090.

18. Thies F, Masson LF, Boffetta P, Kris-Etherton P. "Oats and CVD risk markers: a systematic literature review." *Br J Nutr.* 2014 Oct;112 Suppl 2:S19-30. doi: 10.1017/S0007114514002281.

19. Dimidi E, Christodoulides S, Fragkos KC, Scott SM, Whelan K. "The effect of probiotics on functional constipation in adults: a systematic review and meta-analysis of randomized controlled trials." *Am J Clin Nutr.* 2014 Oct;100(4):1075-84. doi: 10.3945/ajcn.114.089151.

20. Liberato SC, Singh G, Mulholland K. "Zinc supplementation in young children: A review of the literature focusing on diarrhoea prevention and treatment." *Clin Nutr.* 2014 Aug 13. pii: S0261-5614(14)00206-4. doi: 10.1016/j.clnu.2014.08.002.

21. Kruse E, Leifeld L. "[Prevention and conservative therapy of diverticular disease]." [Article in German] *Chirurg.* 2014 Apr;85(4):299-303. doi: 10.1007/s00104-013-2619-4.

22. Tursi A, Brandimarte G, Elisei W, Picchio M, Forti G, Pianese G, Rodino S, D'Amico T, Sacca N, Portincasa P, Capezzuto E, Lattanzio R, Spadaccini A, Fiorella S, Polimeni F, Polimeni N, Stoppino V, Stoppino G, Giorgetti GM, Aiello F, Danese S. "Randomised clinical trial: mesalazine and/or probiotics in maintaining remission of symptomatic uncomplicated diverticular disease—a double-blind, randomised, placebo-controlled study." *Aliment Pharmacol Ther.* 2013 Oct;38(7):741-51. doi: 10.1111/apt.12463.

23. Mathur R, Amichai M, Chua KS, Mirocha J, Barlow GM, Pimentel M. "Methane and hydrogen positivity on breath test is associated with greater body mass index and body fat." *J Clin Endocrinol Metab.* 2013 Apr;98(4):E698-702. doi: 10.1210/jc.2012-3144.

24. de Boer NK, de Meij TG, Oort FA, Ben Larbi I, Mulder CJ, van Bodegraven AA, van der Schee MP. "The scent of colorectal cancer: detection by volatile organic compound analysis." *Clin Gastroenterol Hepatol.* 2014 Jul;12(7):1085-9. doi: 10.1016/j.cgh.2014.05.005.

25. Kjelvik G, Saltvedt I, White LR, Stenumgård P, Sletvold O, Engedal K, Skåtun K, Lyngvær AK, Steffenach HA, Håberg AK. "The brain structural and cognitive basis of odor identification deficits in mild cognitive impairment and Alzheimer's disease." *BMC Neurol.* 2014 Aug 26;14:168. doi: 10.1186/s12883-014-0168-1.

26. Lee SH, Kim YJ. "A comparative study of the effect of probiotics on cariogenic biofilm model for preventing dental caries." *Arch Microbiol.* 2014 Aug;196(8):601-9. doi: 10.1007/s00203-014-0998-7.

27. Huang CB, Alimova Y, Myers TM, Ebersole JL. "Short- and medium-chain fatty acids exhibit antimicrobial activity for oral microorganisms." *Arch Oral Biol.* 2011 Jul;56(7):650-4. doi: 10.1016/j.archoralbio.2011.01.011.

28. Ghasempour M, Sefdgar SA, Moghadamnia AA, Ghadimi R, Gharekhani S, Shirkhani L. "Comparative study of kefr yogurt-drink and sodium fluoride mouth rinse on salivary mutans streptococci." *J Contemp Dent Pract.* 2014 Mar 1;15(2):214-7.

29. Ashwin D, Ke V, Taranath M, Ramagoni NK, Nara A, Sarpangala M. "Effect of Probiotic Containing Ice-cream on Salivary Mutans Streptococci (SMS) Levels in Children of 6-12 Years of Age: A Randomized Controlled Double Blind Study with Six-months Follow Up." *J Clin Diagn Res.* 2015 Feb;9(2):ZC06-9. doi: 10.7860/JCDR/2015/10942.5532.

30. http://www.aboutibs.org/site/what-is-ibs/facts/statistics

31. De Giorgio R, Volta U, Gibson PR. "Sensitivity to wheat, gluten and FODMAPs in IBS: facts or fiction?" *Gut.* 2015 Jun 15. pii: gutjnl-2015-309757. doi: 10.1136/gutjnl-2015-309757. [Epub ahead of print]

32. Ligaarden SC, Farup PG. "Low intake of vitamin B(6) is associated with irritable bowel syndrome symptoms." *Nutr Res.* 2011 May;31(5):356-61.

33. Ghaly S, Lawrance I. "The role of vitamin D in gastrointestinal inflammation." *Expert Rev Gastroenterol Hepatol.* 2014 Nov;8(8):909-23. doi: 10.1586/17474124.2014.925796. Epub 2014 Jul 22.

34. Ananthakrishnan AN. "Environmental Risk Factors for Inflammatory Bowel Diseases: A Review." *Dig Dis Sci.* 2014 Sep 10. [Epub ahead of print]

35. Roberts CL, Keita AV, Duncan SH, O'Kennedy N, Söderholm JD, Rhodes JM, Campbell BJ. "Translocation of Crohn's disease Escherichia coli across M-cells: contrasting effects of soluble plant fibres and emulsifiers." *Gut.* 2010 Oct;59(10):1331-9. doi: 10.1136/gut.2009.195370.

36. Kanai T, Matsuoka K, Naganuma M, Hayashi A, Hisamatsu T. "Diet, microbiota, and inflammatory bowel disease: lessons from Japanese foods." *Korean J Intern Med.* 2014 Jul;29(4):409-15. doi: 10.3904/kjim.2014.29.4.409.

37. Whelan K. "Editorial: The Importance of Systematic Reviews and Meta-Analyses of Probiotics and Prebiotics." *Am J Gastroenterol.* 2014 Oct;109(10):1563-1565. doi: 10.1038/ajg.2014.258.

38. Ford AC, Quigley EM, Lacy BE, Lembo AJ, Saito YA, Schiller LR, Soffer EE, Spiegel BM, Moayyedi P. "Efficacy of Prebiotics, Probiotics, and Synbiotics in Irritable Bowel Syndrome and Chronic Idiopathic Constipation: Systematic Review and Meta-analysis." *Am J Gastroenterol.* 2014 Oct;109(10):1547-1561. doi: 10.1038/ajg.2014.202.

39. Wang ZK, Yang YS, Chen Y, Yuan J, Sun G, Peng LH. "Intestinal microbiota pathogenesis and fecal microbiota transplantation for inflammatory bowel disease." *World J Gastroenterol.* 2014 Oct 28;20(40):14805-14820.

40. Takahata M, Frémont M, Desreumaux P, Rousseaux C, Dubuquoy C, Shimomiya Y, Nakamura Y, Miyake Y. "Evaluation of therapeutic properties of fermented vegetables extract (OM-X) in the model of colitis induced by Citrobacter rodentium in mice." *J Funct Foods,* 2014.10:117–127.

41. Wine E. "Should We Be Treating the Bugs instead of Cytokines and T Cells?" *Dig Dis.* 2014;32(4):403-9. doi: 10.1159/000358146.

42. Wu S, Yoon S, Zhang YG, Lu R, Xia Y, Wan J, Petrof EO, Claud EC, Chen D, Sun J. "Vitamin D receptor pathway is required for probiotic protection in colitis." *Am J Physiol Gastrointest Liver Physiol.* 2015 Jul 9:ajpgi.00105.2015. doi: 10.1152/ajpgi.00105.2015. [Epub ahead of print]

43. Takahata M, Frémont M, Desreumaux P, Rousseaux C, Dubuquoy C, Shimomiya Y, Nakamura Y, Miyake Y. "Evaluation of therapeutic properties of fermented vegetables extract (OM-X) in the model of colitis induced by Citrobacter rodentium in mice." *J Funct Foods,* 2014.10:117–127.

44. Khanna R, MacDonald JK, Levesque BG. "Peppermint oil for the treatment of irritable bowel syndrome: a systematic review and meta-analysis." *J Clin Gastroenterol.* 2014 Jul;48(6):505-12. doi: 10.1097/MCG.0b013e3182a88357.

45. Etxeberria U, Arias N, Boqué N, Macarulla MT, Portillo MP, Martínez JA, Milagro FI. "Reshaping faecal gut microbiota composition by the intake of trans-resveratrol and quercetin in high-fat sucrose diet-fed rats." *J Nutr Biochem.* 2015 Jun;26(6):651-60. doi: 10.1016/j.jnutbio.2015.01.002.

46. Maes M. "Inflammatory and oxidative and nitrosative stress pathways underpinning chronic fatigue, somatization and psychosomatic symptoms." *Curr Opin Psychiatry.* 2009 Jan;22(1):75-83.

47. Frémont M, Coomans D, Massart S, De Meirleir K. "High-throughput 16S rRNA gene sequencing reveals alterations of intestinal microbiota in myalgic encephalomyelitis/chronic fatigue syndrome patients." *Anaerobe.* 2013 Aug;22:50-6. doi: 10.1016/j.anaerobe.2013.06.002.

48. Maes M, Leunis JC. "Normalization of leaky gut in chronic fatigue syndrome (CFS) is accompanied by a clinical improvement: effects of age, duration of illness and the translocation of LPS from gram-negative bacteria." *Neuro Endocrinol Lett.* 2008 Dec;29(6):902-10.

49. Clancy RL, Gleeson M, Cox A, Callister R, Dorrington M, D'Este C, Pang G, Pyne D, Fricker P, Henriksson A. "Reversal in fatigued athletes of a defect in interferon gamma secretion after administration of Lactobacillus acidophilus." *Br J Sports Med.* 2006 Apr;40(4):351-4.

50. Nicolson GL. "Mitochondrial dysfunction and chronic disease: treatment with natural supplements." *Altern Ther Health Med.* 2014 Winter;20 Suppl 1:18-25.

51. Ponikau JU, Sherris DA, Kern EB, Homburger HA, Frigas E, Gaffey TA, Roberts GD. "The diagnosis and incidence of allergic fungal sinusitis." *Mayo Clin Proc.* 1999 Sep;74(9):877-84.

52. Williamson IG, Rumsby K, Benge S, Moore M, Smith PW, Cross M, Little P. "Antibiotics and topical nasal steroid for treatment of acute maxillary sinusitis: a randomized controlled trial." *JAMA.* 2007 Dec 5;298(21):2487-96.

53. Gutierrez-Castrellon P, Lopez-Velazquez G, Diaz-Garcia L, Jimenez-Gutierrez C, Mancilla-Ramirez J, Estevez-Jimenez J, Parra M. "Diarrhea in preschool children and Lactobacillus reuteri: a randomized controlled trial." *Pediatrics.* 2014 Apr;133(4):e904-9. doi: 10.1542/peds .2013-0652.

54. Leyer GJ, Li S, Mubasher ME, Reifer C, Ouwehand AC. "Probiotic effects on cold and influenza-like symptom incidence and duration in children." *Pediatrics.* 2009 Aug;124(2):e172-9. doi: 10.1542/peds.2008-2666.

55. Smith TJ, Rigassio-Radler D, Denmark R, Haley T, Touger-Decker R. "Effect of Lactobacillus rhamnosus LGG and Bifidobacterium animalis ssp. lactis BB-12 on health-related quality of life in college students affected by upper respiratory infections." *Br J Nutr.* 2013 Jun;109(11):1999-2007. doi: 10.1017/S0007114512004138.

56. Song JA, Kim HJ, Hong SK, Lee DH, Lee SW, Song CS, Kim KT, Choi IS, Lee JB, Park SY. "Oral intake of Lactobacillus rhamnosus M21 enhances the survival rate of mice lethally infected with influenza virus." *J Microbiol Immunol Infect.* 2014 Oct 7. pii: S1684-1182(14)00167-4. doi: 10.1016/j.jmii.2014.07.011. [Epub ahead of print]

57. Hao Q, Lu Z, Dong BR, Huang CQ, Wu T. "Probiotics for preventing acute upper respiratory tract infections." *Cochrane Database Syst Rev.* 2011 Sep 7;(9):CD006895. doi: 10.1002/14651858 .CD006895.pub2.

58. Pérez Martínez G, Bäuerl C, Collado MC. "Understanding gut microbiota in elderly's health will enable intervention through probiotics." *Benef Microbes.* 2014 Sep;5(3):235-46. doi: 10.3920/BM2013.0079.

59. Markin D, Duek L, Berdicevsky I. "In vitro antimicrobial activity of olive leaves." *Mycoses.* 2003 Apr;46(3-4):132-6.

60. Borre YE, Moloney RD, Clarke G, Dinan TG, Cryan JF. "The impact of microbiota on brain and behavior: mechanisms & therapeutic potential." *Adv Exp Med Biol.* 2014;817:373-403. doi: 10.1007/978-1-4939-0897-4_17.

61. Collins SM, Kassam Z, Bercik P. "The adoptive transfer of behavioral phenotype via the intestinal microbiota: experimental evidence and clinical implications." *Curr Opin Microbiol.* 2013 Jun;16(3):240-5. doi: 10.1016/j.mib.2013.06.004.

62. Slyepchenko A, Carvalho AF, Cha DS, Kasper S, McIntyre RS. "Gut Emotions - Mechanisms of Action of Probiotics as Novel Therapeutic Targets for Depression and Anxiety Disorders." *CNS Neurol Disord Drug Targets.* 2014 Nov 30. [Epub ahead of print]

63. Steenbergen L, Sellaro R, van Hemert S, Bosch JA, Colzato LS. "A randomized controlled trial to test the effect of multispecies probiotics on cognitive reactivity to sad mood." *Brain Behav Immun.* 2015 Apr 7. pii: S0889-1591(15)00088-4. doi: 10.1016/j.bbi.2015.04.003. [Epub ahead of print]

64. Bravo J, Forsythe P, Chew MV, Escaravage E, Savignac HM, Dinan TG, Bienenstock J, Cryan JF. "Ingestion of Lactobacillus strain regulates emotional behavior and central GABA receptor expression in a mouse via the vagus nerve." *Proc Natl Acad Sci U S A.* 2011 Sep 20;108(38):16050-5. doi: 10.1073/pnas.1102999108.

65. Yang H, Zhao X, Tang S, Huang H, Zhao X, Ning Z, Fu X, Zhang C. "Probiotics reduce psychological stress in patients before laryngeal cancer surgery." *Asia Pac J Clin Oncol.* 2014 Feb 20. doi: 10.1111/ajco.12120. [Epub ahead of print]

66. Schmidt K, Cowen PJ, Harmer CJ, Tzortzis G, Errington S, Burnet PW. "Prebiotic intake reduces the waking cortisol response and alters emotional bias in healthy volunteers." *Psychopharmacology (Berl).* 2014 Dec 3. [Epub ahead of print]

67. Sharma K, Pant S, Misra S, Dwivedi M, Misra A, Narang S, Tewari R, Bhadoria AS. "Effect of rifaximin, probiotics, and l-ornithine l-aspartate on minimal hepatic encephalopathy: A randomized controlled trial." *Saudi J Gastroenterol.* 2014 Jul-Aug;20(4):225-32. doi: 10.4103/1319-3767.136975.

68. Samieri C, Maillard P, Crivello F, Proust-Lima C, Peuchant E, Helmer C, Amieva H, Allard M, Dartigues JF, Cunnane SC, Mazoyer BM, Barberger-Gateau P. "Plasma long-chain omega-3 fatty acids and atrophy of the medial temporal lobe." *Neurology.* 2012 Aug 14;79(7):642-50. doi: 10.1212/WNL.0b013e318264e394.

69. Britton RA, Irwin R, Quach D, Schaefer L, Zhang J, Lee T, Parameswaran N, McCabe LR. "Probiotic L. reuteri treatment prevents bone loss in a menopausal ovariectomized mouse model." *J Cell Physiol.* 2014 Nov;229(11):1822-30. doi: 10.1002/jcp.24636.

70. McCabe LR, Irwin R, Schaefer L, Britton RA. "Probiotic use decreases intestinal inflammation and increases bone density in healthy male but not female mice." *J Cell Physiol.* 2013 Aug;228(8):1793-8. doi: 10.1002/jcp.24340.

71. Villa CR, Ward WE, Comelli EM. "Gut Microbiota-bone Axis." *Crit Rev Food Sci Nutr.* 2015 Oct 13:0. [Epub ahead of print]

72. KawakamI M, Ohhira I, Araki N, Inokihara K, Iwasaki .H, Matsubara T. "The Influence of Lactic Acid Bacteria (OM-X) on Bone Structure." *J Appl Nutr,* 2003;53(1):2-7.

73. Yu Y, Champer J, Beynet D, Kim J, Friedman AJ. "The role of the cutaneous microbiome in skin cancer: lessons learned from the gut." *J Drugs Dermatol.* 2015 May 1;14(5):461-5.

74. Mayes T, Gottschlich MM, James LE, Allgeier C, Weitz J, Kagan RJ. "Clinical safety and efficacy of probiotic administration following burn injury." *J Burn Care Res.* 2015 Jan-Feb;36(1):92-9. doi: 10.1097/BCR.0000000000000139.

75. Groeger D, O'Mahony L, Murphy EF, Bourke JF, Dinan TG, Kiely B, Shanahan F, Quigley EM. "Bifidobacterium infantis 35624 modulates host inflammatory processes beyond the gut." *Gut Microbes.* 2013 Jul-Aug;4(4):325-39. doi: 10.4161/gmic.25487.

76. Kim SO, Ah YM, Yu YM, Choi KH, Shin WG, Lee JY. "Effects of probiotics for the treatment of atopic dermatitis: a meta-analysis of randomized controlled trials." *Ann Allergy Asthma Immunol.* 2014 Aug;113(2):217-26. doi: 10.1016/j.anai.2014.05.021.

77. Humbert P, Bidet A, Treffel P, Drobacheff C, Agache P. "Intestinal permeability in patients with psoriasis." *J Dermatol Sci.* 1991 Jul;2(4):324-6.

78. Scher JU, Ubeda C, Artacho A, Attur M, Isaac S, Reddy SM, Marmon S, Neimann A, Brusca S, Patel T, Manasson J, Pamer EG, Littman DR, Abramson SB. "Decreased bacterial diversity characterizes an altered gut microbiota in psoriatic arthritis and resembles dysbiosis of inflammatory bowel disease." *Arthritis Rheumatol.* 2014 Oct 15. doi: 10.1002/art.38892. [Epub ahead of print]

79. Fry L, Baker B, Powles A, Engstrand L. "Psoriasis is not an autoimmune disease?" *Exp Dermatol.* 2014 Oct 27. doi: 10.1111/exd.12572. [Epub ahead of print]

80. Mohammedsaeed W, McBain AJ, Cruickshank SM, O'Neill CA. "Lactobacillus rhamnosus GG Inhibits the Toxic Effects of Staphylococcus aureus on Epidermal Keratinocytes." *Appl Environ Microbiol.* 2014 Jul 11. pii: AEM.00861-14. [Epub ahead of print]

81. Lauran Neergaard. "Scientists find bacterial zoo thrives in our skin." *Associated Press,* May 28, 2009

82. Roudsari MR, Karimi R, Mortazavian AM. "Health effects of probiotics on the skin." *Crit Rev Food Sci Nutr.* 2013 Dec 23. [Epub ahead of print]

83. Grice EA. "The skin microbiome: potential for novel diagnostic and therapeutic approaches to cutaneous disease." *Semin Cutan Med Surg.* 2014 Jun;33(2):98-103.

84. Dang Y, Reinhardt JD, Zhou X, Zhang G. "The Effect of Probiotics Supplementation on Helicobacter pylori Eradication Rates and Side Effects during Eradication Therapy: A Meta-Analysis." *PLoS One.* 2014 Nov 3;9(11):e111030. doi: 10.1371/journal.pone.0111030.

85. Rosania R, Minenna MF, Giorgio F, Facciorusso A, De Francesco V, Hassan C, Panella C, Ierardi E. "Probiotic multi-strain treatment may eradicate Helicobacter pylori from the stomach of dyspeptics: a placebo-controlled pilot study." *Inflamm Allergy Drug Targets.* 2012 Jun;11(3):244-9.

86. Zwoli?ska-Wcis?o M, Brzozowski T, Mach T, Budak A, Trojanowska D, Konturek PC, Pajdo R, Drozdowicz D, Kwiecie? S. "Are probiotics effective in the treatment of fungal colonization of the gastrointestinal tract? Experimental and clinical studies." *J Physiol Pharmacol.* 2006 Nov;57 Suppl 9:35-49.

87. Karapetian TA, Nikiforova NA, Dorshakova NV, Vinogradova IA. "[Peculiarities of clinical picture of duodenal ulcer in the population of Northern Europe]." [Article in Russian] *Klin Med (Mosk).* 2014;92(4):13-9.

88. Wong RK, Yang C, Song GH, Wong J, Ho KY. "Melatonin Regulation as a Possible Mechanism for Probiotic (VSL#3) in Irritable Bowel Syndrome: A Randomized Double-Blinded Placebo Study." *Dig Dis Sci.* 2014 Aug 5. [Epub ahead of print]

89. Foxman B. "Epidemiology of urinary tract infections: incidence, morbidity, and economic costs." *Am J Med.* 2002 Jul 8;113 Suppl 1A:5S-13S.

90. Borges S, Silva J, Teixeira P. "The role of lactobacilli and probiotics in maintaining vaginal health." *Arch Gynecol Obstet.* 2014 Mar;289(3):479-89. doi: 10.1007/s00404-013-3064-9.

91. Kovachev SM, Vatcheva-Dobrevska RS. "Local Probiotic Therapy for Vaginal Candida albicans Infections." *Probiotics Antimicrob Proteins.* 2014 Nov 2. [Epub ahead of print]

92. Liou AP, Paziuk M, Luevano JM Jr, Machineni S, Turnbaugh PJ, Kaplan LM. "Conserved shifts in the gut microbiota due to gastric bypass reduce host weight and adiposity." *Sci Transl Med.* 2013 Mar 27;5(178):178ra41. doi: 10.1126/scitranslmed.3005687.

93. Alcock J, Maley CC, Aktipis CA. "Is eating behavior manipulated by the gastrointestinal microbiota? Evolutionary pressures and potential mechanisms." *Bioessays.* 2014 Aug 8. doi: 10.1002/bies.201400071. [Epub ahead of print]

94. Lee K, Lee Y. "Production of c9,t11- and t10,c12-conjugated linoleic acids in humans by Lactobacillus rhamnosus PL60." *J Microbiol Biotechnol.* 2009 Dec;19(12):1617-9.

95. Dao MC, Everard A, Aron-Wisnewsky J, Sokolovska N, Prifti E, Verger EO, Kayser BD, Levenez F, Chilloux J, Hoyles L; MICRO-Obes Consortium, Dumas ME5, Rizkalla SW, Doré J, Cani PD, Clément K. "Akkermansia muciniphila and improved metabolic health during a dietary intervention in obesity: relationship with gut microbiome richness and ecology." *Gut.* 2015 Jun 22. pii: gutjnl-2014-308778. doi: 10.1136/gutjnl-2014-308778. [Epub ahead of print]

96. Turnbaugh PJ, Hamady M, Yatsunenko T, Cantarel BL, Duncan A, Ley RE, Sogin ML, Jones WJ, Roe BA, Affourtit JP, Egholm M, Henrissat B, Heath AC, Knight R, Gordon JI. "A core gut microbiome in obese and lean twins." *Nature.* 2009 Jan 22;457(7228):480-4. doi: 10.1038/nature07540.

97. Chacko Y, Holtmann GJ. "Helicobacter pylori eradication and weight gain: has it opened a Pandora's box?" *Aliment Pharmacol Ther.* 2011 Jul;34(2):256. doi: 10.1111/j.1365-2036.2011.04704.x.

98. Riley LW, Raphael E, Faerstein E. "Obesity in the United States - dysbiosis from exposure to low-dose antibiotics?" *Front Public Health.* 2013 Dec 19;1:69. doi: 10.3389/fpubh.2013.00069.

99. Ridaura VK, Faith JJ, Rey FE, Cheng J, Duncan AE, Kau AL, Griffin NW, Lombard V, Henrissat B, Bain JR, Muehlbauer MJ, Ilkayeva O, Semenkovich CF, Funai K, Hayashi DK, Lyle BJ, Martini MC, Ursell LK, Clemente JC, Van Treuren W, Walters WA, Knight R, Newgard CB, Heath AC, Gordon JI. "Gut microbiota from twins discordant for obesity modulate metabolism in mice." *Science.* 2013 Sep 6;341(6150):1241214. doi: 10.1126/science.1241214.

100. Turnbaugh PJ, Ley RE, Mahowald MA, Magrini V, Mardis ER, Gordon JI. "An obesity-associated gut microbiome with increased capacity for energy harvest." *Nature.* 2006 Dec 21;444(7122):1027-31.

101. Núñez IN, Galdeano CM, de LeBlanc Ade M, Perdigón G. "Evaluation of immune response, microbiota, and blood markers after probiotic bacteria administration in obese mice induced by a high-fat diet." *Nutrition.* 2014 Nov-Dec;30(11-12):1423-32. doi: 10.1016/j.nut .2014.03.025.

102. Savcheniuk OA, Virchenko OV, Falalieieva TM, Beregova TV, Babenko LP, Lazarenko LM, Spivak MIa. "[The effect of probiotic therapy on development of experimental obesity in rats caused by monosodium glutamate]." [Article in Ukrainian] *Fiziol Zh.* 2014;60(2):63-9.

103. Wu CC, Weng WL, Lai WL, Tsai HP, Liu WH, Lee MH, Tsai YC. "Effect of Lactobacillus plantarum Strain K21 on High-Fat Diet-Fed Obese Mice." *Evid Based Complement Alternat Med.* 2015;2015:391767. doi: 10.1155/2015/391767. Epub 2015 Feb 23.

104. Hulston CJ, Churnside AA, Venables MC. "Probiotic supplementation prevents high-fat, overfeeding-induced insulin resistance in human subjects." *Br J Nutr.* 2015 Feb 28;113(4):596-602. doi: 10.1017/S0007114514004097.

105. Minami J, Kondo S, Yanagisawa N, Odamaki T, Xiao JZ, Abe F, Nakajima S, Hamamoto Y, Saitoh S, Shimoda T. "Oral administration of Bifidobacterium breve B-3 modifies metabolic functions in adults with obese tendencies in a randomised controlled trial." *J Nutr Sci.* 2015 May 4;4:e17. doi: 10.1017/jns.2015.5.

106. Bjerg AT, Kristensen M, Ritz C, Holst JJ, Rasmussen C, Leser TD, Wellejus A, Astrup A. "Lactobacillus paracasei subsp paracasei L. casei W8 suppresses energy intake acutely." *Appetite.* 2014 Jul 15. pii: S0195-6663(14)00373-0. doi: 10.1016/j.appet.2014.07.016.

107. Brahe LK, Le Chatelier E, Prifti E, Pons N, Kennedy S, Blædel T, Håkansson J, Dalsgaard TK, Hansen T, Pedersen O, Astrup A, Ehrlich SD, Larsen LH. "Dietary modulation of the gut microbiota - a randomised controlled trial in obese postmenopausal women." *Br J Nutr.* 2015 Jul 2:1-12. [Epub ahead of print]

108. Kadooka Y, Sato M, Imaizumi K, Ogawa A, Ikuyama K, Akai Y, Okano M, Kagoshima M, Tsuchida T. "Regulation of abdominal adiposity by probiotics (Lactobacillus gasseri SBT2055) in adults with obese tendencies in a randomized controlled trial." *Eur J Clin Nutr.* 2010 Jun;64(6):636-43. doi: 10.1038/ejcn.2010.19.

109. Zarrati M, Salehi E, Nourijelyani K, Mofid V, Zadeh MJ, Najafi F, Ghaflati Z, Bidad K, Chamari M, Karimi M, Shidfar F. "Effects of Probiotic Yogurt on Fat Distribution and Gene Expression of Proinflammatory Factors in Peripheral Blood Mononuclear Cells in Overweight and Obese People with or without Weight-Loss Diet." *J Am Coll Nutr.* 2014 Jul 31:1-9. [Epub ahead of print]

110. Brahe LK, Le Chatelier E, Prifti E, Pons N, Kennedy S, Blædel T, Håkansson J, Dalsgaard

TK, Hansen T, Pedersen O, Astrup A, Ehrlich SD, Larsen LH. "Dietary modulation of the gut microbiota—a randomised controlled trial in obese postmenopausal women." *Br J Nutr.* 2015 Jul 2:1-12. [Epub ahead of print]

111. Huang EY, Leone VA, Devkota S, Wang Y, Brady MJ, Chang EB. "Composition of dietary fat source shapes gut microbiota architecture and alters host inflammatory mediators in mouse adipose tissue." *JPEN J Parenter Enteral Nutr.* 2013 Nov;37(6):746-54. doi: 10.1177/0148607113486931.

112. Ipar N, Aydogdu SD, Yildirim GK, Inal M, Gies I, Vandenplas Y, Dinleyici EC. "Effects of synbiotic on anthropometry, lipid profile and oxidative stress in obese children." *Benef Microbes.* 2015 Aug 11:1-8. [Epub ahead of print]

113. da Silva ST, dos Santos CA, Bressan J. "Intestinal microbiota; relevance to obesity and modulation by prebiotics and probiotics." *Nutr Hosp.* 2013 Jul-Aug;28(4):1039-48. doi: 10.3305/nh.2013.28.4.6525.

114. Park S, Bae JH. "Probiotics for weight loss: a systematic review and meta-analysis." *Nutr Res.* 2015 May 21. pii: S0271-5317(15)00103-7. doi: 10.1016/j.nutres.2015.05.008. [Epub ahead of print]

115. Le Chatelier E, Nielsen T, Qin J, Prifti E, Hildebrand F, Falony G, Almeida M, Arumugam M, Batto JM, Kennedy S, Leonard P, Li J, Burgdorf K, Grarup N, Jørgensen T, Brandslund I, Nielsen HB, Juncker AS, Bertalan M, Levenez F, Pons N, Rasmussen S, Sunagawa S, Tap J, Tims S, Zoetendal EG, Brunak S, Clément K, Doré J, Kleerebezem M, Kristiansen K, Renault P, Sicheritz-Ponten T, de Vos WM, Zucker JD, Raes J, Hansen T; MetaHIT consortium, Bork P, Wang J, Ehrlich SD, Pedersen O. "Richness of human gut microbiome correlates with metabolic markers." *Nature.* 2013 Aug 29;500(7464):541-6. doi: 10.1038/nature12506.

116. *Death by Medicine,* 2003 Gary Null PhD, Carolyn Dean MD ND, Martin Feldman MD, Debora Rasio MD and Dorothy Smith PhD

Glossary

1. Liu J, Prindle A, Humphries J, Gabalda-Sagarra M, Asally M, Lee DD, Ly S, Garcia-Ojalvo J, Süel GM. "Metabolic co-dependence gives rise to collective oscillations within biofilms." *Nature.* 2015 Jul 22. doi: 10.1038/nature14660. [Epub ahead of print]

2. Carvalho FA, Aitken JD, Vijay-Kumar M, Gewirtz AT. "Toll-like receptor-gut microbiota interactions: perturb at your own risk!" *Annu Rev Physiol.* 2012;74:177-98. doi: 10.1146/annurev-physiol-020911-153330.

About the Author

Martie Whittekin is a board-certified Certified Clinical Nutritionist who has counseled in health and nutrition since the early nineteen eighties. She is the author of the best-seller, *Natural Alternatives to Nexium, Maalox, Tagamet, Prilosec and Other Acid Blockers.* Her other works include *Fat Free Folly* and *Aloe Vera, Modern Science Shed Light on an Ancient Herbal Remedy.* She is a popular lecturer and a frequent guest on national TV and radio programs.

In 1997 Martie began broadcasting a weekly radio health talk show in Dallas, TX, *Healthy by Nature.* The show, which includes interviews with a wide range of experts, is now syndicated. HBNShow.com, her show's website, offers a health Library; a blog, free e-news, radio show archives and information on her television presence.

MS Whittekin graduated from Ohio State University, but has learned at least as much since then by studying with some of the brightest minds in the natural health field. Martie believes that health is a lot more than the absence of a diagnosis—it is having the energy and enthusiasm for life that comes from respecting the body's need for real balance and natural energy starting at the cellular level.

She proudly served on the Board of Trustees for Bastyr University in Seattle (a fully accredited school of natural medicine). Long a champion of preserving freedom of choice in health, she served as President of the National Nutritional Foods Association. (It was the nutrition industry's largest organization representing natural food retailers and manufacturers. It has since been renamed the Natural Products Association.) She served that organization during crucial phases of the effort to pass the Dietary Supplement Health and Education Act and in doing so testified at many congressional hearings. For these efforts she received the NNFA's 2002 "Crusader Award" and before that, the Association of Women in Nutrition's "Woman of the Year."

Martie was a founder and president of Texans for Health Freedom, a group formed to protect a citizen's right to choose alternative medical treatments. Although the battle still rages on, she helped the group achieve at least minimum protection for alternative doctors in the state.

Martie has been married to husband, Bill, since 1978. Together they reared a blended family of 4 terrific kids and are quite proud of their two grandchildren (and many grand dogs).

Index

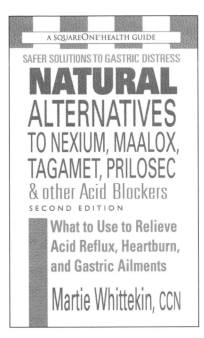

NATURAL ALTERNATIVES TO NEXIUM, MAALOX, TAGAMET, PRILOSEC & OTHER ACID BLOCKERS

Martie Whittekin, CCN

With millions of Americans suffering from heartburn, acid reflux, and other gastric ailments, it's no wonder stomach medications are the best-selling drugstore remedies. Ads for these products claim that they can relieve pain quickly, but what they *don't* tell you is that your pain may indicate a distressed digestive tract. Yes, meds can cover up the symptoms, but they don't treat the cause of the problem. Even worse, they may allow a chronic condition to degenerate. *Natural Alternatives to Nexium, Maalox, Tagamet, Prilosec & Other Acid Blockers* offers safer, more effective alternatives to these popular medications.

Written by Martie Whittekin, an experienced clinical nutritionist, this book examines the underlying causes of acid reflux. It also discusses how acid blockers work and how they can be damaging to long-term health. The author then highlights the most important natural alternatives—both those that provide immediate symptom relief and those that offer long-term relief. You'll find up-to-date product information, as well as recommendations on which natural product (and its proper dosage) is best for you.

If you suffer from the pain of recurrent gastric upset, or if you are currently using an acid blocker, *Natural Alternatives to Nexium, Maalox, Tagamet, Prilosec & Other Acid Blockers* can make a profound difference in the quality of your life.

$7.95 • 272 pages • 4 x 7-inch mass paperback • ISBN 978-0-7570-0210-6

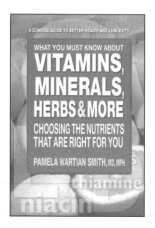

WHAT YOU MUST KNOW ABOUT VITAMINS, MINERALS, HERBS & MORE

Pamela Wartian Smith, MD, MPH

What You Must Know About Vitamins, Minerals, Herbs & More explains how you can restore and maintain health through the wise use of nutrients. Part One of this easy-to-use guide discusses the individual nutrients necessary for good health. Part Two offers personalized nutritional programs for people with a variety of health concerns. People without prior medical problems can refer to Part Three for supplementation plans.

Whether you want to preserve good health or you are trying to overcome a medical condition, this book can help you make the best choices for yourself and your family.

$15.95 • 448 pages • 6 x 9-inch quality paperback • ISBN 978-0-7570-0233-5

THE ACID-ALKALINE FOOD GUIDE
SECOND EDITION

Susan E. Brown, PhD, and Larry Trivieri, Jr.

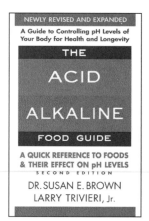

In the last few years, researchers around the world have increasingly reported the importance of acid-alkaline balance. *The Acid-Alkaline Food Guide* was designed as an easy-to-follow guide to the most common foods that influence your body's pH level. Now in its Second Edition, this bestseller begins by explaining how the acid-alkaline environment of the body is influenced by foods. It then presents a list of thousands of foods and their acid-alkaline effects. Included are not only single foods, such as fruits and vegetables, but also popular combination foods, common fast foods, and even international fare. Updated information also explores (and refutes) the myths about pH balance and diet, and guides you to supplements that can help your body achieve a healthy pH level.

$8.95 • 224 pages • 4 x 7-inch mass paperback • ISBN 978-0-7570-0393-6